Neurology in Africa

Neurology in Africa

Clinical Skills and Neurological Disorders

William P. Howlett MB DTM&H FRCPI PhD

Physician and Neurologist, Department of Internal Medicine, Kilimanjaro Christian Medical Centre,
Moshi, Kilimanjaro, Tanzania
Visiting Researcher, Centre for International Health, University of Bergen, Norway

With illustrations by
Ellinor Moldeklev Hoff

Department of Photos and Drawings, University of Bergen, Norway

Layout by
Christian Bakke

Division of Communication, University of Bergen, Norway

CAMBRIDGE
UNIVERSITY PRESS

CAMBRIDGE
UNIVERSITY PRESS

University Printing House, Cambridge CB2 8BS, United Kingdom

Cambridge University Press is part of the University of Cambridge.

It furthers the University's mission by disseminating
knowledge in the pursuit of education, learning and
research at the highest international levels of excellence.

www.cambridge.org
Information on this title: www.cambridge.org/9781107114227

© William P. Howlett 2015

First published 2012 by BRIC
Revised edition published 2015 by Cambridge University Press

Printed in the United Kingdom by Bell and Bain Ltd

A catalogue record for this publication is available from the British Library

Library of Congress Cataloguing in Publication data
Howlett, William P., author.
Neurology in Africa : clinical skills and neurological disorders /
William P. Howlett ; with illustrations by Ellinor Moldeklev Hoff. –
Revised edition.
    p. ; cm.
Includes bibliographical references and index.
ISBN 978-1-107-53485-8 (pbk. : alk. paper)
I. Title.
[DNLM: 1. Nervous System Diseases–Africa South of the Sahara.
2. Neurology–methods–Africa South of the Sahara. WL 140]
RC387.5
362.196800967–dc23   2015017844

ISBN 978-1-107-14422-7 Hardback
ISBN 978-1-107-53485-8 Paperback

DEDICATION
To my son Patrick for the journey together

CONTENTS

PREFACE

The main reason for writing this book is that I have spent many rewarding years working as a physician and neurologist in Africa and would like to pass on some of that experience and knowledge to students there. Neurological disorders are common in Africa and the burden there has increased significantly because of the HIV epidemic and the emerging epidemic of non-communicable diseases. Students often find neurology a difficult subject to approach and there is a need for an easily accessible guide to neurology teaching and education in Africa.

The aim of this book is for students to gain an understanding of neurology, learn the necessary clinical skills and obtain sufficient knowledge to care for patients presenting with neurological disorders. Diagnosis in neurology is based on accurate history and physical examination and this book emphasizes these principles. It is written mostly from the perspective of a general physician practising neurology rather than that of a neurologist.

The book has two sections, the first on clinical skills, with medical students in wards and clinics as its main target group and the second on neurological disorders in adults with students and doctors as its main target group. The order of chapters is based on their importance in Africa, with the most common disorders there; epilepsy, stroke, infections, coma, paraplegia and neuropathies covered in the earlier chapters. The book includes chapters on head and spinal injury and care in neurology, because of their increasing significance within Africa. The choice of content included in each chapter is guided by the experience of the author. It is therefore subjective, selective and restricted by the size of the book. I have earnestly tried to avoid repetition; however in the attempt to make each chapter self-contained some repetition was unavoidable. I have included key points summarizing each section, which I hope will assist students with review. There is also a summary list of useful medical and neurological websites at the end of the book.

The term Africa is used throughout as a handy designation to mean sub-Saharan Africa. The lists of references at the end of each chapter are intended as a general guide to reading about neurology in Africa. For further information I refer the reader to a major neurology textbook.

In writing Neurology in Africa I have borrowed ideas and concepts from a wide range of excellent textbooks of neurology and tropical medicine and I am deeply indebted to their authors. I apologize in advance for any weaknesses and omissions and welcome comments and criticisms. I am reminded daily by students that the Internet is the new medium for education. With that in mind the book is available free online at www.uib.no/cih/en/resources/neurology-in-africa.

NIA was revised and updated in 2014 with information on polio and viral haemorrhagic fevers presented on pages 145 and 146 and also some minor changes throughout the text, mostly spelling corrections

The gap between need and resources is well documented in Africa and it is my experience that neurology is no different. It is my sincere hope that students and doctors in Africa will find this book a useful step towards filling that gap in neurology.

ACKNOWLEDGEMENTS

This book would not have been possible without the help and support of many persons. I am grateful to the many colleagues and friends who have read individual chapters or contributed in any way. These include the following: Mohamed Alwani, John Bartlett, Mike van Beer, Atta Bhatti, Jim Bower, Sam Chong, Glen Crawford, Katia Cikurel, John Crump, Mervyn Dean, Marieke Dekker, Shane Delamont, Tom Doherty, Cathy Ellis, John Eyers, Lars Fadness, Andrew Graham, Henning Grossman, Anthony Hall, Emma Hall, Ben Hamel, Sven Hinderaker, Patrick Howlett, Richard Hughes, Ewan Hunter, Joe Jarvis, Peter Kennedy, Gunnar Kvale, Gabriel Lende, Sean McDermott, Bridget MacDonald, Segni Mekonnen, Odd Morkve, Michael Murati, Ben Naafs, Lina Nashef, Peter Newman, Nikil Rajani, Leone Ridsdale, Tord Ro, Faheem Sheriff, Eli Silber, Ove Stoknes, Jim Todd, Susan Tyzack, Sarah Urasa, Sandeep Velichetii, Richard Walker, Felicity Werrett and Andrea Winkler. I am particularly indebted to the many medical students who have made helpful suggestions. While it is not possible to thank everyone individually I am very appreciative of their contributions.

The photographs used to illustrate the book are from patients attending Kilimanjaro Christian Medical Centre (KCMC) with selected epilepsy images from patients in Hai district. Permission to use photographs for teaching was explicit: where this has not been given, or uncertain, the individual's eyes have been "blanked out". I wish to thank all of them most sincerely. The radiology images are provided by Prof Helmut Diefenthal, Radiology Dept., KCMC. These were carefully collected by him over many years and generously donated for use in the book and I would like to thank him especially. Selected CT & MRI images were kindly provided by the Aga Khan Hospital, Dar es Salaam. The excellent pathological illustrations are provided by Prof Sebastian Lucas, St Thomas Hospital, London and I am particularly indebted to him. My special thanks go to colleagues and staff at KCMC for their continuing support and encouragement. In particular I would like to thank Prof Moshi Ntabaye, Executive Director, Prof Raimos Olomi, Director of Hospital Services, Dr Venance Maro, Head of Internal Medicine, Prof John Shao and Dr Mark Swai.

The writing and publication of this book has been achieved through a long lasting collaboration with the Centre for International Health (CIH) at the University of Bergen (UiB), Norway. I would especially like to thank Prof Rune Nilsen, director of CIH, Prof Gunnar Kvale and friends there for their support. The excellent drawings are by Ellinor Moldeklev Hoff, Department of Photos and Drawings, UiB. I remain especially indebted to her and would like to thank her particularly for this very important contribution. The layout, editing and publishing is by Christian Bakke, Division of Communication at UiB. I am very grateful for his patience, tolerance and professional guidance. The cover design and layout is by Tor Vegard Tobiassen. The scientific editor is Daniel Gibbs, Department of Neurology, Oregon Health and Science University, Portland, Oregon, who works and teaches at KCMC during annual visits there. I am very grateful to him for providing the necessary experience and knowledge to enable me to complete the book.

This book would not have been possible without the practical and financial support of many people for my work in Africa. I am particularly indebted to Dermot Desmond and to the following; The Department of Foreign Affairs, Dublin; Kevin & Bridget O'Doherty; Rory O'Hanlon; David & Stella Gorrod and Stephen Howlett. Finally I would like to thank my family and friends for their loyal support over the years.

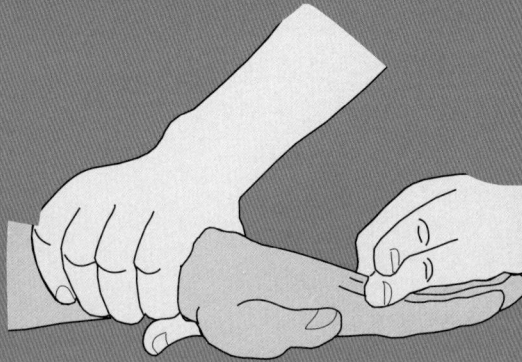

PART 1 – CLINICAL SKILLS

CHAPTER 1
HISTORY AND EXAMINATION

CONTENTS

CHAPTER 1

HISTORY AND EXAMINATION

Introduction

Neurology relies on the fundamental skills of history taking and physical examination. The aim of this section is to help the medical student to learn the basic clinical skills necessary to carry out a neurological history and examination and interpret the findings. Most students find neurology difficult to remember and in particular what to do, how to do it and what it all means. The history is the most important part of neurological evaluation because it is a guide to the underlying disease and also determines which part of the examination needs to be focused on. Indeed many neurological diseases like migraine have symptoms but no abnormal signs. The neurological examination determines abnormal neurological findings and helps to localize the site of the disease (Chapters 2 & 12). The history, examination and localization all together help to determine which disease has occurred at that site. The necessary competence required to carry out these tasks is formed by a combination of knowledge, skills and experience. Neurological knowledge is mostly self learned while clinical skills are taught at the bedside and experience gained over time. The nervous system by its nature is complex but its assessment can be learned with patience, plenty of practice and time.

HISTORY TAKING

Introduction

The history is the most important part of the neurological assessment. The student should aim to be a good listener showing interest and sympathy as the patient's story unfolds. It is important to get the patient's trust and confidence. First introduce yourself to the patient, explain who you are and ask permission to take a history and to carry out an examination. Find out the patient's name, age, address, occupation. Determine handedness by asking which hand do you write with or use more often. Some clinical findings are apparent to the examiner during history taking; these include general state of health and obvious neurological deficits and disabilities. If there is alteration in the level of consciousness or the patient is unable to give a history then it may be necessary to obtain a history and witnessed account from a relative or friend before proceeding directly to neurological examination. The patient's history reveals his personality, intelligence, memory and speech and his body language his attitude and mood. The questions should aim to learn the character, severity, time course and the particular circumstances of each main symptom. The order of history taking is summarized below under key points. While the history is being taken the level of alertness, mental well being and higher cerebral function becomes apparent to the examiner.

Key points in a neurological history

- age, sex, occupation, handedness
- presenting complaints
- history of presenting complaints
- neurology system review questions
- past history
- family history and social history
- drug history
- gynaecological and obstetrical history

Presenting complaint

Start the formal history by asking the patient to state what the problems are and the reason for hospital admission or referral. This could begin with open questions such as "what is the main problem or "tell me about it from the start". Try to let the patient tell the story of the illness as it has happened without any interruption. Make certain that you understand clearly what the patient is describing by their complaints. Determine the order of the presenting complaints, these should ideally not number more than three or four and be in order of importance. For each complaint determine the main site, character, onset, time course, exacerbating and relieving factors, associated symptoms and previous investigations and treatments.

Key points

- what are the problems
- what is the main problem
- when did it start
- site, character, time course, exacerbating & relieving factors, associated symptoms
- previous investigations and treatments

Time course

The time course of symptoms is essential to understanding the underlying cause. Ask the patient to describe the onset, progress, duration, recovery and frequency of each main complaint. In particular ask if the onset was sudden over seconds or minutes as occurs in stroke or more slowly over weeks or months as occurs in mass lesion e.g. tumour. Describe progress whether it was stationary as in a stroke or worsening as in an infection or intermittent as in epilepsy. If the symptoms are intermittent enquire about their frequency and the interval between them. Ask about precipitating or relieving factors, associated neurological symptoms and any particular circumstances in which the symptoms occur.

Key points

- onset
- progress
- duration
- frequency
- recovery

Systems review

A systematic enquiry may reveal symptoms related to the patient's illness. This may include a general medical review in addition to neurological systems review. Carry out a neurological systems review by asking the patient specific screening questions concerning symptoms affecting the various levels of higher cerebral and nervous system functioning. Finally ask if there is anything else that the patient would like to tell you.

Neurology systems review key questions

- change in mood, memory, concentration or sleep
- pain, headache, face or limbs
- loss of consciousness or dizzy spells
- loss of vision or double vision
- loss of hearing or balance
- difficulty speaking or swallowing
- weakness or heaviness in limbs
- difficulty walking
- pins and needles or numbness in arms, legs or body
- difficulty with passing urine, bowels and sexual function

Interpretation

As the history unfolds the examiner begins to hypothesize about the meaning of the history and the cause of the disorder. To reinforce this information it may be necessary to rephrase the questions in different ways or ask some direct questions. The main potential sites of disease are the brain, spinal cord, cranial and peripheral nerves, neuromuscular junction and muscles. It is helpful to attempt to anatomically localize the main site of the disease. Defining an anatomical limit to main symptoms is also helpful e.g. the upper limit of a sensory level in paraplegia, or the motor loss on one side in hemiplegia, or the glove and stocking sensory loss in a polyneuropathy. If the amount of time is limited then it is better to spend time on the history and be selective about the examination concentrating it on the main areas of interest.

Past medical history (PMH)

Enquire about past medical illnesses and accidents including hospitalizations and operations, and record their details in the notes. Where relevant ask specifically about a history of infections, seizures, head injuries, birth and childhood development, diabetes, hypertension and stroke. Enquire if there is a past history of neurological episodes similar to the presenting complaint and outline any investigations, their results and treatments received, and any persisting disabilities.

Family history

Document the patient's first degree relatives i.e. parents, siblings and children including their ages, sex and health. Enquire if there is anyone else in the family with the same illness, if so record the full family tree with their names and ages and indicating any affected family members and any deaths and their causes if known.

Personal & social history

Ask concerning occupation, employment, travel, alcohol intake in number of units per week and smoking in pack years (packs per day times years smoked); if relevant ask concerning the use of recreational drugs. Enquire how the current illness has affected work and social life including time lost from work over the last 6 months. Have a neurological patient describe the home environment, caregivers, community and financial circumstances if relevant.

Drugs, allergies

List the medications the patient is taking including names, duration and dosages. Describe any problems with medications and known allergies.

Menses

Record whether menses are normal and if the patient is pregnant or on the pill.

Key points

- allow the patient time to tell the story of their illness
- listen to the patient
- if patient is unable to give a history obtain it from family or friends
- ask if there "is anything else you wish to tell me"
- history determines the site of interest for neurological examination

General examination

The neurological examination must be performed in the context of a general physical examination. This includes recording the vital signs and examination of the cardiovascular system including listening for carotid bruits, and the respiratory, abdominal, and musculoskeletal systems.

NEUROLOGICAL EXAMINATION

Neurological examination is often considered by the student to be the most difficult part of neurological evaluation. This arises mainly because of technique and uncertainty over what is normal or abnormal. The best way to overcome this is to spend time early on learning the basic neurologic skills and then to practise on colleagues and patients until confident. The main aim is to become familiar with the routine of neurological examination and range of normal findings. The student will then gradually be introduced to abnormal findings in patients with neurological disorders and to what are termed neurological signs. In general, neurological signs are objective, reproducible and cannot be altered by the patient whereas less reliable findings tend to be variable, subjective and less reproducible. The neurological examination may involve an assessment of the level of consciousness, cognitive and mental function, cranial nerves, limbs and gait. Details concerning the clinical examination of level of consciousness and cognitive function are at the end of this chapter. In summary it is wise to listen attentively to the patient's complaints, stick to the routine of a basic neurological examination and to concentrate the neurological exam on the problem area highlighted by the history.

General observations

Observe the patient's general appearance, for any obvious neurological deficit and level of consciousness. The patient's level of consciousness, alertness, higher cerebral function, mental state and ability to give a history become apparent during the history taking. Neurological disorders affecting speech, posture, movement and gait may also become apparent at this stage.

CRANIAL NERVE EXAMINATION

These are tested with the patient in the sitting position.

Olfactory nerve (cranial nerve 1)

The olfactory nerve is responsible for smell. In a routine neurological examination it is sufficient to ask the patient if there is any loss of smell (anosmia). If anosmia is suspected then it should be tested at the bedside. This can be done by simply asking the patient to identify up to four familiar bedside items: e.g. orange peel, cloves, coffee, and soap. Before the test the nasal airway

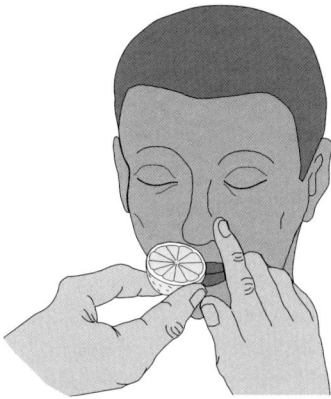

should be shown to be clear by getting the patient to sniff. Explain to the patient to close both eyes and block off one nostril by applying pressure with a finger. In the manner shown in the diagram the item to be identified is then presented to the other open nostril and the patient tries to identify the smell and its source. The procedure is then repeated for each item and on the other side. Patients may only become aware of the loss of smell whilst eating when the perception is often a loss of taste. The most common cause of loss of smell is local disease in the nose or sinuses e.g. head cold, hay fever and smoking.

Figure 1.1 Testing smell

Optic nerve (cranial nerve 2)

Visual acuity

Ask if the patient has any difficulty seeing. Visual acuity (VA) is tested and measured routinely by using a Snellen chart. The patient should stand 6 metres away from the chart and correct for any known refractive error by wearing appropriate glasses. Ask the patient to cover each eye in turn with his hand and find the smallest line that he can read fully without difficulty. VA is expressed as the distance between the chart and the patient over the smallest line completely visible to the patient. The numbers on the chart (below the line) correspond to the distance at which a person with normal vision should be able to see and identify the appropriate line. Below the age of 40 years most should see 6/6 or better. If 6/6 is normal and 36 represents the line that the patient can comfortably read at 6 metres with both eyes then visual acuity for that patient should be recorded as 6/36 in the right (VAR) and left eye (VAL). If VA is 6/60 or less then you can assess the patient's ability to see at 1 meter distance by counting fingers (CF), VA = CF, or seeing hand movements (HM), VA = HM or perceiving light (PL) VA = PL, if unable to perceive light then the patient is blind (NPL). At the bedside setting crude levels of visual acuity can be established by using a small hand held chart e.g. Jaeger chart or by using ordinary newspaper print. Colour vision is not tested routinely, however it can be tested by a using a book of Ishihara plates where at least 15/17 coloured plates identified correctly is considered normal. The most common causes of decreased visual acuity are optical problems, mainly refractive errors in lens, followed by cataracts and lastly diseases involving the retina, macula and optic nerve.

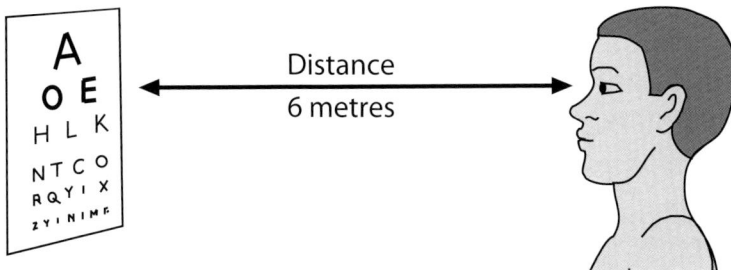

Figure 1.2 Testing visual acuity

Key points

- VA is measured standing 6 metres from a Snellen chart
- VA is distance between patient and chart over the smallest line identified correctly
- VA can be tested at bedside using a small hand held chart or newspaper
- most common causes of decreased VA are refractive errors and cataracts

Visual fields

The organization of the visual pathways means that the pattern of visual field loss varies at different sites along its way. This means that testing for the pattern of visual field loss is useful for localization of lesions along the visual pathway. Visual fields are always described and recorded from the perspective of the patient looking outwards with the fields divided into nasal and temporal halves. At the bedside visual fields are examined by confrontation. The main patterns of loss are homonymous & bitemporal hemianopia, & monocular blindness.

Confrontation

This involves sitting about 1 meter in front of the patient with your eyes at the same horizontal level. Ask the patient to look with both eyes at your eyes (the bridge of your nose). Hold your hands upright halfway between you and the patient held approximately half a meter apart and at about 30 cm above the horizontal. While looking at the patient's eyes first move the index finger tip of one hand (or a 5-7 mm red pin head) and ask the patient to correctly identify which finger moved. The patient should immediately point or indicate the hand on which the finger moved. Do the same with the other hand. Repeat the manoeuvre with the hands held about 30 cm below the horizontal. To examine the visual fields in each eye separately, ask the patient to cover one eye e.g. patient's right eye and the examiner covers the eye opposite, in this case his own left eye. Ask the patient to focus on your uncovered eye. Move your index finger in each of the four quadrants starting in the temporal field followed by the nasal field in same manner as you did on confrontation for both eyes. Repeat for the other eye. Remember that the nose and prominent eyebrows may partially block vision and mistakenly give a field deficit.

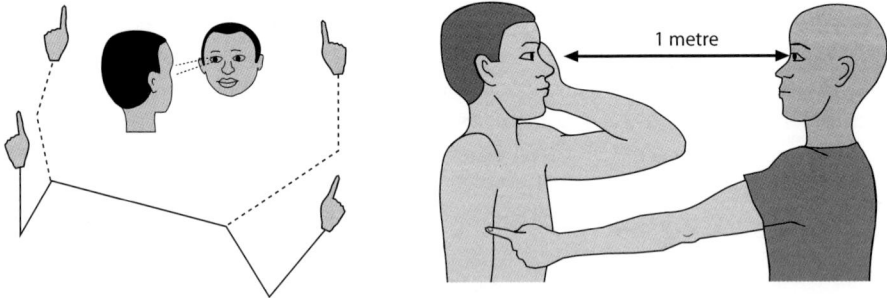

Figure 1.3 Examining visual fields. Testing for visual defects by confrontation.

Field perimetry

Field perimetry can be tested in the same manner using a moving finger tip or a white pin head 5-7 mm target. Start behind the patient's visual field coming forward diagonally in a convex plane from all four quadrants at a 45 degree angle, northeast to southwest and northwest to southeast and the same in reverse asking the patient to indicate as soon as he sees the movement. This establishes the posterior limit of the patient's visual field. The blind spot (optic nerve head) and any central field defects can be easily identified using red pin head moving in the horizontal plane from outside.

Key points

- patients are often unaware of loss of visual fields
- major visual field loss is identified by confrontation
- peripheral visual fields are tested by perimetry examination
- main patterns of loss are homonymous & bitemporal hemianopia & monocular blindness

Ocular fundi

Ocular fundi are tested by fundoscopy. The aim of fundoscopy is to inspect the optic nerve head, arterioles, veins and retina. This is an important part of the neurological examination and is used mainly to exclude papilloedema or swelling of the optic nerve. The main cause of papilloedema in Africa is raised intracranial pressure secondary to CNS infections and mass lesions. Swelling of the optic disc may also be caused by inflammation of the optic nerve and this is called papillitis. The main cause of papillitis is optic neuritis.

How to use an ophthalmoscope

Students and young doctors at first find fundoscopy difficult but the skill comes with training and practice. The most important thing to understand is the position of the optic nerve head within the field of vision you are testing. The optic nerve head lays 15-20 degrees lateral to the point of fixation of the patient's eyes and slightly below the horizontal and corresponds to the blind spot.

The following instructions should be helpful. The patient should fix his gaze straight ahead. Check the focus on the ophthalmoscope is set at zero and the light is bright, then sit opposite the patient and examine the right eye. With the ophthalmoscope in the right hand approach from the patient's right side, look at the patient's right eye from 30 cm away with the ophthalmoscope

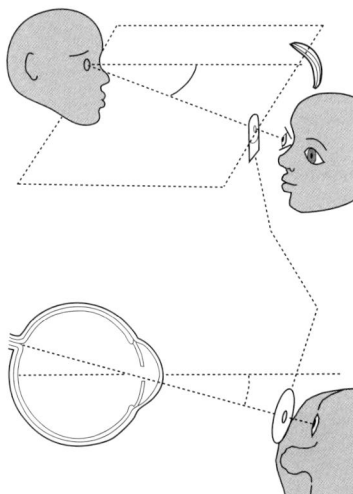

level or slightly below the patient's eye about 15-20 degrees outside or lateral to the patient's line of fixation or direction of gaze. Aim at the centre of the back of head and keep out of the line of sight of the other eye. You should be able to see the pupil as pink in colour; this is the normal retinal or red reflex. Gradually move in towards the eye, encourage patient to continue to look or fixate at a point behind you straight ahead and bring ophthalmoscope to within 1-2 cm of the patient's right eye. It's important to keep patient's eye, point of fixation and ophthalmoscope all on the same plane. Adjust the lens for focus so that you can see the blood vessels clearly and follow blood vessels as they get larger and converge on the disc. Look at the optic disc, blood vessels, retinal background and repeat for the other eye.

Figure 1.4 Fundoscopy

What you find

The normal disc is circular and pale pink in colour, the edge of the disc is clear although not as well demarcated on the nasal side as the temporal side (Chapter 12). The temporal half of the disc is normally paler than the nasal half. The physiological optic cup from which the blood vessels emerge is a well defined depression in the centre of the nerve head. It is pale and occupies about 40-50% of size of the optic disc. The rest of the fundus has an even red background because of blood in the choroid layer. The retina may be darkly pigmented depending on racial background. The macula with a central darker area called fovea lies about one and a half disc spaces from the disc on its temporal side and is free of blood vessels. It can easily be found by asking the patient to look directly at the light of the ophthalmoscope. The arterioles are normally two thirds the sizes of veins and appear a brighter shade of red than veins. The veins on the disc appear to pulsate in 70-80% of normal people in the sitting position, and the absence of pulsation may be an early sign of papilloedema. In papilloedema the whole disc is usually pink red and the veins become distended and lose their pulsation. The optic cup is lost and the edge of the disc and the vessels emerging may appear elevated. Later the whole disc itself becomes indistinct and blurred especially on the nasal side which is normally less distinct and haemorrhages and exudates may be seen on or near its margins and vessels disappearing without an obvious optic disc (Chapter 12). In chronic papilloedema the disc becomes pale as occurs in optic atrophy.

Key points

- approach patient's right eye at same eye level from 30 cm out & 15-20 degrees laterally
- identify red reflex and follow beam of light into eye looking for a normal pale pink disc
- main sign of papilloedema is swelling of the optic disc with blurring of the disc margins
- main sign of optic atrophy is a pale white optic disc
- practise on colleagues and patients with normal eyes

Pupillary reactions

These are examined after the optic nerve and before eye movements. The normal pupillary reactions include the light reflex, the accommodation reflex and the consensual reflex.

Assessing the pupils

Inspect the pupils at rest for size and shape and whether they are equal, central and circular and react to light. It's not always easy to assess pupillary size in a darkened room or in patients with a darkened iris. A difference in pupil size is called anisocoria. It helps to inspect the pupils at rest by shining a torch on the bridge of the patient's nose allowing light to scatter but not affecting the pupils.

Figure 1.5 Testing the light reflex

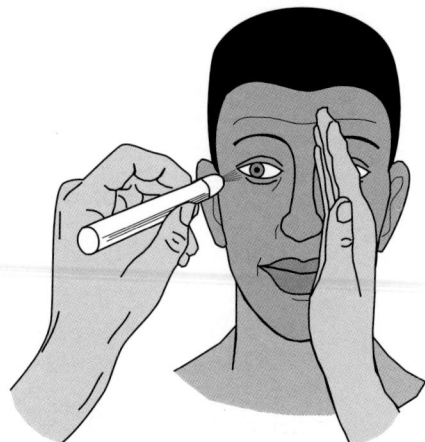

The light reflex

To test the pupillary light reflex, ask the patient to look in the distance and not into direct light. It may help to block off the other eye in the manner shown in the diagram.

Then bring a bright light in from behind or from the side into the patient's field of vision and observe the eye for direct or ipsilateral pupillary constriction. This is called the direct light reflex. Then repeat this again in the same eye now looking for the same response in the other eye. This is called *the consensual reflex*. Check for the same reflexes in the other eye.

The accommodation reflex

The accommodation reflex has two components and is much less clinically important than the light reflex. To test this reflex ask the patient to look in the distance and then at the examiner's finger held 10 cm in front of the patient's nose. As the gaze is shifted from a distant to near object the eyes adduct and pupils constrict. The first component is convergence which requires adduction of both eyes at the same time. The other component involves bilateral simultaneous constriction of the pupils; this combined with adduction is the normal accommodation reflex.

Pupillary disorders

Large and small pupils which react to light and accommodation can occur normally in young and old persons respectively. Pupillary disorders are generally categorized as those resulting in large dilated non or slowly reacting pupils and those resulting in small constricted reacting or non reacting pupils. The main causes of these are to be found in disorders affecting the optic nerve and the iris and its autonomic parasympathetic and sympathetic nerve supply.

Key points

- inspect pupils for size, shape and whether they are equal or not
- **light reflex:** shine a bright light into the eye and watch for pupillary constriction
- **consensual reflex:** inspect the other eye at the same time for pupillary constriction
- **accommodation reflex**: watch eyes adduct & pupils constrict as gaze is shifted to a near object

Oculomotor, Trochlear and Abducens (cranial nerves 3, 4 & 6)

Eye movements

The 3rd 4th and 6th cranial nerves are tested together by examining eye movements. Eye movements are generated in two main ways each of which should be tested separately. Firstly voluntary movements are generated from the frontal lobe; they are also called saccadic because of the rapid jumping movement from one point of fixation to another. These are tested by asking the patient to look rapidly from one side to the other or right and left and are impaired in cortical brain disease. Secondly and more important clinically are pursuit eye or tracking movements which are generated from the occipital lobe when the eyes stay on and follow the point of fixation. These are tested by asking the patient to follow the examiner's moving finger and are impaired in brain stem and cranial nerve disorders. Lastly the cerebellum also plays a main role in controlling eye movements in response to body movements in order to keep the point of fixation. All eye movements are integrated in the brain stem so that the eyes can move together conjugately in all directions. Eye movement abnormalities are usually noted because the patient complains of double vision or diplopia and because the eyes appear to the observer be looking in different directions. When this happens it is called a squint or strabismus. The main causes of diplopia are disorders affecting the function of the 3rd 4th and 6th cranial nerves. The main sites for these disorders are eye muscles, the neuromuscular junction, or the individual nerves and their central connections in the brain stem. The most common causes are vascular and inflammatory disorders affecting the individual nerves and neuromuscular junction respectively.

Testing for pursuit eye movements

Pursuit eye movements are routinely examined during the neurological examination. The examiner tests for horizontal and vertical eye movements by instructing the patient "to follow my finger with your eyes" whilst keeping the patient's head steady. The examiner holds a finger about half a meter away from the patient's face and makes horizontal and vertical movements in the shape of a cross sign being careful not to move the hand too rapidly. The movement is carried out with the index finger held vertically moving horizontally 30-45 degrees right and left from mid point and then repeated in the same way moving vertically with the finger held horizontally. The trochlear nerve is tested by repeating the same movements but this time in the shape of H sign. This should be carried out in each eye field separately to confirm any weakness. Any loss or impairment of normal eye movement or jerkiness (nystagmus) should be noted.

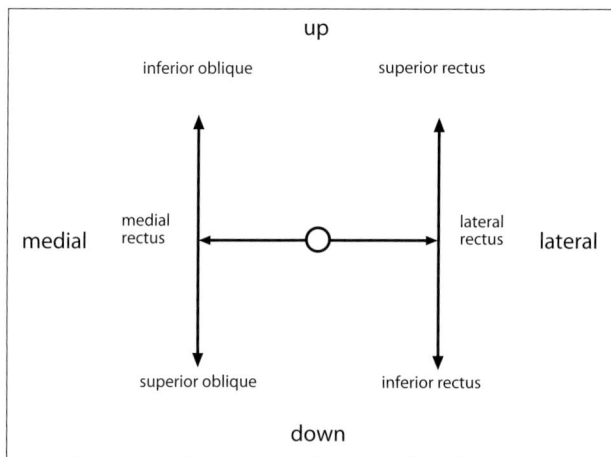

Figure 1.6 Testing eye movements

Nystagmus

Nystagmus is an involuntary rhythmic oscillatory movement of the eyes. Nystagmus is usually asymptomatic. To test for nystagmus ask the patient to follow the examiner's fingers using the same method as when testing for normal eye movements. Nystagmus should be examined in three main positions, at rest, looking right and left horizontally and looking up and down vertically. Be careful not to move the eyes too quickly or too far laterally (not beyond 30 degrees from midline) and note the presence of any nystagmus. Nystagmus is only considered pathological when it is sustained. The characteristics of nystagmus help to localize the site of neurological disease. The main causes of nystagmus are disorders affecting the vestibular system and its central connections, the brain stem, cerebellum and the eye including early onset blindness. It can also rarely be congenital, and then is pendular and multidirectional.

Key Points

- eye movements are tested by following examiner's finger as it traces a cross (+) or (H) sign in the air
- H sign tests the trochlear nerves in addition to the oculomotor and the abducens
- nystagmus is an involuntary oscillatory movement of the eyes
- diplopia is mostly caused by weakness of the ocular muscles

Trigeminal nerve (cranial nerve 5)

The trigeminal nerve has three divisions ophthalmic (V1), maxillary (V2), and mandibular (V3). It is responsible for facial sensation and mastication.

Sensation

To test sensation, first ask if the patient feels any numbness or altered sensation on the face. Then test for light touch (and gentle pinprick and temperature only if necessary) in each of the three divisions of the trigeminal nerve comparing one side with the other. If a sensory loss is found then determine its limits by moving from an abnormal area to normal. Remember that the ophthalmic division extends posteriorly to the vertex and also supplies the cornea and the tip of the nose. The angle of the jaw is supplied by the C2 nerve root rather than the trigeminal nerve. Sensory loss on the face is caused mainly by lesions in the brain stem and the trigeminal nerve.

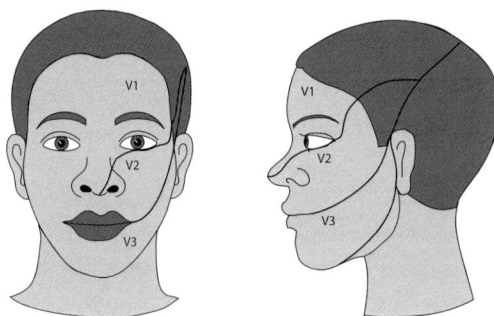

Figure 1.7 Testing facial sensation

Motor

The motor division of the trigeminal nerve can be tested by inspecting for wasting above the zygomatic arch and asking the patient to clench the teeth and to palpate the masseters and pterygoids for force of contraction. Power can be assessed by jaw opening and jaw closure and side to side movements against resistance. Ask the patient to open and close his mouth against the resistance of your hand. In unilateral paralysis the jaw deviates to the weak or affected side. Motor involvement affecting the trigeminal nerve is very uncommon. Causes include myasthenia gravis, motor neurone disease and muscular dystrophy.

Jaw jerk

The jaw jerk is a brain stem stretch reflex which may be absent or present in normal people. To elicit the reflex the patient should let his jaw sag open. Place your finger lightly on the chin. Then tap your finger gently and feel and observe for a brief contraction or movement upwards of the lower jaw. The jaw jerk may be increased in an upper motor neurone lesion and indicates a lesion in the midbrain or above.

Corneal reflex

The trigeminal nerve provides the afferent arc of the corneal reflex. The facial nerve provides the efferent arc. It is a consensual reflex and may be tested by lightly touching the cornea (the coloured part of the eye) with a wisp of cotton wool and observe for reflex blinking in both eyes. The lower lid may be held down while the patient looks up making access to the cornea from below easy. The normal response to touching the cornea is that blinking of both eyes should occur. A unilateral trigeminal nerve lesion therefore results in loss of blinking on both sides whereas a unilateral seventh nerve lesion results in loss of the reflex on the affected side.

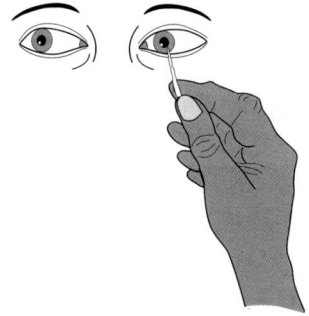

Figure 1.8 Testing the corneal reflex (V and VII)

Key points

- trigeminal nerve supplies sensation to the face and power to the muscles of mastication
- sensation is tested touching in each division of trigeminal nerve & comparing sides
- power is tested by resisting jaw opening, closure & side to side movements
- corneal reflex is tested by touching the cornea lightly from below with a wisp of cotton
- loss of the corneal reflex may be caused by either a 5th or 7th cranial nerve lesion

Facial nerve (cranial nerve 7)

The facial nerve is primarily a motor nerve that is responsible for facial expression, which includes wrinkling of the forehead, eye closure, closure of the lips and smiling. The sensory portion is responsible for special sensation to the anterior two thirds of tongue via the chorda tympani branch. There are also a few sensory fibres to the outer ear canal. In clinical practice there are two types of facial nerve paralysis, a lower motor neurone type which includes Bell's palsy and an upper motor neurone type which is most frequently seen in stroke. It is important to be able to distinguish clinically these two types from each other.

In a lower motor neurone facial palsy there is a complete ipsilateral facial weakness with loss of forehead wrinkling, eye closure, nasolabial fold and drooping of the lips on the affected side. This is in contrast to an upper motor neurone lesion where the facial paralysis affects mainly the lower half of the face with preservation of wrinkling and partial eye closure although they may be reduced.

Examining the facial nerve

To objectively test motor function in the facial nerve start in the upper half of the face by asking the patient to look upwards towards the ceiling by elevating his eyebrows or wrinkling the forehead. Then test eye closure by asking the patient to shut the eyes tightly and assess strength by trying to open patient's eyes with your fingers. If there is a lower motor neurone pattern of weakness there is loss of wrinkling and reduced or no resistance to forced eye opening on the affected side. Movements in the lower half of the face are tested by asking the patient to

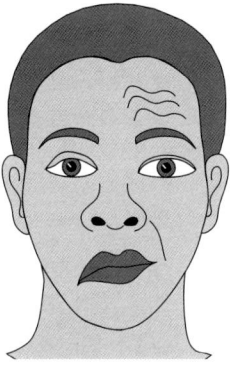

smile, whistle and finally to blow out of the cheeks and to keep the lips closed against the examiner's attempt to open them. Any weakness or asymmetry implies a lesion in the seventh nerve. The reason that both the forehead and eye closure are partially spared in a unilateral upper motor neurone lesion is that they are bilaterally innervated. A bilateral lower motor neurone weakness can be easily missed clinically unless the facial nerves are specifically tested. To assess taste apply a solution of salt, sweet, sour or bitter to the anterior tongue comparing the response on both sides.

Figure 1.9 Testing facial movements. Facial nerve palsy, right (lower motor neurone lesion) Loss of wrinkling of forehead. Loss of nasolabial fold. Drooping of mouth.

Key points

- inspect for drooping of the mouth, loss of nasolabial fold, eye closure and wrinkling
- ask the patient to smile, close their eyes and look up
- a complete facial weakness on one side indicates a lower motor neurone lesion
- facial weakness on one side confined to the lower half indicates an upper motor neurone lesion

Acoustic nerve (cranial nerve 8)

The acoustic nerve has two divisions: the cochlear (hearing) and the vestibular (balance).

Hearing

Hearing is first assessed by asking if the patient has a hearing problem. Hearing can be tested clinically by rubbing the thumb and finger close to the patient's ear and asking if hearing is different between the two sides. Hearing loss is then crudely confirmed by whispering numbers and asking the patient to repeat them whilst standing behind the patient about 60 cm away from the test ear. At the same time hearing in the non affected ear is masked by rubbing fingers close to the tragus or by occluding it with a finger. If the patient cannot hear whispering, then a normal or louder voice is used. The test is then repeated on the other side if necessary. Bedside testing is relatively insensitive and may miss lower levels of hearing loss for which audiometry is required. There are two main types of hearing loss, conductive deafness where there is a failure of transmission of sound (air conduction AC) from the outer to the inner ear or cochlea, and sensorineural deafness or (bone conduction BC) which is due to disease in the cochlea or its neural connections. The Rinne and Weber tuning fork tests can help distinguish whether the hearing loss is conductive or sensorineural in type. The main causes of conductive hearing loss are wax in the outer ear and infection in the middle ear. The main causes of sensorineural hearing loss deafness are ototoxicity, infections, Ménière's disease and presbyacusis.

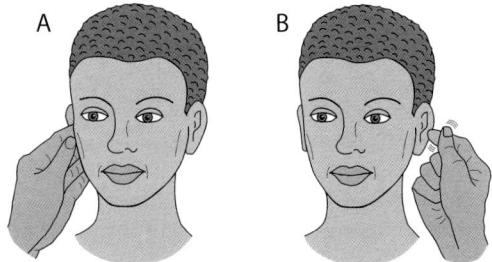

Figure 1.10 Testing hearing

Rinne's test

Use a 256 Hz tuning fork, tap on knee or forearm, then hold the base of beating tuning fork on the mastoid process behind the ear. When the patient stops hearing it then place it beside the external auditory meatus in line with the ear canal. In normal hearing air conduction is greater than bone conduction (AC>BC) so the patient will still hear the tuning fork. In conductive deafness there is impairment of conduction and bone conduction is better (BC>AC). In sensorineural deafness the normal pattern is retained AC>BC but both components are reduced compared to the normal ear.

Weber's test

The base of a vibrating tuning fork is placed on the middle of the forehead or on the top of the head (vertex) and the patient asked in which ear the sound is loudest in, normally the sound is heard equally in both ears or in the middle. If the sound is heard best in the affected ear then there is unilateral conductive hearing loss on that side as only the vibration transmitted directly through bone to the middle ear ossicles can be heard. In contrast if it is heard best in the good ear then there is sensorineural hearing loss in the affected ear.

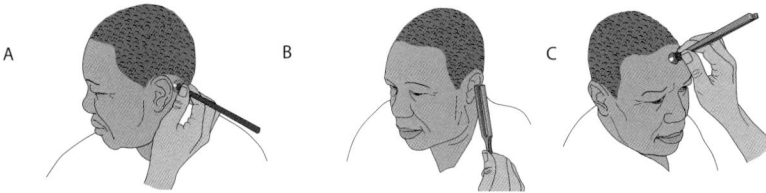

Figure1.11 Distinguishing the type of deafness. The Rinne test A + B. The Weber test C.

Balance

The vestibular portion of the eight nerves transmits sensory information from the vestibular apparatus to the brain stem and cerebellum. Balance depends on normal input from this system in combination with proprioception and eyes. Symptoms and signs suggestive of vestibular dysfunction include positional vertigo, ataxia, nausea, vomiting and nystagmus on looking away from the side of the lesion. Vestibular balance is not routinely tested in a bedside examination but can be tested clinically in disease by the caloric and Hallpike's manoeuvre. The main vestibular causes of loss of balance are benign positional vertigo, vestibular neuronitis and Ménière's disease.

Key points

- hearing is crudely tested by whispering numbers in one ear while blocking the other ear
- conductive hearing loss is failure of transmission through air, BC > AC
- sensorineural hearing loss is failure of transmission through cochlea/neural connections, AC > BC
- Rinne test can discriminate between unilateral conductive and sensorineural hearing loss
- Weber test lateralizes to the affected ear in conductive loss & to normal ear in sensorineural loss

Glossopharyngeal and Vagus nerves (cranial nerves 9 and 10)

Together these supply power to the palate, throat and larynx and are responsible for normal speech and swallowing. The glossopharyngeal nerve supplies ordinary sensation to the posterior pharyngeal wall and sensation to the posterior one third of tongue. The vagus supplies the muscles of the palate, pharynx and larynx. The vagus also has a large autonomic innervation including heart lungs and abdomen.

Testing the gag reflex

Routine testing can be performed by watching the soft palate and uvula move upwards in the midline in response to the patient saying "aah". This is called the voluntary gag reflex. The gag reflex can also be elicited by gently touching each side of the soft palate with an orange stick or tongue depressor and asking the patient if the sensation was the same on both sides and watching the palate rise involuntarily. This is called the involuntary gag reflex. The involuntary gag tests both the afferent glossopharyngeal and the efferent vagus nerve whereas the voluntary gag tests the efferent vagus nerve only. A unilateral paralysis of the palate deviates away from the side of the lesion. It indicates a lower motor neurone lesion of the vagus nerve e.g. a bulbar palsy. An upper motor neurone lesion has to be bilateral to result in any palatal paralysis and then the paralysis of the palate is total e.g. pseudo bulbar palsy. The main causes are brain stem stroke and motor neurone disease.

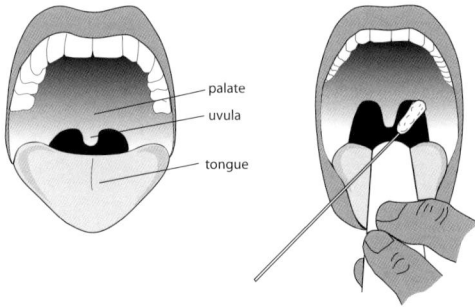

Figure 1.12 Testing the gag reflex. Glossopharyngeal and vagus nerves.

Accessory nerve (cranial nerve 11)

The accessory nerve supplies the sternomastoid and trapezius muscles as shown in the diagrams respectively. Wasting of both muscles should be checked for on inspection. Power is assessed by resisting the movements of both muscles. Note that the right sternomastoid turns the head to the left and vice versa. The strength is gauged by asking the patient to twist the head and the examiner placing a hand on the opposite side of the lower face and resisting the movement. Similarly the strength of the trapezius muscle can be gauged by asking the patient to first elevate or shrug the shoulders and then against resistance. Weakness of these muscles is unusual in clinical practice but does occur mostly in muscle disease and myasthenia gravis.

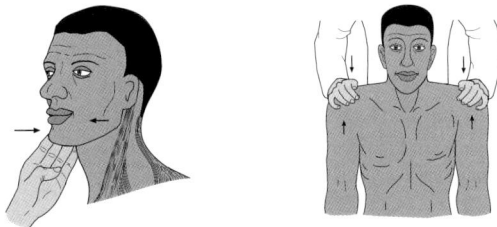

Figure 1.13 Examining the accessory nerve. Testing the sternomastoid and the trapezius.

Key point

· test the sternomastoid and trapezius by resisting head turning and shoulder elevation

Hypoglossal nerve (cranial nerve 12)

The hypoglossal nerve is a purely motor nerve which supplies the muscles of the tongue. Testing the 12th cranial nerve is done by inspecting the tongue at rest and on protrusion. It is first inspected in the floor of the mouth checking carefully for evidence of wasting or fasciculation or spasticity. The mobility and strength of the tongue can be assessed by asking the patient to protrude it in and out quickly as well as from side to side. The strength of the two sides can be assessed by pushing the tongue into either cheek whilst opposing it with your thumb from the outside and comparing the sides. A unilateral lower motor neurone weakness will result in atrophy and fasciculations on the affected side and also deviation towards the same side as the lesion. A unilateral upper motor neurone lesion will result in tongue deviation away from affected side.

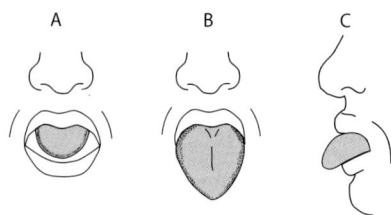

Figure 1.14 Examining the tongue. Hypoglossal nerve.

Key points

- voluntary gag reflex is tested by getting the patient to say "aah"
- involuntary gag reflex is tested by touching the soft palate on both sides
- normal gag reflex causes a symmetrical elevation of the soft palate and uvula
- tongue should be inspected at rest in the mouth, protruded & during movement

EXAMINATION OF THE LIMBS

The arms and legs are examined in the following order, inspection, tone, power, coordination, reflexes and sensation. The upper limbs are examined in the sitting position and the lower in the lying position.

Inspection

The examination starts with bedside observation for obvious deformities, disabilities, postures, contractures or involuntary limb movements or any other abnormality. The way the patient moves to undress for the examination also provides useful information concerning power and coordination. Start the inspection with the patient in the sitting position and the limbs exposed by looking at the skin for scars and trophic changes and the muscles for size, wasting and fasciculation. Compare the right side with the left. Muscle wasting should be looked for in the hands, arms, shoulders, trunk, thighs and legs. In the hands the front and back of the hands, including thenar and hypothenar eminences and the small hand muscles should be checked. Fasciculations are spontaneous rippling movements of muscle motor units and their presence implies a lower motor neurone lesion. They may take a few minutes of continuous observation to see. However they are often benign especially in the calves and after exercise.

Tone

Tone is tested by moving the limbs passively as the examiner feels the degree of resistance. Muscle tone is maintained by the stretch reflex which occurs on passive moving and stretching of muscles around joints. The patient should be relaxed and the joint put through its full range of movement while comparing sides. Tone is categorized as normal, decreased or increased. Decreased tone is uncommon and occurs in lower motor neurone lesions, muscle and cerebellar disease. Increased tone is classified as either pyramidal (upper motor neurone) or as extrapyramidal (Parkinson's disease). In an upper motor neurone lesion increased tone is best appreciated in the arm as a spastic catch on rapid flexing and extending the elbow and on pronation and supination of the forearm. In the leg tone is best appreciated in the lying position with the legs straight by rolling the knee from side to side and on rapid flexing and extending the leg at the knee and ankle joints. The initial resistance and the sudden give away or release is called clasp knife rigidity. This is best appreciated just at the start of flexion at the knee and extension at the elbow. It may be necessary to get the patient to relax by distracting him by asking to count backwards from 100 and to try different speeds of passive movement. A rapid rhythmic persistent contraction and relaxation of the muscles is called clonus. This can be best elicited by dorsiflexing the ankle briskly and maintaining the pressure on the forefoot with the knee flexed to about 90 degrees. Persistent clonus or more than 5 beats is always abnormal and indicates an upper motor neurone lesion. Clonus occurs less commonly around other joints but may be present at the knee and wrist. In extrapyramidal disease the tone is increased and is classified as either lead pipe or cogwheel in type. The rigidity is equally stiff throughout both flexion and extension and is best appreciated by slowly fully flexing and extending the elbow and knee and by pronating and supinating the wrist. It may be increased by distracting the patient by asking him to move the contralateral limb e.g. tapping the thigh at the same time. Cog wheeling represents intrusion of rest tremor into lead pipe rigidity.

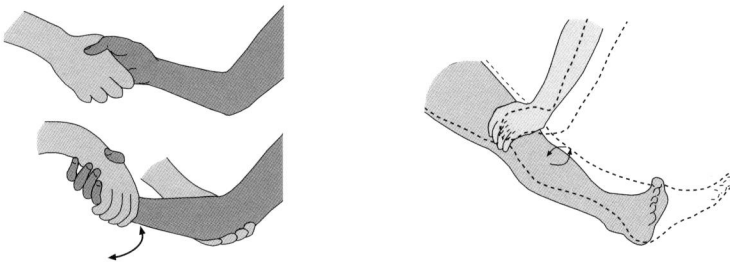

Figure 1.15 Testing tone. Roll the wrist. Roll the knee.

Key points

- patient should be relaxed and the joint put through full range of movement passively
- increased tone is either pyramidal (clasp knife) or extrapyramidal (lead pipe or cogwheel)
- pyramidal rigidity is best appreciated at the start of rapid flexion at the elbow and knee
- extrapyramidal rigidity is best elicited by slow flexion/extension of elbow/knee or rolling wrist
- clonus is elicited by dorsiflexing the ankle briskly & maintaining pressure on the forefoot

Power

Power is tested in a proximal to distal direction comparing sides with the patient in the seated position for the upper limbs and the lying position for the lower limbs. The patient first demonstrates muscle strength by active movements and then the examiner opposes those movements. This is done by the examiner stabilizing the limb proximal to the joint where the movement is being tested and then passively resisting the movement. Recognizing normal power is a matter of experience and allowances have to be made for the sick, old, young and for effort. Power loss is graded as mild moderate or severe or as according to the Medical Research Council (MRC) classification (Table 1.1).

Table 1.1 Measuring strength

MRC Grade	Degree of strength	MRC Grade	Degree of strength
5	normal power	2	moves but not against gravity
4	weakness	1	flicker of movement
3	moves against gravity	0	no movement

In a routine neurological examination it is sufficient to test one proximal and one distal muscle group in the limbs. A screening test for mild loss of power in the upper limbs is the pronator test; this involves holding the arms outstretched with the hands held in supination and eyes closed. If an arm drifts downwards and pronates it suggests mild pyramidal weakness on that side. If the arm rises or deviates outwards it suggests parietal or cerebellar disease. In the ambulant patient walking on the heels is also a good guide to foot drop and walking on toes to weakness of the calf muscles. Rising out of a chair or from the squat position and climbing stairs are the best tests for weakness of the quadriceps and ileopsoas. The trunk muscles should be tested by asking the patient to sit up from the lying position. If the umbilicus moves excessively upwards in paraplegia it is called Beevor's sign.

To test power in the individual muscle groups do the following:
- for shoulder abduction (C5, deltoids), ask the patient to abduct the arms 90 degrees and push upwards against the examiners hands resisting the movement
- for elbow flexion (C6, biceps), ask the patient to extend the elbow 90 degrees and bend or pull the forearm towards his face against resistance
- for elbow extension (C7 triceps), the patient extends (straightens) his forearm 90 degrees against resistance
- for wrist extension (C7, wrist extensors), extension of the patient's wrist with the fist closed is resisted
- for finger extension (C7, 8), the examiner uses two fingers to try to resist the patient extending the fingers
- for finger flexion (C8), the patient's curled fingers of the hand cannot be prised open
- for abduction and adduction of fingers (T1), forceful spread and coming together of the patient's "fingers" is opposed
- for abduction of the thumb (T1), the patient's thumb is brought to a right angle with the palm and the movement opposed

examining for power in the lower limbs starts with hip flexion (L1, L2 ileopsoas)
- for hip flexion the patient flexes the hip and knee to 90 degrees and continues flexing the hip as hard as he can, the examiner places a hand on the lower thigh just above the knee to assess strength
- for hip extension (L5 gluteus maximus), the patient lies flat and pushes down into the bed against the examiner's hand which is placed under his heel
- for knee extension (L3, L4 quadriceps) ask the patient to bend the knee to 90 degrees and to straighten the leg against resistance
- for knee flexion (S1 biceps femoris), ask the patient to flex or bring his knee in 90 degrees towards his bottom while the examiner tries to straighten the leg against resistance

- for foot dorsiflexion (L4, L5 tibialis anterior), ask the patient to extend the foot to 90 degrees while the examiner opposes the movement
- for plantar flexion (S1 gastrocnemius), the patient pushes his foot down towards the ground against resistance

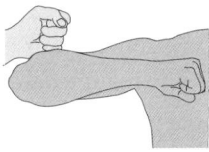

Shoulder abduction
Deltoid
Axillary nerve
C5

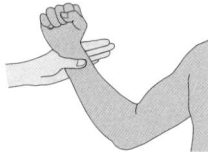

Elbow extension
Triceps
Radial nerve
C7

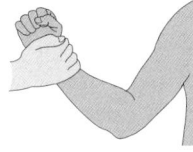

Elbow flexion (forearm midpronated)
Brachioradialis
Radial nerve
C6

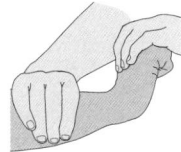

Wrist extension
Extensors
Radial nerve
C7

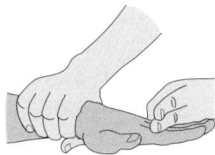

Finger extension
Extensor digitorum
Radial nerve
C7

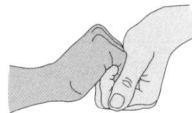

Finger flexion
Flexor digitorum
Median and ulnar nerve
C8

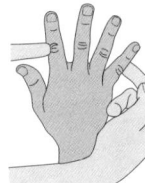

Finger abduction
Dorsal interossel
Ulnar nerve
T1

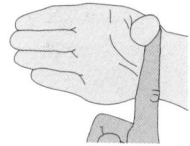

Thumb abduction
Abductor pollicis brevis
Median nerve
T1

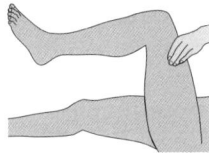

Hip flexion
Iliopsoas
Lumbar plexus and femoral nerve
L1 L2

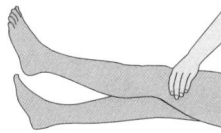

Hip flexion
Quadriceps femoris
Femoral nerve
L3 L4

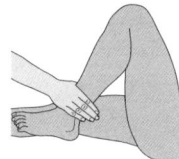

Knee extension
Quadriceps femoris
Femoral nerve
L3 L4

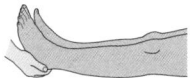

Hip extension
Gluteus maximus
Sciatic nerve
L5 S1

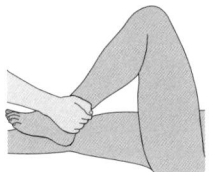

Knee flexion
Hamstrings
Sciatic nerve
L5 S1

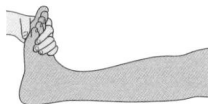

Ankle dorsiflexion
Tibialis anterior
Common peroneal nerve
L4 L5

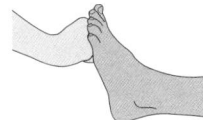

Plantar flexion
Gastrocnemius and soleus
Sciatic nerve
S1 S2

Figure 1.16 Testing power

Key points

- power should be attempted actively by the patient before being examined passively by doctor
- power should be tested proximally before distally
- weakness is graded as mild moderate and severe or 0-5 according to MRC classification
- pattern of muscle weakness is a clue to the underlying disorder

Coordination

The cerebellum and its connections are responsible for the coordination of voluntary movement. These movements depend on normal power and joint position sense. Any significant weakness or impairment of joint position sense invalidates the tests for coordination. Abnormalities of the cerebellar hemispheres produce ipsilateral signs. Cerebellar dysfunction is characterized by incoordination of **speech, limbs and gait**. The speech in cerebellar disease is dysarthric or slow and slurred with a typical scanning quality of getting stuck on the consonants. Nystagmus is a sign of cerebellar disease and is worse on looking to the side of the lesion. The main tests of incoordination are **the finger nose test, the heel shin test** and **gait**. These are carried out with the eyes open. Other clinical features are **dysarthria, nystagmus and hypotonia** of muscles.

The finger nose test

This test is carried out with the arms fully extended horizontally by asking the patient to touch the tip of his nose with the tip of the index finger of his right hand followed by the same with his left hand. An alternative method involves asking the patient to touch the tip of his nose

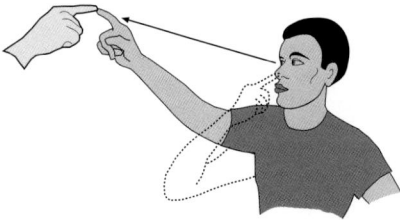

followed by touching the tip of the examiner's index finger. This is called the finger nose finger test and has the advantage of two targets. The examiner's index finger should be held at arm's length away in front of the patient ensuring that the patient has to fully stretch to touch the finger. The examiner should observe the patient for any obvious limb ataxia and intention tremor with increased oscillation on nearing the target.

Figure 1.17 Testing co-ordination. The finger-nose test.

The heel shin test

This is a two step test. The first step is asking the patient to first hold the foot up in the air, then step two to place the heel on the other knee and slowly run it down the shin. Any wobble on reaching the target or side to side or falling off movement on sliding down the shin points to cerebellar disease on the same side.

Figure 1.18 Testing co-ordination. The heel-shin test.

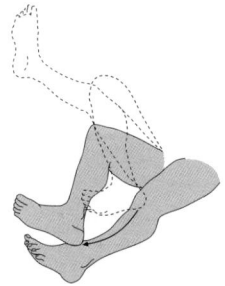

Other tests of cerebellar incoordination are **rapid alternating hand movements** and **dysmetria.** The former is known as dysdiadochokinesia and is demonstrated by rapid tapping the palm of one hand alternately with the palm and back of the other hand and then repeating on the opposite hand. In the normal person the alternate movements are smooth and regular whereas in cerebellar disease they are irregular in amplitude and timing and are jerky. Difficulty judging distance or **dysmetria** is shown by repeatedly tapping the back of one hand with the palm of the other. This can normally be done rhythmically and quickly but in cerebellar disease the movement is uneven and jerky which can be both seen and heard. The **rebound phenomenon** occurs in cerebellar disease where the tapped outstretched hand oscillates before coming back to rest. The **gait** in cerebellar disease is wide based and ataxic and worse on walking a straight line with a tendency to fall to the side of the lesion.

Key points

- finger nose test is performed with the patient sitting & observed for intention tremor
- rapid alternating hand movements (dysdiadochokinesia) is a test of cerebellar disease
- heel shin test is performed with the patient lying flat being observed for ataxia
- the gait in cerebellar disease is wide based and ataxic
- the main signs of cerebellar disease are dysarthria, nystagmus & incoordination

Reflexes

A tendon reflex results from stretching a muscle stretch receptor which in turn discharges via an afferent sensory pathway to an anterior horn cell in the spinal cord. The resulting motor discharge leads to a muscle contraction. These tendon reflexes are easily demonstrable by a blow from a tendon hammer. To elicit a reflex the patient first has to be comfortable and relaxed. The muscle to be tested must be under a degree of stretch and it is normal to test the main reflexes with the arms, knees and ankles flexed at a 90 degree angle. If reflexes are still absent despite relaxation then this should be confirmed with reinforcement, pulling the flexed fingers of two hands tightly together for the lower limbs and clenching the teeth for the upper limbs. Use the whole length of the patella hammer and swing the rubber end on to a tendon or your finger overlying the tendon. The action of the reflex i.e. the contraction of the muscle and the movement that it elicits may be both seen and felt by the examiner (Table 1.2).

Table 1.2 Grading reflexes

Reflexes	Grade	What it means
absent	0	lower motor neurone lesion, neuropathy
absent but present with reinforcement	+/−	normal, but may indicate neuropathy
present	+	normal
brisk	++	may be normal, but may indicate upper motor neurone lesion
very brisk	+++	upper motor neurone lesion

Persistent absent reflexes indicate a lower motor neurone lesion or neuropathy or rarely a myopathy or in the case of a single absent reflex a root lesion. The most common cause of absent reflexes is poor technique with a clumsy or inadequate blow off target. The ankle reflexes may also be absent in the elderly. Increased reflexes may be due to nervousness (or rarely thyrotoxicosis) when in time they will revert to normal and the plantar reflexes are down going. Very brisk reflexes indicate an upper motor neurone lesion in particular when coupled with other signs such as hypertonia, clonus and extensor plantar responses. In order to elicit the main reflexes do as follows:

- elicit the biceps with the arm adducted across the chest wall, put your finger on the biceps tendon and tap it watching the biceps muscle for contraction
- for the supinator reflex, place your finger over the lower third of the radius and hit the finger with a hammer watching the brachioradialis contract
- for the triceps reflex, with the arm in the same position strike the tendon at a 90 degree angle watching for the triceps to contract
- in the legs for the knee reflex, place the free arm under and supporting the knees keeping them flexed to a 90 degree angle. Strike the patella tendon near its origin and watch the quadriceps for contraction

- for the ankle reflex, the knee should be flexed to 90 degrees with the leg in external rotation lying to the side and the medial malleolus pointing upwards. Hold the foot at 90 degree angle exerting gentle pressure on the toes and strike the Achilles tendon and look at the calf muscles for contraction.
- in order to elicit the plantar reflex, explain to the patient what you are going to do. Gently draw a blunt key up the lateral border of the sole of the foot crossing the foot pads or metatarsal heads. Look for the first movement of the big toe at the metatarsophalangeal joint. If the first movement is up going or extensor then this a Babinski sign and indicates an upper motor neurone lesion. In the calloused foot it may be useful to run the stimulus on the outside or lateral aspect of the foot

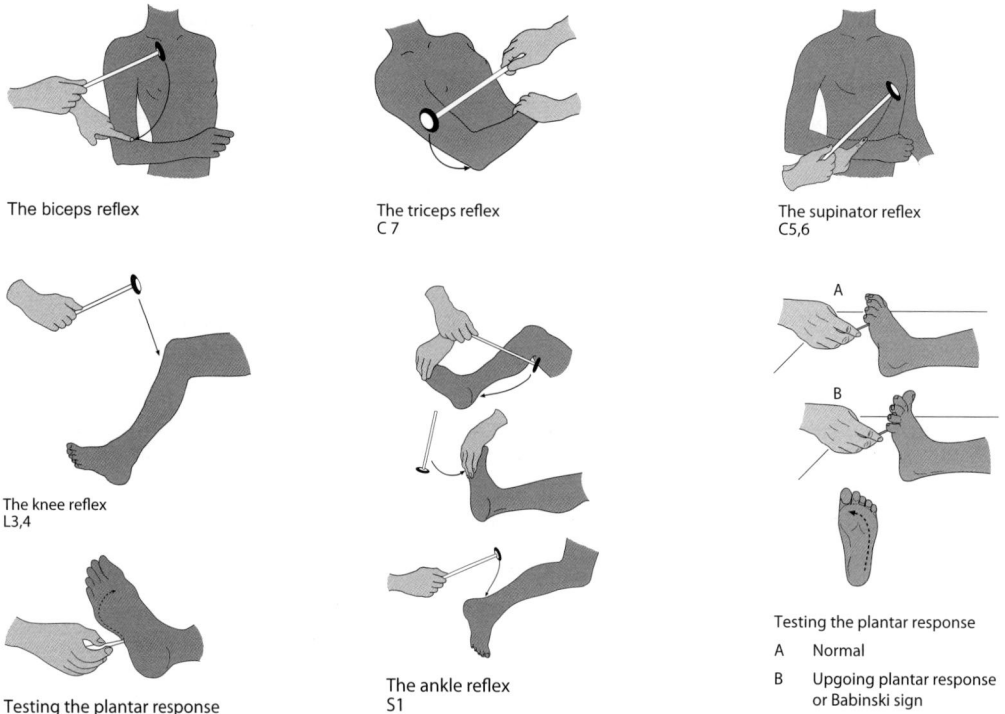

The biceps reflex

The triceps reflex
C 7

The supinator reflex
C5,6

The knee reflex
L3,4

The ankle reflex
S1

Testing the plantar response

Testing the plantar response
A   Normal
B   Upgoing plantar response
     or Babinski sign

A

B

Figure 1.19 Testing reflexes

Key points

- reflexes are elicited in the upper limbs with the patient sitting and in the lower limbs lying
- examiner needs to be skilled in placing finger over appropriate tendons and tapping them
- reflexes are either absent, reduced, normal or increased
- plantar response can be either up going (abnormal), or down going or mute (normal)

Sensation

The sensory examination is often difficult, time consuming and requires the concentration of the examiner and the cooperation of the patient. The technique should be speedy and efficient. The aim of the examination is to detect any loss of sensation and the pattern of loss. There are five main modalities of sensation to test for, these are **light touch, pin prick and temperature (superficial)** and **vibration** and **joint position (deep).** The patient should be instructed about the test being performed and first demonstrate the test you are using on familiar non affected places e.g. the face by asking the patient to say yes every time he feels the stimulus. Then start the examination with the patient's eyes closed by testing from a distal to proximal direction touching main dermatomes and comparing right and left sides. The patient indicates that he has felt the stimulus by saying **"yes"** or by communicating some other way.

Testing superficial sensation

It is usually sufficient to touch each site once varying the timing and moving from an area of abnormal sensation to normal sensation. The same method is applied for testing pain. If the neurological examination is a screening examination to exclude any unsuspected sensory findings then it's enough to use one example of superficial sensation (light touch) and one example of deep sensation (joint position sense) and to test on all four limbs distally. If the patient has noticed an altered sensation in any part of the body then a more detailed sensory examination

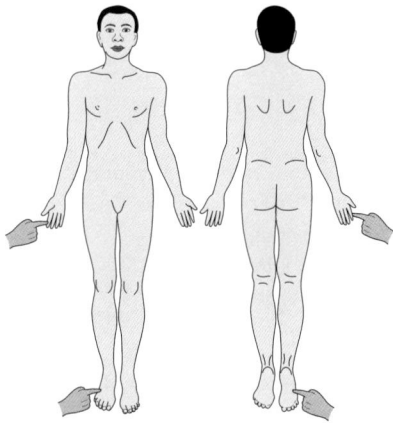

is required, testing the main sensory modalities. Sensory testing begins with testing for **light touch** by using a wisp of cotton wool or a finger tip being careful each time to touch or dab the skin lightly rather than to drag it across the skin. To test for **pain** use a blunt pin or sharp tooth pick taking care not to draw blood. Do not reuse the pin on another patient. **Temperature** is not usually tested in the routine examination. For formal testing it is necessary to fill two test tubes, one with hot and other with cold iced water and ask the patient to tell you which tube is hot or cold on random touching of the limbs, face and trunk.

Figure 1.20 Testing superficial sensation

Joint position

Joint position is first tested on the finger tips and toes. The tip of the digit being tested is held at the sides between the examiner's thumb and the index finger. The patient is shown an upward and downward movement first with his eyes open and told that he will be asked to identify the direction of movement once his eyes are closed. If the patient cannot identify the direction correctly then the next proximal larger joints should be tested until a joint with intact joint position sense is found.

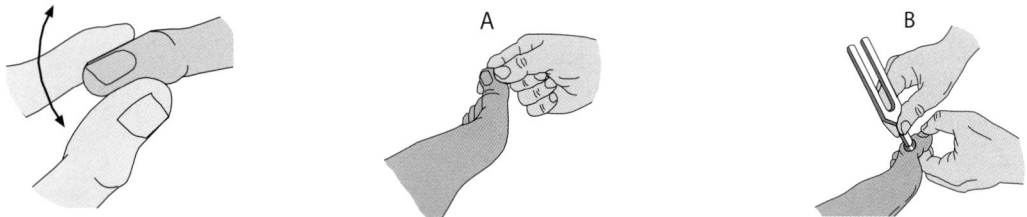

Figure 1.21 Testing deep sensation. Testing joint position in the finger (left).
A) Joint position sense. B) Vibration sense.

Vibration

Vibration sense is tested using a 128 Hz or 256 Hz tuning fork. The beating fork should be first placed on the back of terminal phalanx of the index finger and big toe and the patient asked if he can feel the vibration. If not felt distally it must then be placed on the metacarpal phalangeal joints, wrist, elbow and shoulder in the upper limbs and the medial malleolus, tibial tuberosity in the lower limbs moving onto the anterior iliac crest, rib margin, sternum or clavicle in search of an intact vibration level. Vibration is often lost early on in neuropathies.

Localization

The pattern of sensory loss may indicate the underlying disease. A distal glove and stocking loss of sensation points to a peripheral neuropathy, loss of sensation below a level on the trunk points to a spinal cord lesion, hemisensory loss on the body points to a central brain lesion, loss of temperature discrimination on the face and trunk should suggest a spinothalamic lesion, and a dermatomal loss points to a nerve or nerve root lesion. Details concerning cortical sensory loss including sensory extinction, two point discrimination, graphanaesthesia, and astereognosis can be found in chapter 2.

Key points

- patient should be trained to indicate each stimulus & the direction of movement of the joint
- patient indicates stimulus by saying "yes" and type e.g. "sharp or blunt", "hot or cold"
- testing should be speedy, efficient, starting distally before moving proximally
- routine sensory testing should be restricted to peripheral light touch & joint position
- pattern and type of sensory loss helps to determine the underlying disorder

EXAMINATION OF THE GAIT

The **gait** provides useful clues to the underlying neurological disorder and it is important to examine it. Ask the patient to walk normally with the arms hanging loose by the sides and observe the gait for the following; movement, balance, posture, arm swing, turning and symmetry. If the gait is abnormal note the main characteristic and whether the patient walks unaided or uses a stick or crutch. Note whether the patient is unsteady and if he is able to walk a straight line by putting one foot in front of the other. Gaits can then be categorized as symmetrical or asymmetrical. Examples are the small symmetrical steps of Parkinson's disease and asymmetrical steps of hemiplegic gait. The main abnormal types of gaits are: hemiplegic, paraplegic, cerebellar, Parkinsonian, sensory ataxic, neuropathic and myopathic. These are described in chapter 2.

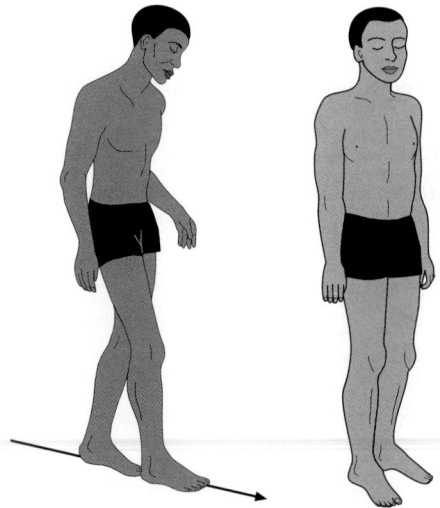

Figure 1.22 Testing gait

Romberg's test

To carry out a Romberg's test ask the patient to stand unsupported with his heels together, toes apart and eyes closed. Reassure the patient that you will catch him if he falls. If he falls or sways repeatedly with eyes closed but not with eyes open this is a positive test indicating impairment of joint position sense in the feet or posterior columns in the spinal cord (proprioception).

Key points in testing gait

· ask the patient to stand with heels together, feet apart and eyes closed
· observe for swaying or falling
· ask the patient to walk normally with arms hanging loosely by the sides
· observe for balance, posture, arm swing and unsteadiness
· if ataxia is still suspected, ask the patient to walk a straight line & place one foot in front of the other

CONSCIOUSNESS

Consciousness is a state of awareness of self and environment and any alteration or impairment requires objective measurement. In neurology patients the level of consciousness may range from being awake and fully conscious which is normal through confusion to altered consciousness and coma (Table 1.3). The level of alertness or confusion can be measured by checking for orientation in time, person and place. Coma can be measured using the Glasgow Coma Scale (GCS) (Table 1.5). Their value is that they produce objective measurement of the patient's level of alertness (orientation) and consciousness (coma) which are important for the assessment and ongoing care of the patient.

Table 1.3 States of consciousness

Level	Clinical features	Measurement scale
Normal	awake and fully conscious	
Confused	inability to think and speak clearly with lack of attention and memory and disorientation	orientation in time, person and place (10/10)
Coma	altered level of consciousness	Glasgow Coma Scale (15/15)

Table 1.4 Testing for orientation 10/10*

Time	Person	Place
time	name	hospital
day	age	town/district
month	year of birth	country
year		

* score one for each correct answer

Table 1.5 Glasgow Coma Scale

Activity	Best response	Score
Eye opening	- spontaneously	4
	- to speech	3
	- to pain	2
	- nil	1
Motor response	- obeys commands	6
	- localizes stimulus	5
	- flexes withdrawal	4
	- flexes weak	3
	- extension	2
	- nil	1
Best verbal	- oriented fully	5
	- confused	4
	- inappropriate	3
	- incomprehensible (sounds only)	2
	- nil	1
Maximum score		15

when assessing record, eye opening (E4), motor (M6), & best verbal response (V5) patients are considered comatose if GCS ≤8/15

Mental state

The general physical state, appearance and behaviour of the patient is also helpful e.g. a recent onset of confusion points to an organic cause whereas a chronic unkempt unconcerned patient with a thought disorder is more likely to be non organic or psychiatric. Patients with psychiatric disorders should be referred for psychiatric evaluation. However an organic cause may need to be excluded first.

Cognitive function

The level of patient cooperation and insight into the illness are also important factors. Patients presenting with confusional states or delirium may need further cognitive evaluation. This initially involves simple bedside clinical tests for attention and concentration. These include testing for orientation in time and place, checking the ability to repeat a set of up to 6 numbers or to count back from 20 or recite the months of the year backwards or other learned abilities. In chronic organic brain disease states e.g. dementia or localized brain disease a more detailed evaluation of cognitive function may be helpful. This involves additional cognitive testing including tests for registration, memory, calculation and language. These can be formally measured by the Mini mental state examination (MMSE) (Chapter 17).

Key points

- patient's general appearance & performance are indicators of neurological & mental health
- a detailed assessment of mental state & higher cerebral function is done when the history indicates
- level of alertness and orientation are used to monitor the confused patient
- Glasgow Coma Scale is used to monitor level of consciousness in the semi or unconscious patient

Other neurological signs

- Signs of meningism
- Frontal lobe release signs
- Superficial reflexes
- Straight leg raising test

Signs of meningism

These signs are found in patients with meningitis, subarachnoid haemorrhage and other causes of meningism. However be aware that the neck may be stiff or rigid in other conditions such as cervical spondylosis, Parkinsonism and tetanus giving rise to a false positive sign of meningism.

- neck stiffness
- Kernig's sign
- Brudzinski's sign

Neck stiffness

The patient should be lying flat. The head should be supported by placing your hands under the patient's occiput until the weight of the head is carried in the hands indicating the patient has relaxed. Neck flexion should be induced slowly by gently lifting the head off the bed whilst at the same time feeling for tone or resistance to the movement. In the normal person the neck flexes easily without resistance with the chin usually reaching the chest. Neck stiffness is present when the neck is rigid or resists any attempt to passively flex the neck. This will result in failure to bring the chin onto the chest. Neck stiffness is the most sensitive of the signs of meningism.

Figure 1.23 Examining for neck stiffness. Use your fingers to flex the neck whilst assessing the degree of resistance.

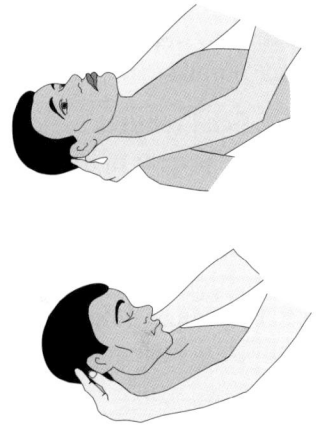

Kernig's sign

The patient should be lying flat. This is elicited by passively attempting to straighten the leg after flexing both the thigh and knee to an angle of greater than 90 degrees. In meningitis this is met by pain and resistance in the lumbar area as a result of stretching of inflamed nerve roots. In patients with meningeal irritation the sign is positive on both sides.

Figure 1.24 Testing for meningism. Kernig's sign.

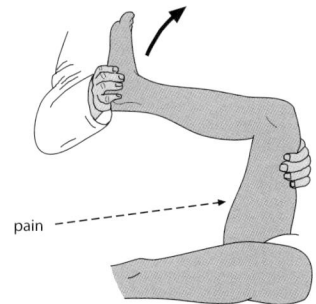

Brudzinski's sign

Whilst examining the patient for neck stiffness observe whether forward flexing of the neck induces any involuntary hip and knee flexion. Involuntary lower limb flexion indicates meningeal irritation. This is a sensitive test for meningitis in young children but not in adults.

Frontal lobe release signs (FLRSs)

These signs may be present infrequently in normal persons. However they occur more frequently and are usually exaggerated in frontal lobe disorders and other diffuse mainly cortical neurological disorders.

Snout reflex

This is elicited by pressing or tapping on the closed lips in the midline with a patella hammer or closed knuckle. In positive cases this elicits a puckering of the lips (orbicularis oris) and occasionally a contraction of the chin (mentalis muscle).

Palmomental reflex

Scratch the palm of the hand at the base of the thumb in a distal direction with a key. In positive cases there is a contraction of the chin (mentalis muscle) on the same side as the stimulus.

Grasp reflex

Place your fingers in the palm of the patient's hand and stroke it gently whilst pulling your hand away. In positive cases the patient's hand will involuntarily curl and grasp the examiner's hand. A unilateral grasp reflex indicates contralateral frontal lobe pathology.

Superficial reflexes

These are present in healthy persons but are absent in an UMNL. The abdominal reflexes may also be absent in obese persons and after pregnancy and after abdominal surgery.

Abdominal reflex

Test by stroking lightly with the sharp end of the patella hammer in each of the four quadrants of the abdomen from the outside in a diagonal or horizontal approach. The abdominal wall contracts in each quadrant in the normal patient.

Cremasteric reflex

This is performed in men. The inner aspect of the upper thigh is stroked lightly from below upwards. In the normal male this results in an elevation of the testis on the same side. Its absence may indicate an UMNL above the level of L1.

Straight leg raising test

This is a test for entrapment of the lumbar and sacral nerve roots. With the patient lying flat after placing a hand under the patient's heel lift the fully extended or straightened leg. An angle of 90 degrees is normal but may be less in older patients. Limitation of movement with pain suggests nerve root entrapment on the affected side. Note the angle achieved and the difference if any between the two sides. The most common cause is herniation of an intervertebral disc.

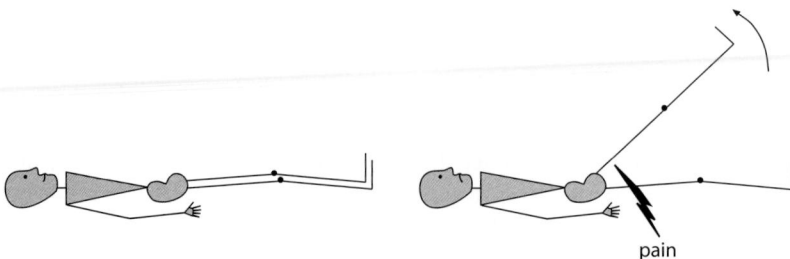

pain

Figure 1.25 Testing for sciatica. Lift leg to 90 degrees with leg fully extended.

KEY TO BASIC NEUROLOGICAL EXAMINATION

GENERAL ASSESSMENT	assess for alertness, orientation, level of consciousness
CRANIAL NERVES	
Visual acuity	can you see normally, if vision is decreased then check VA
	first cover one eye & read letters on this chart, repeat for other eye
Visual fields	tell me when you see my finger tip moving, test on each side
Fundoscopy	look at the optic disc and fundus
Pupils	shine bright light in each eye, look for pupillary constriction
Eye movements	follow my finger moving right left and up down
	check for diplopia and any loss of eye movements
Facial sensation	with your eyes shut, say "yes" when you feel me touching your face
Facial movements	inspect the face
	look up at the ceiling
	close your eyes tightly & don't let me open them
	smile or show me your teeth
Hearing	can you hear normally, if not examine each ear
	"repeat numbers I am whispering or speaking"
	use tuning fork tests only if deafness is confirmed
Palatal movement & tongue	open your mouth and say "aah", inspect gag reflex
	inspect tongue at rest, protruded and on movement
Neck/shoulders	turn your head against my hand
	shrug your shoulders against my hands
LIMBS	
Inspection	look for wasting and fasciculation in arms, legs & trunk
Tone	bend and straighten the patient's elbow & knee
Power: Arms	hold elbows out from your sides & push upwards
	bend & straighten your elbow
	bend your wrist & fingers upwards
	separate your fingers sideways
	bend your thumb upwards
Power: Legs	push your thigh upwards
	bend & straighten your knee
	push your foot down & upwards towards your face
Co-ordination	touch tip of your nose with tip of your index finger
	hold foot in the air, touch knee with heel & run it down the shin
Reflexes	tap briskly the biceps, triceps, supinator, knee and ankle tendons
	elicit the plantar response
Sensation (eyes closed)	say "yes" or "indicate" when you feel me touching you
	"I am moving your finger/big toe. Tell me is it up or down"
GAIT	
	observe standing, heels together & toes separated (eyes closed)
	observe walking normally, straight line, heel to toe

Selected references

Ginsberg Lionel, *Neurology, Lecture Notes*. Blackwell Publishing 8th edition 2005.

Wilkinson Iain & Lennox Graham, *Essential Neurology*. Blackwell Publishing 4th edition 2005.

Harrison Michael, Neurological *Skills, A guide to examination and management in Neurology*. Butterworth's 1st edition 1987.

Fuller Geraint, *Neurological examination made easy*, Churchill Livingstone. 3rd edition 2004.

Donaghy Michael, *Neurology*. Oxford University Press 1st edition 1997.

Turner, Bahra, Cikurel, *Neurology*. Crash Course, Elsevier Mosby 2nd edition 2006.

O'Brien MD. *Aids to the examination of the peripheral nervous system*. Saunders 1st edition 2000.

PART 1 – CLINICAL SKILLS

CHAPTER 2
LOCALIZATION

CONTENTS

CHAPTER 2

LOCALIZATION

The site of the lesion

The nervous system can be divided into the central (CNS) and peripheral (PNS) nervous system. In the CNS the main sites of disease are the *cerebral hemisphere, basal ganglia, cerebellum, brain stem and spinal cord* (Fig. 2.1). In the PNS the main sites of disease are the *cranial* and *peripheral nerves*. Diseases of the neuromuscular junction and muscle are included by convention. The main aim of this chapter is to localize abnormal neurological findings to their main site of origin within the nervous system. After reading the chapter the student should aim to distinguish between an upper and lower motor neurone lesion and to be able to localise neurological disorders to their main site of origin. Details concerning localization and the cranial nerves are outlined in Chapter 12.

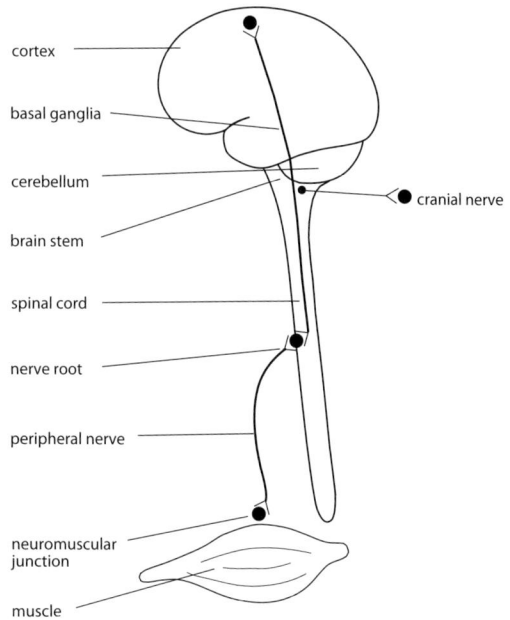

Figure 2.1 Main sites of neurological disorders

MOTOR SYSTEM

CNS

The motor system in the CNS consists of the brain and spinal cord, beginning in the motor cortex and extending down the brain stem and spinal cord to end at the lower border of L1. The motor tract begins in the frontal lobe, descends via the corona radiata on the same side to become the internal capsule. It then descends into the brain stem as the pyramidal tract and mostly (85%) crosses at the lower end of the medulla to the opposite side. From there it descends into the spinal cord as the lateral corticospinal tract and finally synapses with the anterior horn cells at the front (anterior) of the spinal cord on the same side (Fig. 2.2). A lesion anywhere along this pathway in the brain or spinal cord results in an upper motor neurone lesion (UMNL). The neurological signs of an UMNL are *loss of power, increased tone (hypertonia), clonus, increased reflexes (hyper-reflexia)* and *extensor plantar response (up going toes or Babinski sign)*. The presence of these signs localise the site of the lesion to the CNS. The main UMN disorders presenting with these signs are hemiplegia arising from lesions in the brain and quadriplegia arising from lesions in the brain stem. The other main UMN disorders are quadriplegia and paraplegia arising from the spinal cord depending on the level of the lesion.

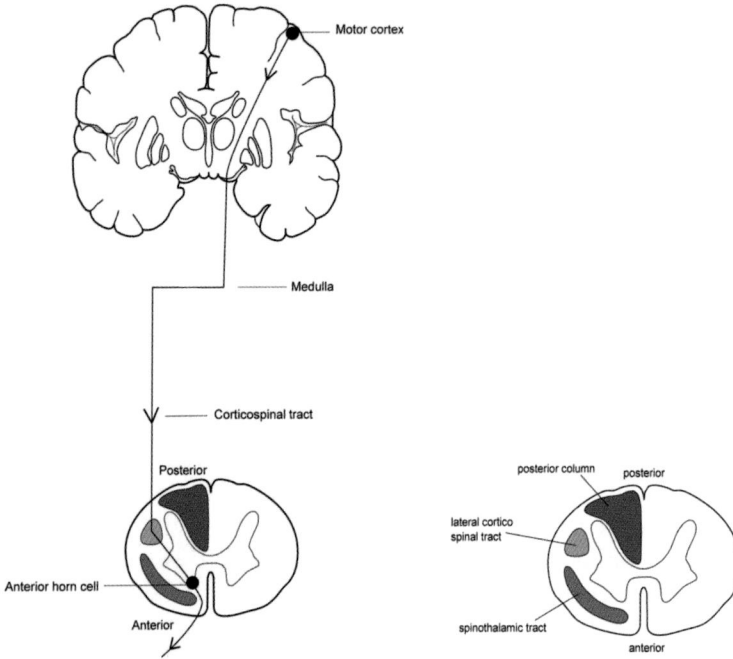

Figure 2.2 The corticospinal tract (left). Spinal cord section. Main motor and sensory tracts (right).

PNS

The motor system in the PNS consists of cranial and peripheral nerves, extending from their nerve nuclei in the brain stem and anterior horn cells in the spinal cord to the neuromuscular junction in muscle (Fig. 2.3). A lesion anywhere along this pathway is called a lower motor neurone lesion (LMNL). The neurological signs of a LMNL are *loss of power, muscle wasting, fasciculation, decreased tone (hypotonia)* and *decreased* or *absent reflexes (hyporeflexia or areflexia)*.

The presence of LMN signs localise the site of the lesion to the peripheral nervous system. The main clinical disorders causing these signs are peripheral neuropathies, mononeuropathies and cranial nerve palsies.

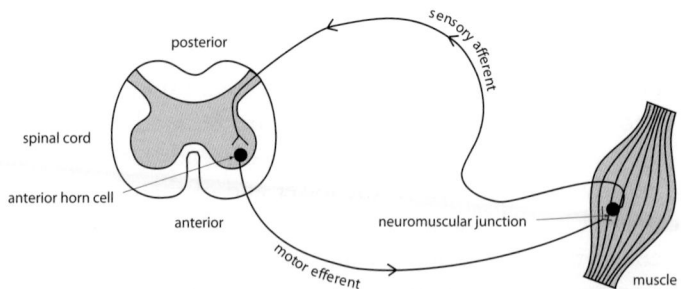

Figure 2.3 The peripheral reflex pathway

The diagram "**the peripheral reflex arc**" outlines the pathway of a peripheral reflex. It is essential to be able to distinguish clinically between an UMNL and a LMNL, in order to be able to correctly localise a neurological disorder to its main site of origin. It is important to note that loss of power is common to both and therefore does not help to distinguish between them, and that these signs may not all be present in any one individual patient. The main differences between them are summarized in the table 2.1 below.

Table 2.1 Key differences between UMNL & LMNL

Neurological findings	UMNL*	LMNL*
wasting		yes
fasciculations		yes
tone		
increased	yes	
decreased		yes
clonus	yes	
reflexes		
increased	yes	
decreased/absent		yes
Babinski sign	yes	

a blank space means no

SENSORY SYSTEM

The sensory system comprises of nerves and tracts which carry stimuli arising from the periphery including skin, joints, muscle and viscera via the peripheral nervous system (PNS) to the brain. In the CNS there are two main sensory pathways, *the dorsal columns* and *the spinothalamic tracts* (Fig. 2.4). The dorsal columns transmit joint position sense, vibration sense and light touch. The peripheral nerves transmitting these sensations enter via enter the posterior roots of the spinal cord and ascend in the dorsal columns to the lower end of the medulla, where they synapse. They then cross the midline and ascend to reach the thalamus, from where a further relay goes to the sensory cortex in the parietal lobe of the brain on the same side. Sensory symptoms arising from the posterior columns are *numbness, tingling* and *loss of co-ordination*. The spinothalamic tract transmits pain, temperature and crude touch. These enter the posterior spinal cord ascend a few segments, and then cross the midline to ascend in the anterolateral spinothalamic tract via second order neurones to the ipsilateral thalamus, and finally to the parietal lobe on the same side. The main sensory symptoms arising from disorders of the spinothalamic tract are *pain* and *dysaesthesia*. Sensory symptoms arise from disease at different levels in the nervous system. The main sensory sites of clinical interest are at the level of *peripheral nerves, spinal cord* and *brain*.

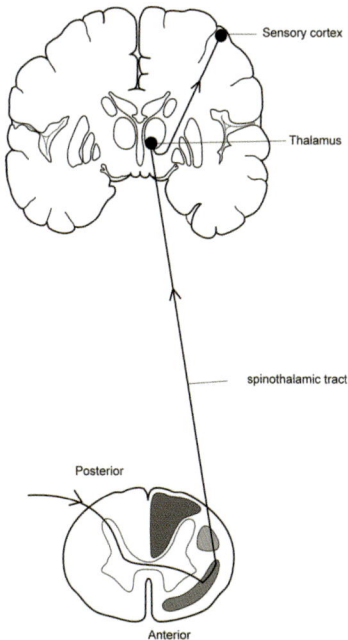

Figure 2.4 The spinothalamic tract (left).

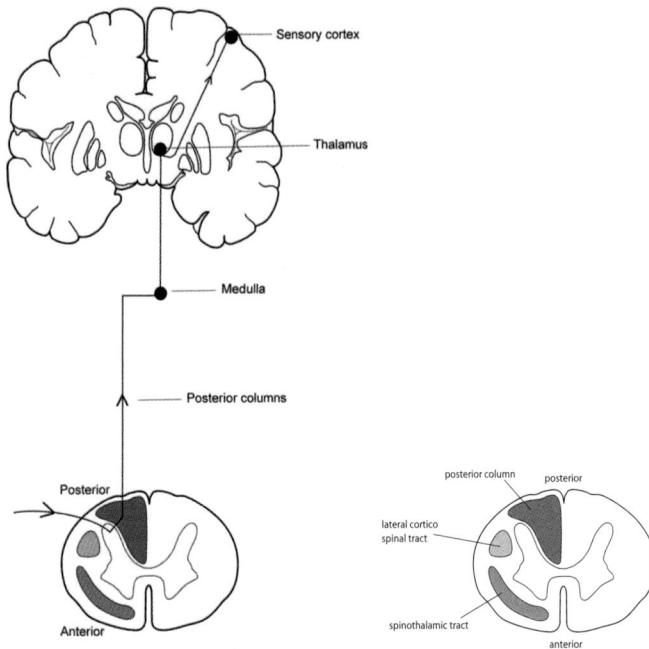

Figure 2.4 continued Spinal cord section. Main motor and sensory tracts (right). The posterior columns (left).

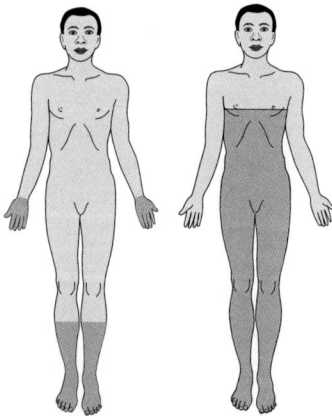

The anatomical pattern of sensory loss helps to localise the site of the underlying disorder. The main patterns of sensory loss are outlined in the following figures 2.5–7.

Figure 2. 5 Sensory loss in peripheral neuropathy glove and stocking distribution (left)

In **peripheral nerve disorders** the most common pattern of loss is that seen in peripheral neuropathies where the *loss* is mainly *distal* and affects *the feet* and *hands* in a *glove* and *stocking distribution*. The main causes of this are HIV and diabetes mellitus.

Figure 2.6 Sensory loss in paraplegia (right)

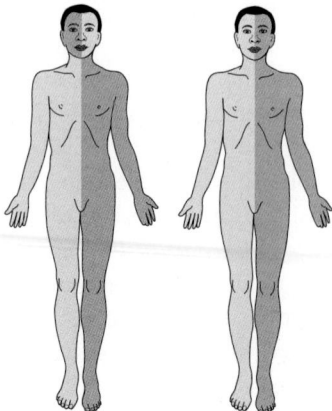

In **spinal cord disorders** the *loss involves* the *limbs* (usually the legs) and the *trunk below* the *level* of the *lesion*. The extent and pattern of loss depends on the underlying lesion, e.g. complete or partial cord involvement resulting in paraplegia. The main causes are trauma and infection.

Figure 2.7 Sensory loss in brain stem lesion (left). Sensory loss in hemiplegia (right).

In **brain disorders** sensation is *lost* or more commonly *altered* on the *side of the body opposite* the site of *lesion*. The main causes are vascular and space occupying lesions.

CEREBRAL HEMISPHERES

The brain has two hemispheres, each containing a frontal, parietal, temporal and occipital lobe, each lobe with their own distinctive functions. The main neurological signs indicating a lesion on one side of the brain are a *loss of power* or less frequently *sensation* on one side of the body, *a loss of speech* if the dominant hemisphere is involved and *a loss of vision* to one side if the optic pathway is involved. The presence of these focal neurological signs help to localize the site of the lesion to a cerebral hemisphere on one side and also to an individual lobe within that hemisphere (Fig. 2.8).

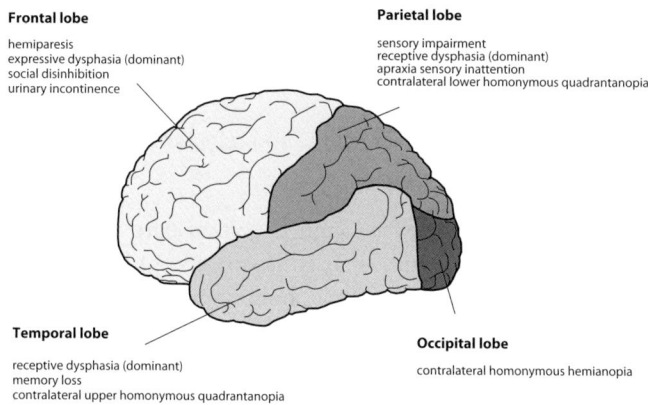

Frontal lobe
hemiparesis
expressive dysphasia (dominant)
social disinhibition
urinary incontinence

Parietal lobe
sensory impairment
receptive dysphasia (dominant)
apraxia sensory inattention
contralateral lower homonymous quadrantanopia

Temporal lobe
receptive dysphasia (dominant)
memory loss
contralateral upper homonymous quadrantanopia

Occipital lobe
contralateral homonymous hemianopia

Figure 2.8 Cerebral hemispheres

Frontal lobe

The frontal lobe contains the motor cortex, which is responsible for motor function and movements of the opposite half of the body. Disorders affecting either frontal lobe result in *weakness* or a *loss of power* involving the opposite side of the body and also a *loss* or *impairment (dysphasia) of speech (aphasia, expressive),* if the speech area (Broca's area) in the dominant hemisphere is affected. *Personality changes* with features of *social disinhibition* and *urinary incontinence* may also occur. *Frontal lobe release signs,* including the grasp reflex may also be present.

Parietal lobe

The parietal lobe contains the sensory cortex whose main function is discriminatory sensation involving the opposite half of the body. Patients with lesions in the parietal lobe have subtle sensory impairments, which require higher sensory testing to demonstrate. They have an *inability* to *recognise familiar shapes, textures* and *numbers* and an *impairment of fine touch* when tested on the opposite hand on either side. Lesions involving the dominant hemisphere result in *difficulty* with *calculation, writing* and *apraxia (difficulty performing task related movements)* and a *receptive dysphasia* if the dominant hemisphere is affected (Wernicke's area). Lesions involving the non dominant hemisphere result in a lack of *visuo-spatial awareness* with *hemi-neglect* of the opposite side of the body. This can result in an inability to dress or wash on the affected side. A lesion in either parietal lobe may result in an *inferior quadrantic visual field defect* or a loss of the lower half of the visual field coming from the opposite side.

Temporal lobe

The temporal lobe contains Wernicke's receptive speech area in the dominant hemisphere. Damage to it results in loss of understanding of speech and writing *(aphasia, receptive)* and *loss of memory. Seizures* originating in the temporal lobe may begin with a characteristic *hallucinatory prodrome* of *smell, taste, vision, hearing* or *emotion*. A lesion in either lobe may result in a *superior quadrantic visual field defect* or loss of the upper half of the visual field coming from the opposite side.

Occipital lobe

The occipital lobe is responsible for vision. Lesions of the occipital lobe may result in a *contralateral homonymous hemianopia* or loss of the visual field coming from the opposite side.

SPEECH DISORDERS

There are three main types of speech disorder: *dysphonia, dysarthria* and *dysphasia.*

Dysphonia

This is a *disorder* of *voice production* of *sound* as air goes through the vocal cords. It results in inability to produce a normal volume of speech or sound. It is usually recognized during the history taking, because the sound the voice generates is low, hollow or hoarse. It arises from failure of adduction of the vocal cords due either to paralysis or to local disease in the larynx. It can be suspected by asking the patient to cough, when instead of the normal sharp explosive cough there is a characteristic husky or bovine like cough. The diagnosis is confirmed by inspection of the larynx and vocal cords. The main causes are a local lesion e.g. a tumour, recurrent laryngeal nerve paralysis, and myasthenia gravis.

Dysarthria

This is an *inability* to *coordinate* the *movements* of *tongue, lips* and *pharynx* to *articulate* or produce understandable sounds. This makes words sound slow and slurred and leads to difficulty in their understanding. Any neurological disorder which affects the muscles or movements involved in speech production can produce a dysarthria. The main causes are stroke, cerebellar disease, and cerebral palsy.

Dysphasia

This is a *disorder of language production* resulting in either a *loss* of *understanding* or *expression* of words or *both*. It arises because of damage to the speech areas in the brain in the dominant hemisphere. The main speech centres are situated on the left side of the brain in >90% of right handed people and also in about two thirds of left handed people. Dysphasia and aphasia are clinically classified as either receptive, expressive or global.

Key points

- listening determines the type of speech disorder
- it can be dysphonia, dysarthria or dysphasia
- pts with dysphonia can't make the sounds
- pts with dysarthria can make the sounds but the words don't sound normal
- pts with dysphasia cannot either understand or say words normally or both

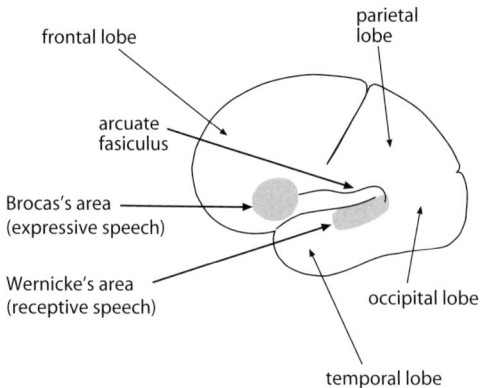

Figure 2.9 Main speech areas of the brain

Key points

- establish whether the patient is right or left handed and his/her language
- listen to speech for fluency, content & meaning
- assess reception by simple commands/questions e.g. "close your eyes"
- assess expression by asking the patient to name 3 familiar objects; e.g. pen, watch & glasses

Receptive

A patient with receptive aphasia *loses understanding* for both the *spoken* and *written word,* and is unable to follow even simple bedside questions and commands. The speech content is fluent but meaningless and many words are either incorrect or newly created. It is caused by a lesion in Wernicke's area (Fig. 2.9).

Expressive

A patient with expressive aphasia understands normally but *has difficulty* in *finding* the *words.* In this type of aphasia there are often great gaps between the words, with non fluent telegraphic or monosyllabic speech and lack of rhythm. Writing may be poor. The patient is usually aware, though frustrated and may use gestures to try to help to express. It is caused by a lesion in Broca's area in the dominant frontal lobe (Fig. 2.9).

Global

This occurs when the patient is neither able to *understand* the *spoken* or *written word* or able to *express* himself. It is caused by an extensive lesion of the dominant hemisphere, affecting both temporal and frontal speech areas. The main cause of aphasia is stroke.

Key points

- pts with receptive aphasia do not understand
- pts with expressive aphasia cannot express the right words
- pts with global aphasia can neither understand nor express the right words

BASAL GANGLIA

The basal ganglia and their connections control movement. Diseases affecting them cause movement disorders, which are characterised by either too *little* or too *much movement*. Parkinson's disease (PD) causes too little movement. The main clinical features of which are *bradykinesia, rest tremor, rigidity* and *gait disorder*. Disorders that result in too much movement include *dystonia* and *chorea*. The main causes are medications and stroke.

CEREBELLUM

The cerebellum and its connections coordinate voluntary movement. Disorders affecting the cerebellum cause incoordination. The main symptoms and signs of cerebellar disease are *dysarthria, nystagmus* and *incoordination* of the *limbs* and *gait*. Hypotonia and pendular reflexes are additional signs but may not always be present. Cerebellar signs are localizing and the presence of unilateral cerebellar signs help to localise a lesion to the cerebellum to the same side. The main causes are stroke, drugs including alcohol, hereditary disorders, tumours and forms of neurodegenerative disease.

BRAIN STEM

The brain stem (Fig. 2.10) comprises the midbrain, pons and medulla. It is responsible for the lower ten cranial nerves, the ascending motor and descending sensory tracts, integrating co-ordination and balance and the central regulation of heat, respiration, circulation and consciousness. The clinical features of a brain stem disorder will depend on the site and the extent of the lesion. In general a brain stem lesion is suggested when *cranial nerve palsies* and *ataxia* occur on *one side* of the *head* and *a loss of power* and *sensation* occurs on the *opposite half* of the *body*. An alteration or loss of consciousness and quadriplegia occurs with extensive brain stem lesions. The main causes are stroke, trauma and mass lesions.

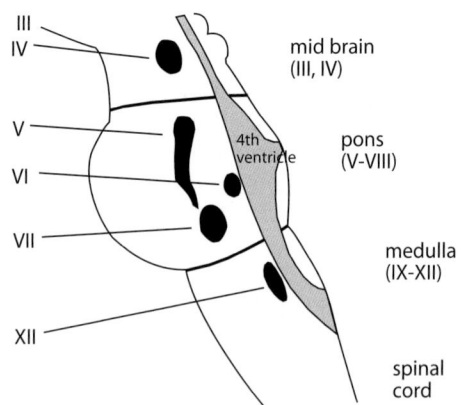

Figure 2.10 Brain stem. Main cranial nerve nuclei in the brain stem

SPINAL CORD

The spinal cord (CNS) extends from the top of C1 vertebra down to the end of L1. It is then continuous with the cauda equina (PNS) which extends from L1 down to S5 (Fig. 2.11).

The spinal cord is surrounded by three layers, a thick dura, an arachnoid and a pia which is adherent to the cord. The subarachnoid space contains cerebrospinal fluid and extends down to S5. The cord is made up of a large H shaped grey area in the centre containing many nerve cells and a peripheral white area which contains the ascending and descending axons or tracts (Fig. 2.12).

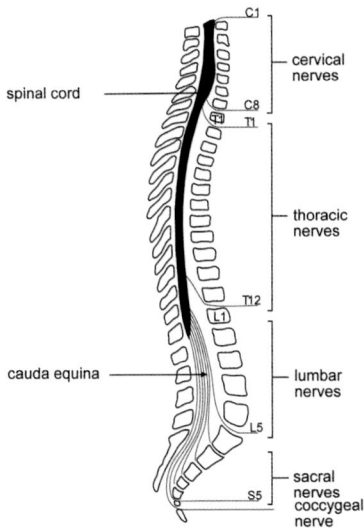

Figure 2.11 Spinal cord.
Spinal nerve and vertebra coloumn

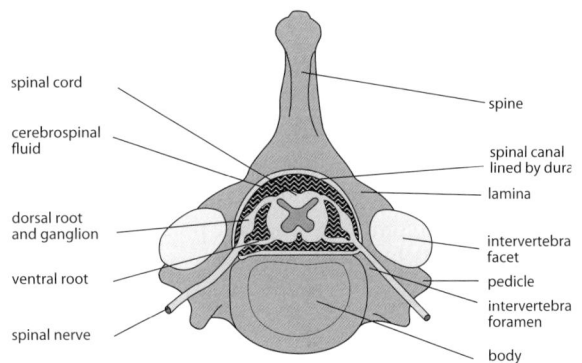

Figure 2.12 Vertebra showing spinal cord, nerve roots and spinal nerves

The main ascending tracts are the *spinothalamic* and *dorsal columns* (Fig 2.4) and the main descending tracts are the *corticospinal tracts* of which the *lateral* (LCST) is the main one (Fig 2.2). These main tracts all cross the spinal cord to supply the opposite side. The spinothalamic tract crosses shortly after entry and the posterior columns and the corticospinal tract cross at the lower end of the medulla. Any lesion affecting the spinal cord may result in *loss of motor, sensory* and *autonomic function below* the *level* of the *lesion.* Disorders affecting the spinal cord result in either a *quadriplegia* or *paraplegia,* depending on the site and level of injury or disease. The main causes are trauma, TB, infections, myeloneuropathies and peripheral neuropathies.

Paraplegia

Paraplegia means *paralysis of the legs.* This results from a lesion affecting either the spinal cord or the cauda equina. It can very rarely arise from a lesion within the brain. When the lesion affects the spinal cord above the level T12, L1 the clinical findings are those of *spastic paraplegia.* These **UMNL** signs are almost always combined with loss of sensation at and below the level of the lesion. The *sensory level* below which sensation is lost or reduced is very important as its upper limit usually indicates the site of the lesion. When the lesion affects the spinal cord below the level L1 it involves the cauda equina and the neurological findings are those of a *flaccid* *paraplegia.* In this case the findings are all **LMNL** signs which when combined with upper limit of sensory loss in the legs and perineum will help to determine the site of the lesion.

Quadriplegia

Quadriplegia indicates *paralysis* of all *four limbs.* The clinical findings are the same as for paraplegia except in this case all four limbs are involved. When the site of the lesion is in the lower half of cervical cord there may be radiculopathy or lower motor neurone signs involving the arms (C5-T1) at the level of the lesion and upper motor neurone signs and sensory loss below the level of the lesion. Both spastic and flaccid forms of quadriplegia and paraplegia are associated with loss of bladder and bowel control.

Bladder

The bladder is innervated by the autonomic and somatic or voluntary nervous system. The autonomic supply comprises of the parasympathetic fibres from S2-4 which are involved in emptying the bladder and the sympathetic fibres from T11-L2 which are involved with urine retention. The voluntary nerve fibres (S2-4, pudendal nerve) supply the external bladder neck sphincter. Loss of control of bladder function or neurogenic bladder arises primarily because of lesions in the spinal cord or cauda equina. Patients with spinal cord lesions present with a spastic paraparesis and spastic bladder with frequency, urgency and incontinence. They may develop satisfactory reflex bladder emptying or require intermittent self-catheterization and anticholinergic drugs. Patients with cauda equina lesions present with flaccid paraparesis and flaccid bladder with urine retention and usually require a permanent urinary catheter. Constipation is a feature of both types of paraplegia.

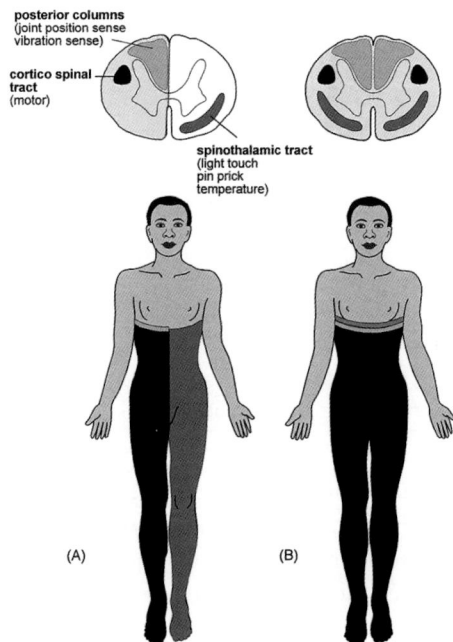

Figure 2.13 Sensory loss associated with spinal cord lesions. A: Hemisection of cord. B: Complete transverse section of cord

Localization

A lesion affecting one half of the spinal cord results in a hemi section or a *Brown-Sequard syndrome* (Fig. 2.13). This has three main and diagnostic neurological features all occurring below the level of the lesion. These are a *loss* of *power (UMNL)* and a *loss* of *joint position sense* and *vibration* occurring on the ***same side*** as the ***lesion*** and a *loss of pain* and *temperature* on the ***opposite side*** the ***lesion***. A lesion causing a complete transverse section of the cord results in a *total loss of power* and *feeling **below** the **level** of the **lesion*** and *loss of bowel* and *bladder control* (Fig. 2.13).

PERIPHERAL NERVOUS SYSTEM

Peripheral nerves

The peripheral nervous system is made up of mixed motor and sensory fibres comprising the cranial and peripheral nerves. Details concerning cranial nerve disorders and localization are presented later in chapter 12. In general disorders affecting the peripheral nerves are divided into two main groups called neuropathies: *mononeuropathies* which involve single nerves and *polyneuropathies* which involve all nerves. The main causes of these are HIV, diabetes and leprosy.

The diagrams below are to help to remind the student of the following, a typical peripheral *reflex arc* using the knee jerk as an example (Fig. 2.14), the main *segmental motor movements* and their nerve roots (Fig. 2.15), the main *peripheral reflexes* and their *nerve root* of origin (Fig 2.16), and the main *sensory dermatomes* (Fig. 2.17).

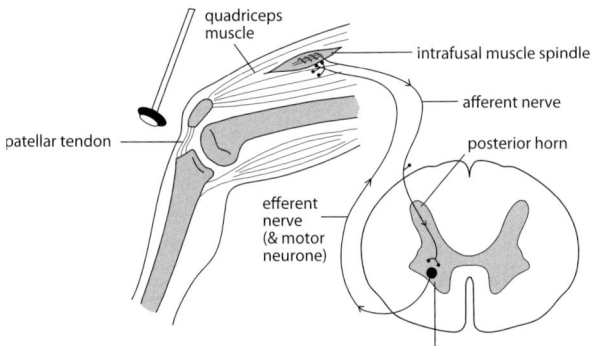

Figure 2.14 The knee reflex

The diagram entitled "the segmental limb movements" shows the main movements tested during motor neurological examination and their *nerve roots innervations*.

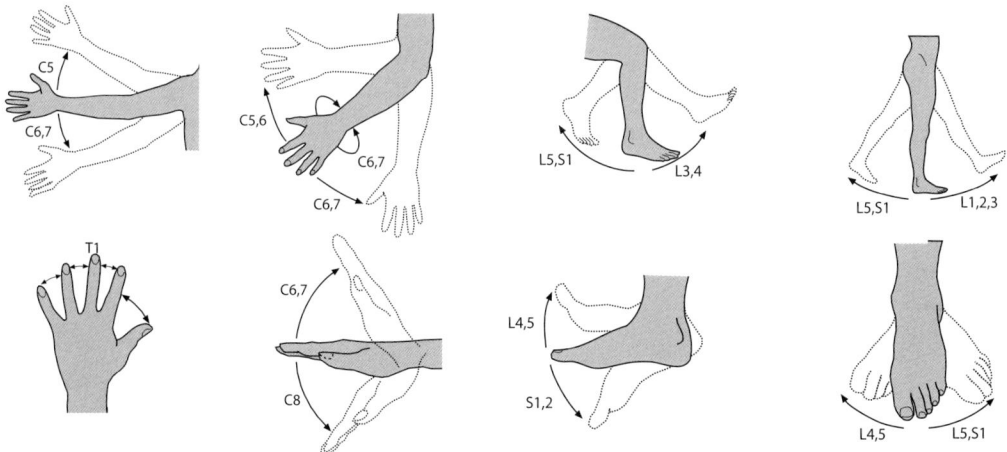

Figure 2.15 The segmental limb movements

The diagram marked *"reflexes"* shows a simplified method of remembering the nerve root origins of the main peripheral reflexes. This is done by "counting from 1 to 8 from below up".

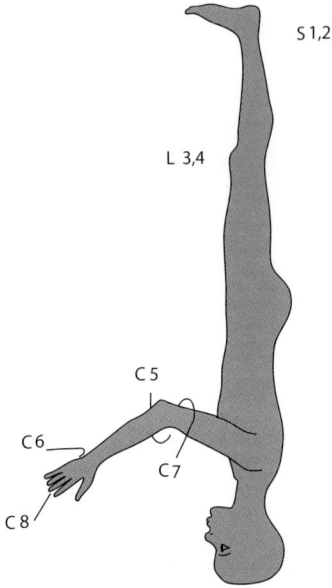

Figure 2.16 Reflexes. Count from the ankle

The diagram marked skin territories shows the *main sensory dermatomes* and their nerve root origin.

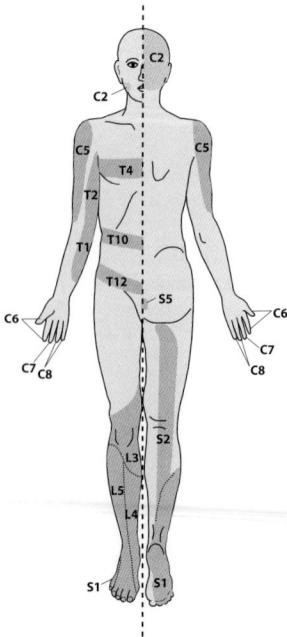

Figure 2.17 Skin territories of landmark nerve roots

The main sites of neurological disorders and the resulting patterns of motor and sensory loss are summarized in Tables 2.2 & 3.

Table 2.2 Main sites and patterns of motor loss

Site	Pattern of motor loss (weakness)
CNS (UMNL)	
hemisphere	hemiparesis
brain stem	cranial nerve palsies one side & hemiparesis on other side. quadriparesis & LOC*
spinal cord (C1-T12)	quadriparesis paraparesis
PNS (LMNL) *spinal cord (L1-S5)*	paraparesis
anterior horn cell	localised/generalized
nerve root	root distribution
nerve plexus	>one nerve root
mononeuropathy *(cranial or peripheral)*	single peripheral nerve
polyneuropathy	feet and legs > hands and arms

* loss of consciousness, these may occur in an extensive brain stem lesion

Table 2.3 Main sites and patterns of sensory loss

Site	Sensory loss
PNS	
single nerves	nerve distribution
all peripheral nerves	glove and stocking
spinal nerve roots	dermatomal
cauda equina	both legs & perineum
CNS **Spinal cord**	
complete transection	all below level of the lesion
hemisection *(Brown Sequard Syndrome)*	joint position/vibration/light touch on same side & pain/temperature on opposite side
Brain	
brain stem	face on same side as lesion & limbs on side opposite lesion
*parietal lobes**	on side opposite the lesion a. numbness b. agnosia c. loss of two point discrimination d. astereognosis e. graphanaesthesia f. sensory inattention

* cortical sensory testing

Cortical sensory testing: Definitions

agnosia: abnormality of perception despite normal sensory pathways

two point discrimination: ability to determine whether one or two points are being applied at the same time (normal discrimination on finger tips: 2-3 mm)

astereognosis: inability to recognise familiar shapes and textures when felt in either hand with both eyes shut

graphanaesthesia: inability to identify numbers drawn on the palms with both eyes shut

sensory inattention: inability to correctly recognise and report a stimulus (visual or tactile) coming from the side opposite the lesion when the two stimuli are presented together to both sides at the same time

NEUROMUSCULAR JUNCTION

Neuromuscular disease results in a pattern of weakness which is characteristically *fatigable* on repeated testing. The neurology examination is usually normal apart from the muscle weakness. The degree of weakness ranges from *drooping* of the *eye lids* and *diplopia* in mild cases to *difficulty* to *talk, swallow, breathe, move eyes* and *limbs* in severe cases. The main cause of neuromuscular junction weakness is myasthenia gravis.

MUSCLE

Muscle disease results in weakness and sometimes muscle wasting. Neurology examination is normal apart from the muscle weakness and reflexes are usually preserved until late in the disease when they may be lost. The clinical characteristic of myopathic weakness is that the *proximal muscles* are more involved than the *distal ones*. This is most obvious whilst asking the patient to repeatedly elevate the arms over the head or whilst attempting to stand up from a seated position on the ground or in a chair. The main causes of muscle weakness are myopathy, polymyositis and muscular dystrophy.

GAIT DISORDERS

A normal functioning gait requires the coordinated action of an intact sensory and motor system, which in turn relies on normal balance and muscles. Neurological causes of gait disorder may arise from any one or all of these. Gait disorders are classified on the basis of their *main clinical presentation*. The main types of abnormal gait are outlined below in Table 2.4. The site of abnormality is suggested by the characteristic gait and confirmatory neurological signs.

Table 2.4 Common gait disorders seen in clinical practice

Gait disorder	Clinical features
Hemiparetic gait	arm adducted, leg extended, stiff & circumducting
Spastic paraparesis	slow, stiff, jerky with scissoring/adduction at knees & dragging of toes
Cerebellar	wide based & unsteady, can't walk a straight line
Parkinson's	slow & stiff with small & shuffling steps, neck & trunk & limbs semi flexed & decreased or no arm swing
Sensory ataxic	high stepping gait with stomping feet
Neuropathic	high stepping with foot drop
Myopathic	waddling or rolling

Key points

- neurological history & examination are essential
- most important question is whether the lesion is in the CNS or PNS
- neurological findings help to correctly localize the site of the lesion
- localization determines the likely cause, investigations & management

Selected references

Fitzgerald M.J.T. & Folan-Curran Jean, *Clinical Neuroanatomy and related neuroscience.* 4th edition. Elsevier Harcourt Publishers Ltd, 2002.

Wilkinson Iain & Lennox Graham, *Essential Neurology.* Blackwell Publishing 4th edition 2005.

Harrison Michael, *Neurological Skills, A guide to examination and management in Neurology.* Butterworth's 1st edition 1987.

Fuller Geraint, *Neurological examination made easy.* Churchill Livingstone, 3rd edition 2004.

O'Brien MD, *Aids to the examination of the peripheral nervous system.* Saunders 1st edition 2000.

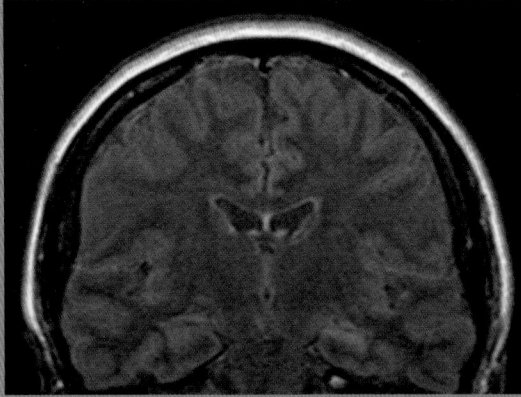

PART II – NEUROLOGICAL DISORDERS

CHAPTER 3
PUBLIC HEALTH

CONTENTS

CHAPTER 3

PUBLIC HEALTH

Global burden of neurological disorders

Public health is about the prevention of disease and the promotion of healthy living. Public health necessarily focuses on the community and groups of people; this is in contrast to the doctor who focuses on the patient. However, they both represent two ends of the same spectrum, one dealing with disease at population level, and the other dealing with disease at individual level. This chapter briefly outlines some of the basic principles of public health and their relationship to neurological disorders and health care delivery. The student should aim to be able to define incidence, prevalence and mortality rates and to understand disease burden and its measurement and prevention with particular regard to neurological disorders.

MEASUREMENT OF DISEASE

Disease occurrence

The simplest measurement of any disease is how common it is or the frequency of the disease in a community. In order to answer that question accurately, public health has first to be able to define and diagnose the disease, according to certain criteria and then measure its frequency in relation to the size of population in which the disease occurs or cases arise. This information is essential for public health planning and implementation. The science and art of gathering such information are the instruments of public health, much in the same way as the neurology history and examination are the instruments used for clinical neurology. The parameters used most frequently to report information on disease are the incidence, prevalence and mortality rates.

Incidence rate

Incidence rate is the most accurate method of measuring the frequency of a disease. The incidence rate is the number of new cases occurring in a defined population over a period of time. Measuring incidence over a period of time in a defined population gives an accurate measurement of disease frequency. Incidence measured over a year can be used to obtain the annual incidence of the disease. The annual incidence of the disease will include all new cases, or events occurring in the defined population during one year, including those who die soon after getting the disease, and those who recover from their disease. Incidence is measured as a rate, since it is always necessary to specify the time of observation. Incidence rate is often expressed as the number of new cases per 1000 person-years, 10,000 person-years, or 100,000 person-years, according to how common the disease is. For very common diseases, like diarrhoea or the common cold, or for diseases where epidemics occur over a short period of time, the incidence rate can be expressed as number of new episodes per 1000 person-months, or 10,000 person-months. In contrast some neurological disorders are expressed per 100,000 person-years because they are uncommon or rare like myasthenia gravis or Guillain Barre Syndrome GBS.

Prevalence rate/ratio

Prevalence measures the number of cases of a particular disorder in a defined population at a fixed point in time. This includes all cases, not just new cases. Prevalence is expressed as a ratio of the number of cases per 1000, 10,000 or 100,000 of the population. Prevalence is used mostly to measure the frequency of chronic diseases and disabilities that accumulate in the community over time. A disease with a short duration can have low prevalence despite a high incidence, whereas a disease with a long duration may have a high prevalence despite a relatively low incidence rate. Many neurological diseases have long durations and despite relatively low incidence rates, they can still have relatively high prevalence. These include chronic diseases like epilepsy, paraplegia, leprosy and stroke. Some neurological disorders have a particularly high prevalence e.g. migraine 5-10,000/100,000 of the population. When a disease is this common its frequency can be expressed more simply, as the proportion or percentage of the population affected, in the case of migraine 5-10%. Though epilepsy is ten times less common its prevalence can still be expressed more simply as 0.5-1% of the population affected.

Mortality rate

Mortality is expressed as the total number of deaths in a defined population over a defined period of time, usually during one year. Mortality rates are often expressed as the number of deaths per 1000, 10,000 or 100,000 of the population per year, according to how high the mortality is. The overall or crude death rate for all causes is often given as the total number of deaths per 1,000 of the population occurring during one year. The crude mortality rate for all causes in Sub-Saharan Africa is around 18/1,000 per year in contrast to around 9/1,000 per year in high income countries. However this does not mean that the risk of dying is just twice as high in Africa. In fact the risk is higher because crude death rate is heavily dependent on the age structure and life expectancy of a population. As the population in Africa is mainly young (50% <12 yrs) and average life expectancy short (<50 yrs) then the figure 18/1000 actually represents a much higher overall risk of death in Africa. Crude mortality rates are therefore a better guide to a change in overall risk within a population than to the comparison of risk across populations in different countries.

Mortality rate can be calculated for specific age groups, e.g. 0-1 year, 1-4 years, 5-14 years, 10 years e.g. 20-29 years & 15-49 years. Such age-specific rates can be used to validly compare mortality across population groups within countries and across different countries. During emergency situations e.g. epidemics of cholera a shorter study time period of a day, week or month may be used when calculating mortality rates.

Case fatality ratio

Case-fatality ratio or proportion can be defined as the number of deaths from a disease divided by all cases of that disease that occurred over a period of time. It is usually expressed as a percentage. The case fatality for rabies is 100% and for tetanus is over 50%, in contrast the case fatality for tension headache is zero.

Definitions

- Incidence rate: number of new cases of a disease occurring in a population during a specified time period
- Prevalence rate: total number of cases present in a defined population at a point in time.
- Prevalence ratio: proportion of a population affected by a disease at a given point in time
- Mortality rate: the total number of deaths in a population during a specific time period
- Case fatality ratio: the number of deaths divided by the number of cases diagnosed during a specific time period

DISEASE BURDEN

Disability-adjusted life years (DALYs)

WHO uses the term disability adjusted life years (DALYs) lost to measure disease burden. This approach combines the number of years of healthy life lost (YLL) as a result of premature death, and the years lost through disability or (YLDs). The combined sum of YLLs and YLDs is called DALYs which is defined as the number of healthy years lost due to disability and premature death. This provides a measure of the number of years of healthy life which are lost as a result of a particular illness or disease. Burden of disease measurements like DALYs are particularly useful for measuring the community burden of neurological disorders, many of which are chronic, disabling and eventually shorten life.

Disability is counted in terms of years, but because it is not the same for every disorder, e.g. the degree of disability with paraplegia is much greater than that with headache, it needs to be adjusted depending on the type of the disability and also the age of the patient. The disability severity varies on a scale between 0 and 1 and this disability weight reflects the average degree of disability associated with each disorder. The years lived with a disability are multiplied by the disability weight for the condition in question to get the years lost due to the disability. The disability weight scale assigned to the different neurological disorders is available through WHO.

The gold standard assumes an expected healthy life of 82.5 years. For example if a man dies at the age of 30 years as a complication of a paraplegia which resulted from a RTA which happened when he was 20 years old then the number of years of expected life lost (YLLs) due to his premature death are 82.5 - 30 = 52.5 years. The number of DALYs lost is even greater as it includes the 10 years of life lived with paraplegia that has a disability weight of **0.671**. This will then correspond to 10 x 0.671 = 6.7 life years lost due to disability, and the sum of DALYs lost will be: 52.5 + 6.7 = 59.2 years.

Definitions

- YLLs: years of life lost due to premature death
- YLDs: years lived with a disability
- DALYs: the sum of life years lost due to premature death and disability

The burden of neurological disorders in Africa

The burden of deaths and disability attributable to neurological disorders in Africa is presented below according to WHO estimate 2005.

Death

Neurological disorders are an important cause of mortality and constitute about 12% of all deaths worldwide, with stroke alone accounting for 85% of all neurologic deaths. In Africa the proportion of all deaths (**YLLs**) attributable to neurological disorders is **4.6%** (Fig 3.1). This is comprised of **stroke 3.2%, infections 1.0% and epilepsy 0.4%**. The main reasons for this relatively lower proportion are the younger population distribution with high rates of fatal non neurological infections and also notably the burden of neurological deaths related to human immunodeficiency virus (HIV) infection are not included in this figure.

Deaths attributable to neurological disorders in Sub-Saharan Africa (4.6% of all deaths)

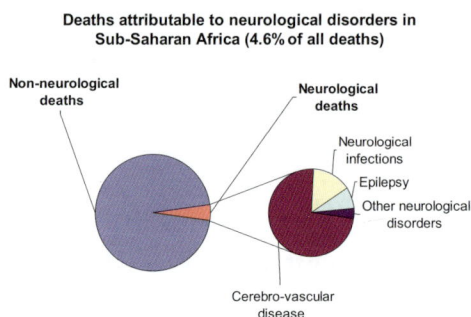

Non-neurological deaths
Neurological deaths
Neurological infections
Epilepsy
Other neurological disorders
Cerebro-vascular disease

Figure 3.1 Deaths caused by neurological disorders

Disability

Disability can be defined as a physical or mental impairment that substantially limits one or more major life activities. Disabilities can be caused by disease, trauma or other health conditions and may require ongoing medical care. Many neurological diseases result in disability, and lasting disability is the most common outcome after a neurological illness or injury. The main neurological disabilities are impairment of motor or cognitive functions. These include a wide range, from loss of mobility in stroke and paraplegia to cognitive impairment in head injury. Other lasting disabilities include epilepsy and loss of sight or hearing. Disability may be a fixed disability as occurs in head injury or progressive as in dementia. Neurological disorders contribute >**14%** of the total burden of **YLDs** in Africa. (Fig. 3.2). The causes include **infections 4.2%, nutrition/neuropathies 4%, head injuries 3.6%, epilepsy 0.9%, migraine 0.6%, stroke 0.4%,** and **neurodegeneration 0.4%**.

Mental Disease

Neuropsychiatric disorders including **depression, psychoses, alcohol abuse** and **substance use** account for significant proportion of global disease burden >**14%** of **YLDs**. These frequently coexist with neurological disorders but are not covered in this textbook. Neurological and mental disease together account for >**28%** of total **YLDs** in Africa.

Disability (YLDs) attributable to neurological disorders in Sub-Saharan Africa (14.17%)

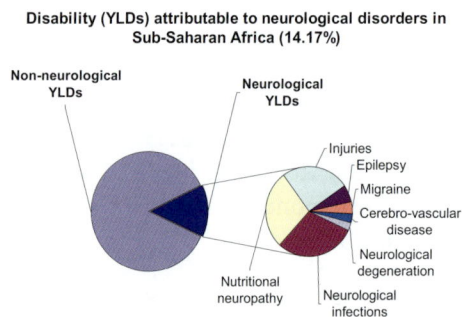

Non-neurological YLDs
Neurological YLDs
Injuries
Epilepsy
Migraine
Cerebro-vascular disease
Neurological degeneration
Nutritional neuropathy
Neurological infections

Figure 3.2 Disability caused by neurological disorders

Death and disability (DALYs)

Globally neurological disorders contribute >**6%** of the total DALYs. In Africa NDs account for about **3%** of total burden of disease as measured by DALYs. The main neurological disorders contributing to DALYs in Africa are **stroke 1.1%, infections** (mostly tetanus & meningitis) **0.9%,** and **epilepsy 0.5%**. However this is an underestimate as the burden of HIV related neurological disorders is not included in this category by WHO estimate. **HIV/AIDS** on its own accounts for over **5%** of total DALYs worldwide, most of which occurs in SSA.

HEALTH PROMOTION AND DISEASE PREVENTION

Health promotion can be defined as the process of enabling people to increase control over their health and its determinants, and thereby improve their lives. The primary means of health promotion occurs through developing a healthy public policy that addresses the prerequisites of health such as income, housing, food, water, security, employment, transport and quality working conditions.

Disease prevention (preventive medicine or preventive care) refers to measures taken to prevent illness or injury, rather than curing them. The major preventable risk factors for global disease are outlined below in Table 3.1. Prevention strategies are designed to decrease morbidity and mortality and are categorised as primary, secondary and tertiary prevention (Table 3.2). These strategies are aimed either at the general population or targeted at selective subgroups of the population. Specific examples of prevention strategies in neurology are presented in Table 3.3.

Table 3.1 Major preventable risk factors for disease globally, WHO

Risk factor	% global disease burden
Under nutrition	15
Over nutrition	13
Unsafe sex	6
Tobacco	4
Alcohol	4
Unsafe water/sanitation/hygiene	4

Primary prevention strategies intend to avoid the development of a disease. Primary prevention stops a disease from happening or stops individuals from becoming at risk. Most population-based health promotion activities are primary preventive measures. General or population based prevention is designed to stop or reduce known risks in the whole population. Examples are to vaccinate all infants at birth in order to prevent tetanus and to promote healthy eating and exercise to prevent non communicable diseases.

Selective or targeted primary prevention normally targets high risk groups and may require some form of screening test in order to identify those at increased risk. Examples are preventive programmes targeted towards high risk groups, identified after screening for non communicable diseases or HIV.

Secondary prevention activities are aimed at early disease detection and treatment, thereby increasing opportunities for interventions to prevent disease progression and the emergence of symptoms. Secondary prevention aims at decreasing disease severity through the early detection, diagnosis and treatment of the disease. Examples of this include diagnosing and treating hypertension to prevent stroke or treating HIV with ARTs to prevent AIDS.

Tertiary prevention reduces the negative impact of an already established disease by restoring function and reducing disease-related complications. Thus tertiary prevention involves treating and managing disease complications which have already occurred, in order to prevent death and reduce disability. Examples of this in neurology are rehabilitation of stroke and paraplegia. Rehabilitation is an active process by which those affected by injury or disease achieve a full or optimum recovery, in all aspects of life. It is one of the key components of health care, along with prevention and treatment.

The distribution and determinants of risks in a population have major implications for which type of public health intervention is used. Decreasing a small risk in a large number of people usually results in more cases being prevented than decreasing a larger risk in a smaller number. Thus, general prevention strategies aiming at reaching the whole population are often more cost-effective than prevention targeted to high risk groups only. However, combining population-based and high risk strategies can be even more effective.

Table 3.2 Prevention of disease

Primary	preventing a disease before it happens
Secondary	decreasing disease severity through early detection, diagnosis and treatment
Tertiary	treating & managing disease complications to increase quality of life, reduce disability & prevent death

Table 3.3 Examples of prevention strategies in neurological disorders in Africa

Prevention strategies	Measures	Expected outcome
Primary prevention	vaccination	prevents tetanus
	increased exercise healthy diet low salt diet stop smoking reduce cholesterol	combined with secondary measures decreases stroke by 70%
	wearing seatbelts/helmets	decreases death/head injury by 40-50%
Secondary prevention (screening, early diagnosis and treatment)	treating epilepsy	decreases mortality, morbidity >70% seizure free
	treating hypertension	decrease stroke, heart and renal failure
	ART and OI prophylaxis	decreases mortality/morbidity in HIV
Tertiary prevention (rehabilitation & palliative care)	rehabilitation hospital and community based	improved quality and independence of life
	palliative care	stops/decreases pain and other symptoms

HEALTH DELIVERY

Governments, departments of health and health care planners define health policies and implement disease prevention and care strategies. They are supported by non government organizations and voluntary organizations. The debate in health care in Africa as elsewhere in the world is "where to get the best value for your money". In general where resources are limited it is the public health based population primary prevention interventions that have the greatest priority and potential to save lives (Table 3.3). However, within health delivery there needs to be a balance between prevention and care as the successful implementation of both are linked and interdependent. In neurology successful examples of primary prevention include vaccination to prevent tetanus and meningitis and bed nets to prevent cerebral malaria.

Examples of secondary prevention include treating epilepsy, ART, prophylaxis of opportunistic infections in HIV and treatment of hypertension to prevent stroke. Both approaches are complementary to health care policy in Africa.

Neurological service provision

Adequate health systems are a prerequisite for health care. These are the institutions and organizations within a country that provide and deliver the health services. The basic resources needed to provide these services are staff, facilities, equipment and medications. Staff includes the ministry of health and the health care workers (HCW) including traditional practitioners. The services which they provide are delivered at three main levels in Africa (Table 3.4).

Primary care is the first point of contact of the health service with the patient. Health care is delivered at this level by primary health care workers (PHCW), mainly medical assistants and nurses working at dispensaries and health care centres. The most common neurological disorders encountered in primary care are headache and epilepsy. Limitations to the successful delivery of neurological service at this level include the lack of adequate education and training in neurology, cultural barriers and practical constraints both financial and geographic. Any long term measures designed to improve services at this level must be targeted on education and be culturally appropriate, sustainable and adequately resourced.

Secondary care is provided at district, regional and mission hospitals. The main health care workers (HCW) involved in secondary care are nurses, medical assistants and doctors. Available facilities at this level include general inpatient and outpatient services, paediatric, medical, surgical and obstetrical care in addition to laboratory, radiological and some rehabilitation services. Public health and some HCW training are sited at regional and also at some mission hospitals. The balance and make up of each facility depends on the type of hospital and where it is. However diagnostic neurology facilities including a CT scanner or electrophysiology facilities (EEG) are usually not available at this level. Patients presenting with major neurological disorders often present at this level for the first time. The most common disorders include epilepsy, stroke, infections, paralysis and coma and are the subject of individual chapters in this book.

Tertiary care is provided at referral or teaching hospitals. These specialist hospitals act as referral and care centres serving large areas of the country with populations involving many millions. The HCWs providing the service at this level are nurses, occupational and physiotherapists, doctors and specialists. The main aim in neurology is to provide a specialist diagnostic, treatment and management service. However because of the lack of trained specialists, mainly neurologists and neurosurgeons there is frequently only a limited service available. Diagnostic facilities usually available at these centres include neuroimaging, a CT scanner (occasionally MRI), electrophysiology facilities including EEG, and rehabilitation services including physiotherapy and occupational therapy. These centres also provide national facilities for undergraduate and postgraduate teaching and training and also for research into neurological disorders. The aim of this book is to support neurological education and training in Africa.

Table 3.4 Health care level and activities in Africa

Level	Site/population	Staff (HCW)	Activities
Primary health care	dispensary/health care centre (2000-5000)	nurses/medical assistants	immunization, maternal and child, family planning, treatment of common diseases including epilepsy
Secondary health care	district/mission hospital (100,000-200,000)	nurses/medical assistants and 1-2 doctors	emergency and curative services
	regional hospital (0.5-1 million)	nurses/medical assistants and doctors	care, preventative and training
Tertiary health care	consultant hospital (millions)	nurses/doctors and specialists	care, teaching, research

Selected references

Bergen DC. *Preventable neurological diseases worldwide.* Neuroepidemiology. 1998;17(2):67-73.

Bergen DC, Silberberg D. *Nervous system disorders: a global epidemic.* Arch Neurol. 2002 Jul;59(7):1194-6.

Birbeck GL. *A neurologist in Zambia.* Lancet Neurol. 2002 May;1(1):58-61.

Birbeck GL, Munsat T. *Neurologic services in sub-Saharan Africa: a case study among Zambian primary healthcare workers.* J Neurol Sci. 2002 Aug 15;200(1-2):75-8.

Bower JH, Howlett W, Maro VP, Wangai H, Sirima N, Reyburn H. *A screening instrument to measure the prevalence of neurological disability in resource-poor settings.* Neuroepidemiology. 2009;32(4):313-20.

El Tallawy HN, Farghaly WM, Rageh TA, Shehata GA, Metwaly NA, Abo Elftoh N, et al. *Epidemiology of major neurological disorders project in Al Kharga district, New Valley, Egypt.* Neuroepidemiology. 2010;35(4):291-7.

Haimanot RT, Abebe M, Mariam AG, Forsgren L, Holmgren G, Heijbel J, et al. *Community-based study of neurological disorders in Ethiopia: development of a screening instrument.* Ethiop Med J. 1990 Jul;28(3):123-37.

Janca A, Prilipko L, Saraceno B. A *World Health Organization perspective on neurology and neuroscience.* Arch Neurol. 2000 Dec;57(12):1786-8.

Menken M, Munsat TL, Toole JF. *The global burden of disease study: implications for neurology.* Arch Neurol. 2000 Mar;57(3):418-20.

Neurological Disorders: *public health challenges.* WHO 2006

Osuntokun BO, Adeuja AO, Schoenberg BS, Bademosi O, Nottidge VA, Olumide AO, et al. *Neurological disorders in Nigerian Africans: a community-based study.* Acta Neurol Scand. 1987 Jan;75(1):13-21.

Prince M, Patel V, Saxena S, Maj M, Maselko J, Phillips MR, et al. *No health without mental health.* Lancet. 2007 Sep 8;370(9590):859-77.

Siddiqi OK, Atadzhanov M, Birbeck GL, Koralnik IJ. *The spectrum of neurological disorders in a Zambian tertiary care hospital.* J Neurol Sci. 2010 Mar 15;290(1-2):1-5.

Singhal BS. *Neurology in developing countries: a population perspective.* Arch Neurol. 1998 Jul;55(7):1019-21.

Jamison DT, Feachem RG, Makgoba MW, et al., editors. *Disease and Mortality in Sub-Saharan Africa.* 2nd edition. Washington (DC): World Bank; 2006.

PART II – NEUROLOGICAL DISORDERS

CHAPTER 4
EPILEPSY

CONTENTS

CHAPTER 4

EPILEPSY

Introduction

Epilepsy is a predisposition to recurrent unprovoked seizures. Seizures are caused by attacks of sudden, excessive, abnormal electrical discharges arising mainly from the neurones in the cortex of the brain. The site, spread and pattern of electrical discharges determine the clinical features of epilepsy. The seizures may range from a brief awareness of sensation lasting only seconds to a sudden loss of consciousness associated with involuntary stiffening and jerking body movements. The latter is termed **generalized tonic-clonic epilepsy** and historically was called **grand mal**. Epilepsy is the most common community based major neurological disorder and the individual case history and description of the seizure are crucial to the diagnosis of epilepsy. This chapter outlines the main epilepsy syndromes, their classification, causes, clinical presentation diagnosis and management. The student should aim for an overall understanding of epilepsy and in particular its burden, diagnosis, management and treatment.

EPILEPSY SYNDROMES

Epilepsy is classified according to cause and clinical seizure type. **Idiopathic** epilepsy (60-70%) occurs where no known cause is found or suspected and many of these are most likely genetic in origin. **Symptomatic** epilepsy (30-40%) occurs when there is an underlying structural abnormality in the cerebral cortex such as a scar or tumour or another condition predisposing to seizures. Seizures in epilepsy may be classified according to their clinical presentation and their site of electrical origin in the brain (Table 4.1). If seizures arise focally from one site within the brain these are termed as the **partial onset seizures**. These can present with motor, sensory, autonomic and psychological symptoms. If the electrical discharge remains focal and consciousness is fully retained, these are classified as **simple partial seizures**. If the electric discharge arises focally and consciousness is altered, these are classified as **complex partial seizures**. If the electrical discharge arises focally and spreads to involve the rest of the entire cerebral cortex, this results in a **generalized tonic-clonic seizure**. These are classified as **secondary generalized tonic-clonic seizures (grand mal)** and are the most common type of seizure disorder **(70%)**. Seizures may also arise from electrical discharges deep within the brain spreading equally rapidly to all parts of the cortex at the same time. These are termed as **generalized onset seizures (30%)**. These include **"absence" seizures (petit mal) myoclonic seizures, tonic-clonic seizures (grand mal)** and **atonic seizures**. Epilepsy may also be described as active or inactive, controlled or uncontrolled depending on the degree of remission and response to treatment.

CLASSIFICATION

Table 4.1 Classification of Seizures

Category	Seizure type	Consciousness
Partial onset seizures *(70%)*	simple partial complex partial secondary generalized tonic–clonic	not impaired impaired loss of consciousness
Generalized onset seizures (30%)	absence myoclonic primary generalized tonic-clonic	impaired not clinically impaired loss of consciousness

EPIDEMIOLOGY

Epilepsy is defined as the tendency to have recurrent seizures. It affects 0.4 to 0.6% of the world's population at any point in time, with a larger proportion of the general population (3-5%) having one or two non-recurrent isolated seizures throughout their life which do not develop into epilepsy. The global burden of epilepsy is estimated to be >50 millions of whom 80% live in low or middle income countries. Estimates of the frequency in Africa vary widely and studies from there have in the past suggested that active epilepsy is 2-3 times higher than in high income countries with a median frequency of 15/1000 (1.5%). However methodological difficulties make it difficult to compare most studies. A recent multicentre study from five sites in East Africa which reproduces strict methodology suggests a median frequency there of <0.5% which is similar to other parts of the world. The criteria used to diagnose active epilepsy were 2 or more unprovoked seizures during the previous 12 month period. There are two peak age groups when epilepsy occurs, the first one is in childhood and adolescence during which both birth related and genetic causes are typically found and the second peak occurs in older adults (>65 years) when there is usually an underlying structural cause in the brain.

AETIOLOGY

The aetiology is unknown or idiopathic in about two thirds of cases of epilepsy in Africa. This may in part be a function of under investigation due to lack of resources. Epilepsy has many causes and it is likely that genetic and historical causes account for a significant proportion of these. The main causes and their estimated frequencies in Africa are presented in Table 4.2. Genetic predisposition and brain injury are both known risk factors for epilepsy. Genetic factors are indicated by a positive family history of epilepsy. The underlying mechanisms of epilepsy are not known but a chronic pathological process as a result of tissue injury or some other common mechanisms seems likely in many cases. Pre and perinatal brain injuries arise largely as a result of hypoxia and hypoglycaemia because of intrauterine infections e.g. toxoplasmosis, rubella, HIV etc and because of poor obstetric care. Febrile convulsions (FC) as an infant or young child are a significant risk factor for scarring in the temporal lobe and epilepsy in later life.

A history of previous CNS infection is a major risk factor for epilepsy in Africa. This is particularly the case for infants, children and younger adults. The main infections are meningitis, cerebral malaria, neurocysticercosis, encephalitis and brain abscess. Malaria is the most common cause of acute symptomatic seizures in children in malaria endemic parts of Africa. HIV is the most common cause in young adults. However it is important to remember that single seizures or those occurring during a febrile illness are not classified as epilepsy. Helminthic infections are an important cause of epilepsy in parts of Africa, in particular where free-range pig rearing is practised resulting in neurocysticercosis. Traumatic head injury mainly as a result of road traffic accidents and falls are increasingly a cause of epilepsy in young adults. Brain tumours and cerebrovascular disease account for a proportion of epilepsy mainly affecting adults.

Table 4.2 Main causes of epilepsy in Africa & their estimated frequency

Cause	% of total	(range)
genetic	40	(6-60)
pre & perinatal	20	(1-36)
infections & febrile convulsions	20	(10-26)
cerebrovascular disease	10	(1-42)
head injury	5	(5-10)
brain tumour	5	(1-10)

Ref Preux & Druet-Cabanac Lancet Neurol 2005; 4: 21-31

Key points

- active epilepsy affects at least 0.5% of the population in Africa
- peak age groups affected are young children, teenagers & older adults
- cause is unknown in up to two thirds of cases
- genetic factors may account for a sizable proportion
- pre & perinatal brain injury & infections are main causes in young persons
- stroke, head injury and tumour are main causes in older age groups

COMMON FORMS OF SEIZURES

Generalized tonic-clonic seizure (GTCS)

This is the most common form of epilepsy in adults. Typically it involves consecutive clinical phases including tonic-clonic limb movements, loss of consciousness, frothing from the mouth, tongue biting, incontinence and post ictal confusion. If the origin of the seizure is focal as in secondary or **partial onset epilepsy** an aura may be present at the onset. In contrast there is no aura in **primary** or **generalized onset epilepsy.**

Aura phase

The clinical type of aura depends on the site of origin of the seizure. This phase typically lasts a few seconds or less and consists of a brief recurring stereotyped episode. The episode is characterized by an awareness of a familiar, typically epigastric feeling or the hallucination of a smell, taste but rarely hearing, usually coupled with automatisms if the origin is in the temporal lobe. If the origin is the parietal lobe, the episode is sensory, if in the frontal lobe it is motor and if in the occipital lobe it is visual. The aura phase of a partial onset GTCS may be forgotten because of retrograde amnesia.

Tonic phase

The tonic-clonic phase starts suddenly with loss of consciousness; the patient may make a loud noise or a cry and fall to the ground. There is a brief stiffening and extension of the body due to sustained tonic muscle contraction lasting about 10 seconds but which can last a minute.

During this tonic phase breathing stops and cyanosis may be recognised by observers. Urinary incontinence and less frequently faecal incontinence may occur at the end of this stage.

Clonic phase

The tonic phase is followed by the clonic phase characterized by repeated generalized convulsive muscle spasms. These are violent, sharp, rhythmical, powerful, jerky movements involving the limbs, head, jaw and trunk. The eyes roll back, the tongue may be bitten and frothing from the mouth may occur due to excess salivation as the result of excessive autonomic activity. This phase typically lasts a minute or two but may be more prolonged. The patient remains unconscious.

Coma phase

When the jerking has stopped normal breathing pattern returns but is shallow, the limbs are now flaccid and the patient remains unconscious and cannot be roused. The duration of unconsciousness ranges typically from about 5-20 minutes and reflects the extent and duration of the seizure. Then there is a gradual return of consciousness.

Post-ictal phase

On recovery of consciousness there may be confusion accompanied by a headache, drowsiness and typically sleepiness for a variable period sometimes lasting for up to several hours. Over the following days, there is usually some muscle stiffness and soreness and evidence of any injury sustained during the attack. Patients have retrograde amnesia for the seizure but may sometimes remember the aura phase before loss of consciousness.

Diagnostic features of a GTCS

- witnessed convulsion
- loss of consciousness
- tonic-clonic limb movements
- incontinence
- tongue biting
- postictal confusion

Absence seizures

This is the most common form of primary generalized onset epilepsy. It affects mainly children usually <10 yrs, (4-12 yrs) and is more common in girls. An attack occurs without warning. Usually parents or teachers note that the child suddenly stops what he or she is doing for a few seconds but does not fall down or convulse. The eyes remain open staring blankly ahead with occasionally blinking or eyelid fluttering. There is no response to an outside stimulus during the attack which ends as suddenly as it starts, usually with the child resuming activities unaware of what has happened. The attacks are brief lasting, typically between 5-15 seconds and can reoccur several times daily. The EEG shows a characteristic 2-3 per sec generalized symmetrical slow and spike wave discharges. Both attacks and EEG changes can be provoked by hyperventilation. The attacks respond well to treatment with low dose sodium valproate or ethosuximide. Children usually grow out of these attacks in their late teens but some few may develop into generalized onset TCS.

Diagnostic features of absence seizures

- mainly a childhood disorder & more common in girls
- stereotyped recurring episodes of loss of awareness or absences
- child goes blank, switches off for few seconds, stares ahead & may blink
- unresponsive during attack but does not convulse or fall down

Myoclonic seizures

These are another form of primary generalized onset seizures which are characterized by sudden, brief involuntary jerky limb movements lasting a few seconds. These seizures typically occur in young teenagers in the mornings after waking, with consciousness being preserved. Simple myoclonic jerks, which are generally benign, must be distinguished from **juvenile myoclonic epilepsy (JME)**. **JME** consists of the triad of myoclonic jerks on waking occurring in all patients, generalized onset TCS in >90% of patients and typical day time absences in about one-third of patients. Absences may sometimes be an early feature, they begin in childhood and early teens and myoclonic jerks follow usually at around the age of 14-15 years. GTCS usually appears a few months after the onset of myoclonic jerks typically occurring shortly after waking. Occasionally JME may start or become clinically identified in adult life as 'adult myoclonic epilepsy'. The EEG in JME shows typical polyspikes and slow wave discharges and may show photosensitivity. Treatment with low dose sodium valproate is usually very successful.

Diagnostic features of juvenile myoclonic epilepsy

- simple myoclonic jerks are benign and may not need treatment
- JME consists of morning myoclonic jerks, daytime absences & GTCS on waking

Partial onset seizures

If the site of electrical discharge is restricted to a focal area of the cortex in one cerebral hemisphere, then the patient will have partial onset seizures. The main causes include infections, infarcts, head injuries, tumours and hippocampal sclerosis, the latter due to frequent febrile convulsions in childhood. The clinical features depend on the site of the cortical focus and thus may be sensory or motor and involve alteration in consciousness. If there is no accompanying alteration of consciousness, then it is classified as a simple partial motor or sensory seizure. If there is alteration or clouding of consciousness, then it is a complex partial seizure. If the electrical spread becomes generalized, then it is classified as a secondary GTCS. Any patient presenting with new partial onset seizure disorder should be investigated with a brain scan to exclude a focal underlying cause.

Temporal Lobe epilepsy (TLE)

Complex partial seizures arise mainly in the temporal or frontal lobes. Temporal lobe epilepsy (TLE) is the commonest type of complex partial seizure disorder. The temporal lobe structures, particularly the hippocampus, are susceptible to injury during febrile convulsions, which may result in mesial temporal sclerosis (Fig. 4.6) and later TLE. The clinical features reflect the functions of the temporal lobe which include memory, speech, taste and smell. Seizures present as stereotyped episodes characterised by subjective experiences and movements. The subjective experiences include blank spells or absences, a sense of fear or déjà vu (an indescribably familiar feeling "that I have had this before"), or an inexplicable sensation rising up in the abdomen or chest. They may also include memories rushing back and hallucinations of smell, taste, hearing or images. To an observer the patient may appear confused and exhibit repeated stereotyped movements or automatisms including chewing and lip smacking. The attack typically lasts seconds to minutes depending on the extent and cause of the lesion. Attacks can be still more complex and if the electrical activity spreads to the rest of the brain then a GTCS may occur.

Diagnostic features of TLE

- stereotyped episodes lasting seconds
- déjà vu, depersonalization, rising sensation in epigastrium
- hallucination of mainly taste or smell
- movements, automatisms: lip smacking, chewing
- confusion and altered emotion
- may develop into a GTCS

Motor seizures (Jacksonian epilepsy)

This is a partial onset motor seizure disorder which occurs as a result of a focal lesion in the frontal lobe in or near the motor cortex. The convulsive movement begins typically in the corner of the mouth or in the index finger or big toe and then spreads slowly proximally to involve the leg, face, and hand (Jacksonian march) on the side of the body opposite the lesion. There may also be clonic movements of the head and eyes to the side opposite the lesion. The attack may develop into a secondary GTCS, and may infrequently result in a temporary limb paralysis (Todd's paralysis).

Diagnostic features of focal motor seizures

- clonic movements begin focally in the corner of mouth or finger or toe
- spreads slowly to involve face, hand, arm, foot & leg on the same side
- may develop into a secondary GTCS
- may result in a temporary limb paralysis

Febrile convulsions

Febrile convulsions are seizures in children which typically occur between the ages of 3 months and 5 years as a result of fever from any cause. They are mostly GTCS in type and are a known risk factor for epilepsy in later life, and in particular TLE. They can cause damage to the temporal lobe that subsequently causes epilepsy. The scarring is mainly in the mesial temporal lobe and can be seen on MRI. The worldwide risk of epilepsy after childhood febrile convulsions is estimated to be 2-5%. In Africa this risk increases to around 10%, particularly after a history of repeated convulsions in malaria. Convulsions complicating malaria are one of the most common reasons for children presenting to clinics and hospitals in Africa. Convulsions occurring in uncomplicated malaria tend to be brief and non recurrent, whereas those occurring with complicated and cerebral malaria are more prolonged, multiple and recurrent, and carry a higher subsequent risk of epilepsy.

Clinical diagnosis

The diagnosis of epilepsy is mainly clinical. Epilepsy is difficult to diagnose and there is both under and over diagnosis of the condition. The first principle of diagnosis is to obtain a clear history from the patient and an eye-witnessed account of the episode. This involves the context in which the attack occurs, the details of the minutes or seconds leading up to and what happened during and after the attack. An attack of a GTCS is diagnostic if it includes a description of the convulsion, incontinence, tongue biting (Fig. 4.1) and post ictal confusion. All of these may not be present in any one patient. The description may alternatively be that of the typical vacant episodes of absence seizures or the aura of a partial onset seizure or of any another type of seizure disorder. If a patient cannot describe what happened, very often it is necessary to interview and record an eye-witnessed account or review a video of the attack if available.

The history from the patient or family should include current illnesses and specific questions concerning known risk factors for seizures including perinatal injury, febrile convulsions, infection, head injury, alcohol consumption and drugs. A detailed family history is helpful particularly in suspected cases of primary generalized seizures. There should be a thorough general and neurological examination. Look for evidence of seizures including tongue biting, scars and evidence of injuries. Patients who have had a single non recurrent seizure are not considered to have epilepsy, they should however be investigated to exclude an underlying cause e.g. toxoplasmosis in HIV, a vascular cause or tumour. The differential diagnosis of epilepsy includes any cause of syncope or loss of consciousness including, pseudoseizures, hypoglycaemia, hyperventilation and transient ischaemic attacks (Chapters 5 & 9). The main differences between epileptic and or non epileptic attacks (pseudoseizures) are summarised below in Table 4.3.

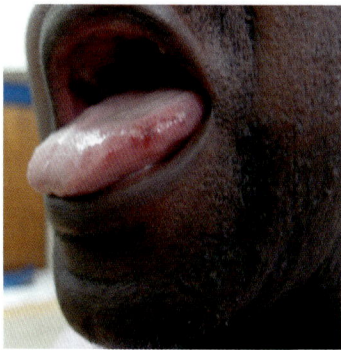

Figure 4.1 Tongue biting

Key points

- obtain a clear history from the patient
- get an eye witnessed account of the episodes
- check past & family for any risk factors for epilepsy
- do a general & neurological examination
- look for stigmata of seizure/epilepsy

Pseudoseizures (non epileptic dissociative attacks)
Some patients have unexplained GTCS like episodes of loss of consciousness either consciously or subconsciously. The diagnosis should be suspected if there are atypical episodes of loss of consciousness occurring in a teenager or young adult, often female, lasting longer than 5 minutes. These episodes resemble seizures and are considered to be psychogenic or non epileptic in origin and are a major cause of misdiagnosis of epilepsy. There are no absolute criteria to distinguish between pseudoseizures and epileptic attacks clinically (Table 4.3). The attacks can mimic a GTCS and can occur in association with known epilepsy. In high income countries as many as one third of patients with known epilepsy may suffer from a non epileptic attack at some time. During a typical attack there is no tonic phase, there may be shouting and coordinated limb movements particularly involving hyperextension of the back, pelvic thrusting and repeated side to side head turning. There is no post-ictal confusion phase and the patient typically reports no awareness during the attack or memory of the episode afterwards. The

vital signs and neurological reflexes remain normal during the episode. Definitive assessment of a suspected case requires simultaneous co-registration of both the clinical attack and an EEG using telemetry. Management includes reassurance and in particular the avoidance of unnecessary antiepileptic medications. A psychiatric opinion may be helpful in persistent cases.

Table 4.3 Differences between epileptic and non epileptic attacks

Clinical features	Epileptic	Non epileptic
Sex	any sex	females > males
Age group	any	teenagers/young adults
Duration	minutes	prolonged
Vital signs	abnormal	normal
Tonic/post ictal phases	present	absent
Body movements	repetitive	stereotyped
Plantar response	may be up going	normal
EEG	abnormal	normal

INVESTIGATIONS

The diagnosis of epilepsy is primarily based on a clinical description of the seizures. The main aim of investigations is to confirm or exclude the diagnosis, to establish a cause and to classify the type of epilepsy. Routine investigations including full blood count, serum glucose, renal and liver function tests are rarely helpful in screening for causes of epilepsy. However other screening tests should include HIV and other possible local causes of seizures in sub Saharan Africa (SSA) including cysticercosis. Electroencephalography (EEG) and brain imaging are the main methods of investigation of epilepsy.

Electroencephalography

The EEG is extremely useful in the diagnosis and classification of epilepsy. It is particularly useful if recorded during an epileptic attack, where the finding of epileptiform activity (spikes and sharp waves) confirms the clinical diagnosis. However the majority of EEGs are recorded interictally (between the attacks) when the EEG may be normal (Fig. 4.2). Only about 50% of persons with proven epilepsy have an abnormal first interictal EEG. This percentage can be increased to around 85% with repeated EEG testing, using provocation tests (hyperventilation and flashing lights) and by doing sleep recordings. The finding of a normal interictal EEG therefore does not exclude the diagnosis of epilepsy. By the same token more than 10% of normal persons may have non-specific EEG abnormalities and approximately 1% may have epileptiform paroxysmal activity without clinical seizures. The prevalence of these abnormalities is higher in children, with about 2-4% having functional spike discharges. The EEG is particularly useful in children and young adults where a diagnosis of either primary or secondary seizure disorder is suspected. This is especially true for absence seizures when the characteristic symmetric 3 per second spike and wave pattern is seen in all leads (Fig. 4.3). In partial onset seizures the EEG frequently reveals sharp wave abnormalities originating focally from one area of the brain (Fig. 4.4). In generalized seizures the EEG shows electrical discharges in all leads (Fig. 4.5).

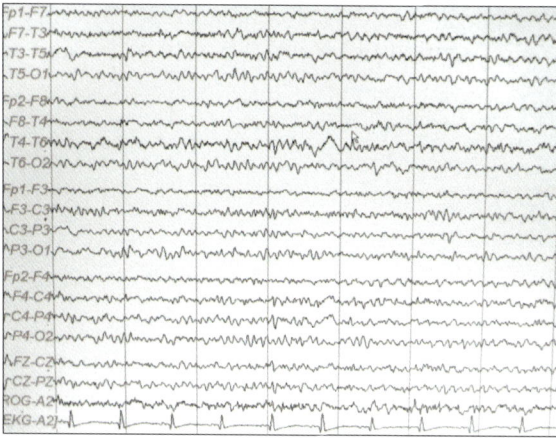

Figure 4.2 EEG normal

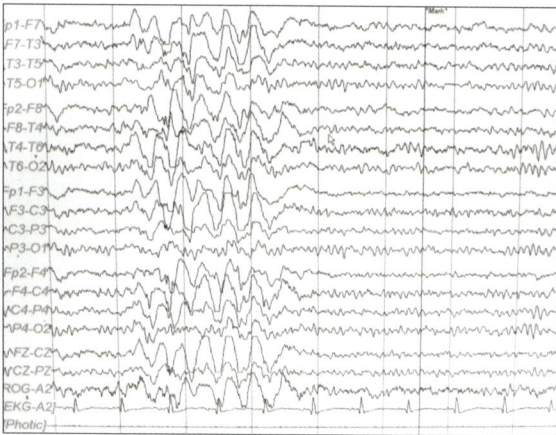

Figure 4.3 EEG absence seizure. Two to three per second spike & wave.

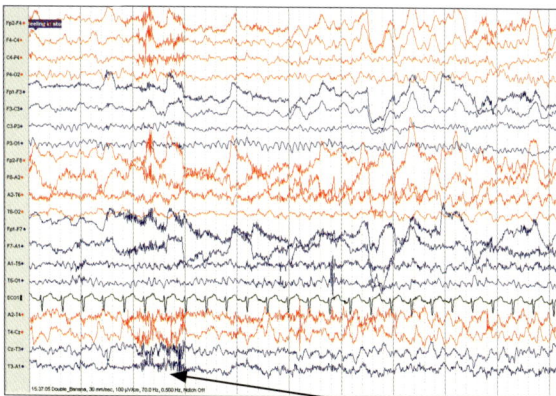

Figure 4.4 EEG focal seizure. Unilateral right sided electrical discharge.

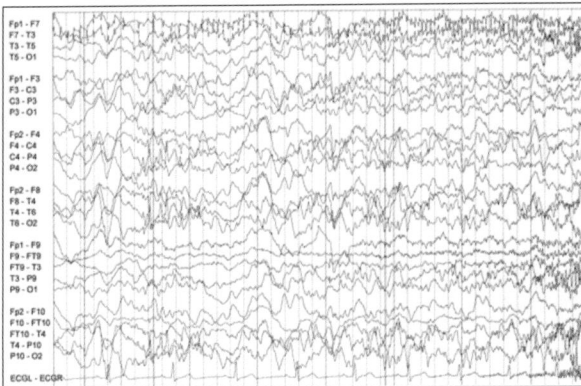

Figure 4.5 EEG generalized seizure. Bilateral electrical discharge.

Brain imaging

Brain imaging with CT or MRI is helpful when a focal cause of epilepsy is suspected, particularly in partial onset epilepsies. This is even more so the case in epilepsies of later age onset, 25 yrs or greater because of their likely focal onset. Brain imaging is expected to be normal in most generalized onset epilepsies which occur in a mainly younger age group e.g. teenagers. MRI scanning is more sensitive than CT, and may be necessary to show the underlying lesion e.g. mesial temporal sclerosis (Figure 4.6) in some partial onset seizure disorders.

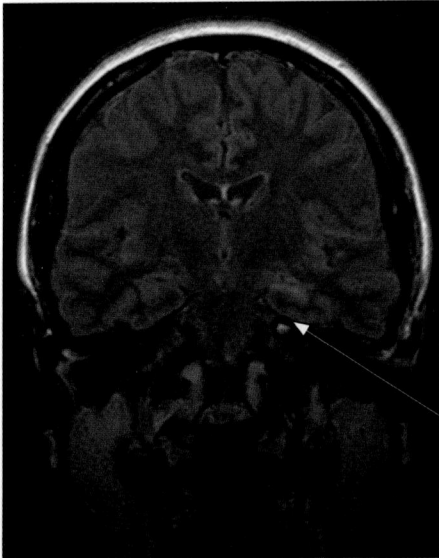

Figure 4.6 MRI T1. Mesial temporal sclerosis. Sclerosis & contracted hippocampus (left).

Key points

- aim is to confirm the clinical diagnosis, find the cause & classify epilepsy
- EEG & imaging are indicated in recent new onset seizure disorders
- EEG may be normal initially & need repeating with provocation testing & sleep
- EEG can distinguish between partial & generalized onset seizure disorders
- brain imaging is mostly indicated in new onset partial seizure disorders in adults

MANAGEMENT OF EPILEPSY

General advice

Remember that epilepsy has a bad name and has been falsely attributed to witchcraft, spirits, and demonic possession and to contagion in Africa. The sudden unpredictable attacks, the need to take medications every day for years and their side effects and obvious restrictions on social life and occupation make patients feel stigmatized. It is important therefore to listen to patient's and family's anxieties and to explain the nature of epilepsy and its management. Antiepileptic drugs (AED) are usually advised when two or more unprovoked seizures have occurred within the previous 12 months. Patients may require medication for years and sometimes for life, and all the AEDs have side effects. It is important to explain that about two thirds of patients with epilepsy suppress their attacks completely by using a single AED in adequate doses and also that young people with primary generalized onset seizure disorders tend to grow out of their epilepsy in their late teens or early twenties.

The patient should be made aware of the potential triggering effect on seizures of fatigue, sleep deprivation, alcohol, infections and also flashing lights if photosensitive. Driving may be legally restricted nationally and some jobs may be off limits including bus, lorry and train drivers, airline pilots, and the armed forces. Some activities are obviously dangerous to the patients with epilepsy and precautions are necessary, these include fishing, boating, swimming, working at heights, near moving machinery and open fires. Remember that most patients in Africa will visit the traditional healer and receive advice and treatment. Patients with epilepsy are most probably safer when they are with other people.

Key points

- epilepsy is a very stigmatizing disease
- listen to worries of patient & family & explain the nature of epilepsy
- AED treatment is advised if two or more unprovoked seizures occur within the last 12 months
- explain the hazards & restrictions & that AED treatment may need to be taken for life
- 60-75% become seizure free on single AED if taken in adequate doses

First aid for seizures

Most tonic-clonic seizures do not require emergency drug treatment. Firstly, avoid injury by removing the patient from any immediate danger e.g. fire, road traffic, water etc. See the scars from burns and scalds in Fig 4.7. Do not attempt to force anything between the teeth. Wait until the tonic-clonic phase is over, and then make certain that the airway is clear by extending the neck. Then place the patient on his side in the recovery position to avoid aspiration if he vomits. If the seizure stops and there is a previous history of seizures, then no further medical action is required. If the seizure does not cease spontaneously, emergency medical treatment is needed. In children with febrile convulsions, it is important to lower the temperature and treat the underlying cause.

Upper Limbs

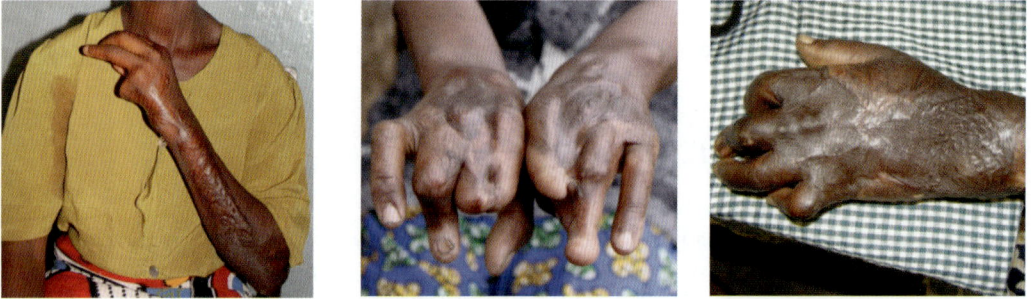

Lower Limbs

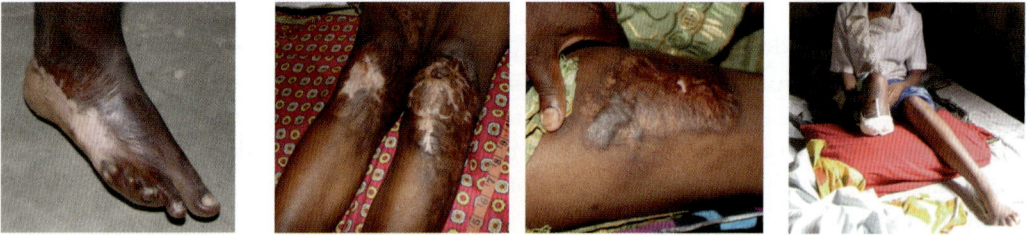

Trunk and face

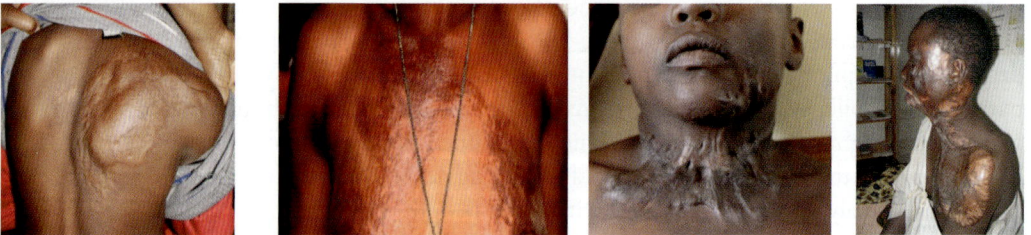

Figures 4. 7 Scars & deformities as a result of burns & scalds

DRUG TREATMENT

The aim of drug treatment is to make the patient seizure free. The choice of drug is determined mainly by the type of epilepsy. Every effort should be made early on to find the single best drug (monotherapy) available using the smallest dose with the fewest side effects. The main drugs, their indication, dosage and side effects for treatment of epilepsy in Africa are outlined in Table 4.4. Treatment is started at low dose and increased slowly as necessary to an effective maintenance dose, when seizures are controlled or the patient develops intolerable side effects. The single most common reason for failed drug treatment is using insufficiently high doses of medication where necessary. One of the main limiting factors in epilepsy treatment is the side effects of medication. Other reasons for treatment failure include non-compliance due to lack of accessibility and availability of drugs, their cost, and life style including alcohol. However, if seizures still persist despite using an adequate dose of an appropriate single AED, then another first line drug is added withdrawing the first drug only after establishing seizure control. Treatment is always aimed at making the patient completely seizure-free but this may not be possible in up to one third of patients. Reasons include refractory epilepsy and underlying cause. In these situations when monotherapy is ineffective a group of epilepsy patients will require two and possibly even three drugs in combination (polytherapy). Deaths directly attributed to the AEDs are uncommon (<1:50,000) and are usually caused by early idiosyncratic reactions.

Key points

- using one drug start slow & aim low
- if seizures are stopped, do not increase the dose any further
- if seizures are not controlled, increase dose as long as no or few side-effects
- if seizures still persist add a second AED
- all drugs prescribed should be available locally

Drugs

Phenobarbitone (PHB): This is indicated for all types of epilepsies and is widely available and used in Africa. WHO recommends it as the first line drug for the treatment of epilepsy in Africa in both children and adults. Phenobarbitone is usually used in previously untreated patients and is particularly useful in status epilepticus because with an adequate loading dose it has a quick effect. It has a long half life and may be used in a single daily dose often taken at night just before sleep. The starting dose for teenagers and adults is usually 60 mg, it can be increased by 30 mg weekly to a usual maximum maintenance dose of either 180 mg once daily or 90 mg twice daily. For children the dose should be calculated by weight at 5 mg/kg. Any reduction in dosage needs to be particularly slow (every 2 weeks) and gradual because of the risk of withdrawal seizures and status epilepticus. The main side effects are sedation, photosensitivity and cognitive/behavioural dysfunction in children. Phenobarbitone is a potent microsomal liver enzyme inducer and decreases the half life of other drugs metabolised in the liver. This becomes particularly relevant clinically with concomitant use of the oral contraceptive pill, where the dose of the pill has to be increased to be effective.

Carbamazepine (CBZ): This is used in all types of epilepsy except in absences and myoclonus. It is the drug of first choice for partial onset epilepsies and is very effective. The starting dose is low at 100 mg twice daily increasing slowly by 200 mg increments every 2 weeks until seizures are controlled. The usual therapeutic dose is between 400-1600 mg daily in divided doses. The maximum dose is 2,400 mg daily. Most people respond to a daily dose of 2-400 mg twice or three times daily. The main side effects are drowsiness, ataxia and dizziness which are dose dependent and decrease with time but may limit the dose. The onset of rash and hypersensitivity allergic reaction usually within the first two weeks of starting treatment requires immediate stopping of the medication. CBZ is the least teratogenic of the main AEDs and has a liver enzyme induction effect similar to phenobarbitone.

Phenytoin (PHT): This is used to treat all types of epilepsy except absence seizures. Its advantages are that it can be given once daily as a single dose usually at night. Loading with phenytoin is possible in previously untreated patients and in status epilepticus for a quick effect. The usual loading dose is 900 mg and the usual oral starting dose is 200-300 mg daily. The main disadvantage is that it has a narrow therapeutic range and dose adjustments may produce large changes in plasma concentrations and intoxication. Therefore any increase in dosage should be by small increments of 25-50 mg every 2 weeks up to a usual maximum dose of 400-450 mg daily. If available, the measurement of drug levels can guide dosage. The main side effects are ataxia, drowsiness and dizziness which are dose dependent. The chronic toxicity effects of hirsutism, gum hypertrophy, facial skin thickening and acne limit its long term usage over years particularly in young persons. Liver enzyme induction occurs similarly to phenobarbitone.

Sodium valproate (SVP): This is the drug of first choice for idiopathic and generalized onset epilepsies and is also used in partial onset secondary generalized seizures. The starting dose is 200 mg twice daily increasing by 200-400 mg increments if necessary every 2 weeks up to a maximum of 1.4 gm twice daily. The main side effects are nausea, vomiting, tremor, weight gain, hair loss, polycystic ovary syndrome and teratogenesis all of which are dose dependent. Hepatotoxicity is idiosyncratic and may very rarely be fatal. It displaces phenytoin from plasma protein binding which may lead to phenytoin toxicity.

Ethosuximide: This is indicated for generalized absence seizures only. It is given twice daily and the starting dose is 250 mg daily increasing weekly to a maintenance dose of 750-1500 mg in divided doses. The main side effects are nausea, drowsiness, headache and ataxia. Rare idiosyncratic reactions include lupus like syndrome and blood dyscrasias.

Newer drugs for epilepsy

These include **lamotrigine, levetiracetam** and **topiramate** amongst many others. They are used in people who have not responded or tolerated standard AEDs. **Levetiracetam** is a particularly useful first and second line drug in adults with uncontrolled focal and generalized epilepsies. Information on these drugs is available in larger textbooks and online.

Table 4.4 Drug treatment of epilepsy in Africa

Drug	Main indications	Dosage starting	Dosage maintenance	Main side effects
Phenobarbitone	all epilepsies	60 mg/po/daily	180 mg/daily	**sedation**, ataxia, photosensitivity, **cognitive/ behavioural dysfunction**
Carbamazepine	partial onset epilepsies	100 mg/po/bd	2–800 mg/bd	**ataxia/sedation** (dose dependent), **rash**, allergic reaction
Phenytoin	partial onset/ secondary generalized seizures	200–300 mg/ po/nocte	3–450 mg/daily	**ataxia, drowsiness**, dizziness (dose dependent) hirsutism, **gum hypertrophy, facial skin thickening** and acne
Sodium Valproate	primary generalized and partial onset epilepsies	200 mg/po/bd	400–1400 mg/bd	**nausea**, vomiting, **tremor, weight gain**, hair loss, **polycystic ovary syndrome**, hepatotoxicity, teratogenesis (dose dependent),
Ethosuximide	absence seizures only	250 mg/po/od	250–750 mg/bd	**nausea, drowsiness**, headache, ataxia, **blood dyscrasia**

Discontinuing of AEDs

AEDs may be effectively withdrawn in some patients who have been seizure free for 2-5 years. This will largely depend on the type of epilepsy, the implications for recurrence and the side effects of medications. There is an increased risk of recurrence in adults particularly between

1 and 2 years after stopping. This risk is greatest in partial onset seizures which are severe. Children who have been seizure free for 2 years off medication tend to remain so. The final decision to withdraw medication must be made by the patient or family and be carried out slowly over months with gradually decreasing doses because of the risk of provoking seizures by too rapid a withdrawal.

AEDs AND WOMEN

There are some special precautions when using AEDs in women. Carbamazepine, phenytoin and phenobarbitone are all liver enzyme inducers that decrease blood levels of oestrogen and progesterone. In patients taking these AEDs, the dose of oestrogen in the contraceptive pill needs to be increased from 25mg to at least 50 mg in order to be effective and even then contraceptive efficacy is reduced. Depot preparations are less affected by concomitant AED usage. The use of AEDs in women with epilepsy is associated with increased risk of teratogenicity. Women should be counselled about the risks of taking AEDs before becoming pregnant. The rate of major malformations born to mothers taking **valproate, carbamazepine, phenytoin** or **phenobarbitone** is **4-8%**. This risk increases proportional to number of AEDs and the dosage used. Valproate is the most inclined to cause malformations and these defects include the neural tube defects, anencephaly and spina bifida, hole in the heart, hare lip and cleft palate. In order to decrease this risk the total recommended daily dose of valproate in childbearing women is **<1000 mg** or switch to Levetiracetam or Lamotrogine monotherapy.

Best practice is to use a single drug in the lowest effective dose and to offer folic acid prophylaxis before conception. A dose of **folic acid** of 5 mg daily has been shown to decrease incidence of neural tube defects in women not taking AEDs. Note that this dose is higher than the usual prophylactic dose (0.4mg) prescribed with ferrous sulphate in early normal pregnancy. The dose of AEDs may have to be increased in pregnancy particularly during the third trimester and just before delivery because of an increased risk of seizures which happens in about one quarter of patients. Any dose increase can be reversed 6 weeks after delivery.

Vitamin K is routinely recommended in patients taking enzyme inducing AEDs starting one month before delivery and also to the baby at delivery. Seizures occurring in late pregnancy or in the immediate postpartum period should suggest the possibility of eclampsia. In eclampsia, **magnesium sulphate** is the drug of choice in a dose of 3-4 gm iv stat (max 20 gm daily).

Key points

- oestrogen dose should be increased to 50 mg in some women on AEDs and the pill
- AEDs increase risk of teratogenesis, SVP is the most teratogenic & CMZ is the least
- folic acid 5mg before conception decreases the risk of neural tube defects
- dose of AEDs may need to be increased in the 3rd trimester
- vitamin K is given to mother & all infants if on enzyme inducing AEDs

STATUS EPILEPTICUS

Status epilepticus is defined as continuous seizures or two or more repeated attacks of GTCS without recovery of consciousness between attacks or an attack lasting longer than 30 minutes. It is a medical emergency with a mortality rate of 10-20% in Africa. Permanent brain damage can occur as a result of hypoxia and acidosis if repeated or single seizures last longer than 30 minutes. The main risk factors in Africa are a history of epilepsy, current infection, suddenly stopping AEDs in particular phenobarbitone, mental handicap and an underlying structural brain disorder.

Management

The drug treatment of status is outlined in Table 4.5. General measures include ensuring a clear airway with adequate oxygenation (> 95% oxygen saturation) and ensuring an adequate circulation (pulse & BP) and establishing iv access (Chapter 9). A blood glucose should be checked and if low (<2.5 mmols) treated with 50 ml of 50% glucose. Infections are treated. If there is a history of alcohol abuse or poor nutrition then thiamine 100-250 mg should be given iv slowly. Reasons for failure to respond to emergency treatment include inadequate doses of phenytoin or phenobarbital, failure to continue adequate maintenance therapy and the presence of acidosis or an underlying medical disorder.

Table 4.5 Drug treatment of status epilepticus

Stage	Drug/route/rate	Comment
early status (0-30 mins)	**diazepam** 10 mg/iv bolus over 2 minutes *or* **lorazepam** 4 mg (0.1 mg/kg) iv bolus over 2 minutes	if seizures continue after 5 mins either one can be *repeated* just once but may cause respiratory depression
established status (30-60 mins) *(if seizures continue & patient is not on phenytoin or phenobarbitone)*	**phenytoin** iv n. saline infusion of 15 mg/kg (900-1,000 mg total dose) @ 50 mg/min/iv (in N/S over 20 mins) *or* **phenobarbitone** infusion iv 10 mg/kg/@100 mg/min/ over 7-10 minutes (adult total dose is 700 mg)	if iv is unavailable, give phenytoin via nasogastric tube, *(absorption is excellent)* if patient is already on phenytoin or phenobarbitone then use half the usual full loading dose if seizures stop continue with *maintenance* oral phenytoin or phenobarbitone
refractory status (>60 mins) *(if seizures still continue)*	involve anaesthesia & proceed to ventilation, Rx **thiopentone** or **midazolam** or **propofol**	if seizures are stopped for >24 hours; stop ventilation & continue daily maintenance dose of phenytoin or phenobarbitone & reinstate regular AEDs

PROGNOSIS

The standardised mortality rate worldwide in patients with epilepsy is 2-3 times higher than in the general population and studies suggest that mortality is much higher in Africa, possibly 5-6 times. Some of this is explained by the underlying cause at diagnosis but most is related to the epilepsy itself, its severity and the lack of diagnosis and treatment in Africa. Risk factors for increased mortality include age group, seizure type, frequency and drug compliance. The main causes of mortality and morbidity due to seizures include accidents, drowning, falls and burns. Status epilepticus and sudden unexpected or unexplained death which occurs in epilepsy **(SUDEP)** may each account for 5-10% of all epilepsy related deaths.

Driving and epilepsy

Patients with epilepsy must not drive unless their seizures are completely controlled by medication. Generally driving is not allowed until the newly diagnosed and treated seizure patient has been seizure-free for at least three months. When AEDs are discontinued, driving again is forbidden until the patient has been seizure-free for at least three months after the last dose of medication. Legal restrictions on driving with epilepsy vary between countries and should be researched and followed.

TREATMENT GAP

In Africa the vast majority of people with epilepsy (75-80%) do not receive any or adequate treatment for their disease. This is called the treatment gap. Among the reasons for this are the social stigma, poor medical infrastructure, insufficient supply and cost of and accessibility of AEDs, and the scarcity of well informed or trained medical personnel. There are also higher levels of cognitive impairment among the patients with epilepsy. Future plans for intervention must prioritise and find novel ways to encourage the diagnosis and treatment of epilepsy in the community. This is supported by first raising the level of awareness of epilepsy and ensuring that adequate supplies of the first line AEDs are available with clear guidelines concerning their use. These AEDs should be free or affordable and available at sites which are convenient and accessible to the patient. There is also a need to provide and train health care workers and to involve traditional health care workers and patient's supporters and families in the care of the patient.

Key points

- epilepsy is the most common major community based neurological disorder
- majority do not receive or get adequate treatment
- reasons include stigma, lack of education, resources, manpower & infrastructure
- there is a great need to improve the care of epilepsy in Africa

Selected references

Baskind R, Birbeck GL. *Epilepsy-associated stigma in sub-Saharan Africa: the social landscape of a disease.* Epilepsy Behav. 2005 Aug;7(1):68-73.

Birbeck GL. *Seizures in rural Zambia.* Epilepsia. 2000 Mar;41(3):277-81.

Birbeck GL, Hays RD, Cui X, Vickrey BG. *Seizure reduction and quality of life improvements in people with epilepsy.* Epilepsia. 2002 May;43(5):535-8.

Birbeck GL, Kim S, Hays RD, Vickrey BG. *Quality of life measures in epilepsy: how well can they detect change over time?* Neurology. 2000 May 9;54(9):1822-7.

Burton K, Rogathe J, Whittaker RG, Mankad K, Hunter E, Burton MJ et al. *Co-morbidity of epilepsy in Tanzanian children: a community-based case-control study.* Seizure. 2012 Apr;21(3):169-74.

Burton KJ, Rogathe J, Whittaker R, Mankad K, Hunter E, Burton MJ, et al. *Epilepsy in Tanzanian children: association with perinatal events and other risk factors.* Epilepsia. 2012 Apr;53(4):752-60.

Diop AG, de Boer HM, Mandlhate C, Prilipko L, Meinardi H. *The global campaign against epilepsy in Africa.* Acta Trop. 2003 Jun;87(1):149-59.

Diop AG, Hesdorffer DC, Logroscino G, Hauser WA. *Epilepsy and mortality in Africa: a review of the literature.* Epilepsia. 2005;46 Suppl 11:33-5.

Feely M. *Fortnightly review: drug treatment of epilepsy.* BMJ. 1999 Jan 9;318(7176):106-9.

Kariuki SM, Ikumi M, Ojal J, Sadarangani M, Idro R, Olotu A, et al. *Acute seizures attributable to falciparum malaria in an endemic area on the Kenyan coast.* Brain. 2011 May;134 (Pt 5):1519-28.

Mac TL, Tran DS, Quet F, Odermatt P, Preux PM, Tan CT. *Epidemiology, aetiology, and clinical management of epilepsy in Asia: a systematic review.* Lancet Neurol. 2007 Jun;6(6):533-43.

Mani KS, Rangan G, Srinivas HV, Srindharan VS, Subbakrishna DK. *Epilepsy control with phenobarbital or phenytoin in rural south India: the Yelandur study.* Lancet. 2001 Apr 28;357(9265):1316-20.

Mushi D, Burton K, Mtuya C, Gona JK, Walker R, Newton CR. *Perceptions, social life, treatment and education gap of Tanzanian children with epilepsy: a community-based study.* Epilepsy Behav. 2012 Mar;23(3):224-9.

Ngoungou EB, Preux PM. *Cerebral malaria and epilepsy.* Epilepsia. 2008 Aug;49 Suppl 6:19-24.

Preux PM, Druet-Cabanac M. *Epidemiology and aetiology of epilepsy in sub-Saharan Africa.* Lancet Neurol. 2005 Jan;4(1):21-31.

Sander JW, Shorvon SD. *Epidemiology of the epilepsies.* J Neurol Neurosurg Psychiatry. 1996 Nov;61(5):433-43.

Tomson T, Beghi E, Sundqvist A, Johannessen SI. *Medical risks in epilepsy: a review with focus on physical injuries, mortality, traffic accidents and their prevention.* Epilepsy Res. 2004 Jun;60(1):1-16.

Winkler AS, Blocher J, Auer H, Gotwald T, Matuja W, Schmutzhard E. *Epilepsy and neurocysticercosis in rural Tanzania-An imaging study.* Epilepsia. 2009 May;50(5):987-93.

Winkler AS, Mayer M, Schnaitmann S, Ombay M, Mathias B, Schmutzhard E, et al. *Belief systems of epilepsy and attitudes toward people living with epilepsy in a rural community of northern Tanzania.* Epilepsy Behav. 2010 Dec;19(4):596-601.

Yemadje LP, Houinato D, Boumédiène F, Ngoungou EB, Preux PM, Druet-Cabanac M. *Prevalence of epilepsy in the 15 years and older in Benin: a door-to-door nationwide survey.* Epilepsy Res. 2012 May;99(3):318-26.

PART II – NEUROLOGICAL DISORDERS

CHAPTER 5
STROKE

CONTENTS

CHAPTER 5

STROKE

Introduction

Stroke is a major medical disorder caused by interruption of blood supply to the brain which results in a loss of neurological function. It usually occurs suddenly without warning and frequently results in death or disability. The two main mechanisms are blocking of the arteries causing ischaemia and rupture of the arteries causing haemorrhage. The aim of management of stroke is to try to limit the area of damage in the brain, assist recovery and prevent any recurrence. The management of stroke in high income countries over the last two decades has witnessed marked improvement with the creation of dedicated stroke care units in hospitals and a more active approach to the management and prevention of stroke. This chapter presents an overview of the main characteristics of stroke. The student should aim for an overall understanding of stroke, including its increasing burden, main causes and prevention, and in particular to be able to diagnose and manage a patient presenting with stroke.

Definition: Stroke is a sudden neurological deficit lasting more than 24 hours with no explanation other than a vascular cause. If the patient recovers fully within 24 hours without any neurological deficit, then this is classified as a transient ischaemic attack (TIA).

Epidemiology

Stroke is the third most common cause of death worldwide after heart disease and cancer. It is reported to be the leading neurological cause of death in Africa (Chapter 3). The annual incidence of stroke in high income countries is 2-3 per 1000 persons and the prevalence reaches 0.5 to >1% of the population in older age groups (>65 yrs). A similar high incidence rate has been reported recently in one study in Tanzania. The overall prevalence of stroke is reported to be lower in Africa with age adjusted rates being less than half that in high income countries. However with increasing urbanization and life style changes the burden of stroke is steadily increasing and it is now one of the leading causes of neurological admissions and death in urban hospitals throughout Africa.

AETIOLOGY

Stroke occurs as a result of ischaemia or haemorrhage

Ischaemia

Ischaemia accounts for >80% of strokes worldwide and for 60-80% in Africa. Ischaemia is caused by thrombosis or embolism resulting in loss of blood supply to part of the brain (Fig. 5.1). Thromboembolism is the main cause and arises from atheromatous plaques situated in the major blood vessels in the neck and brain (Fig. 5.5). This is termed athero-thromboembolism. It results in occlusion of the arteries supplying the brain, most commonly the middle cerebral artery (Figs. 5.2 & 3). A smaller number of ischaemic strokes arise from occlusion of the small end arteries arising from the larger blood vessels deep within the brain. These are called lacunar strokes. Ischaemia is also caused by cardioembolism. This arises mainly from mitral valve disease, atrial fibrillation, cardiomyopathy and much less frequently, recent myocardial infarction. Less common causes of ischaemic strokes are sickle cell disease, HIV infection, vasculitis and venous sinus thrombosis.

Haemorrhage

About 10-20% of strokes worldwide are caused by haemorrhage. This percentage is higher in Africa (20-40%) probably because of the high burden of untreated or inadequately treated hypertension. Haemorrhagic stroke occurs when there is sudden release of blood into the brain. The main types are intracerebral haemorrhage (ICH) and subarachnoid haemorrhage (SAH) (Figs. 5.4 & 6). Hypertension is the major cause of ICH and is also a risk factor for SAH. The sources of bleeding in chronic hypertension are ruptured Charcot-Bouchard micro aneurysms which form on small perforating end arteries deep in the brain. Less common sources of bleeding are arteriovenous malformations (AVMs), tumours, trauma and amyloid. The most common site affected is the internal capsule area which usually results in a complete hemiparesis. When the source of bleeding is in the brain stem, or cerebellum there is usually quadriparesis with cranial nerve palsies, ataxia and coma. Subarachnoid haemorrhage (SAH) is mainly caused by a ruptured underlying intracranial saccular (berry) aneurysm arising from the circle of Willis and less frequently AVM.

Key points

- stroke is a leading cause of death in adults in Africa
- the main causes are ischaemia & haemorrhage
- ischaemia is caused by atheroma & embolism
- haemorrhagic strokes arise from ICH or SAH
- main causes are hypertension & aneurysms

Pathogenesis

When the blood supply to the brain is lost acutely either as a result of ischaemia or haemorrhage, a core area of the brain will undergo infarction/necrosis. This core area of the brain is irreversibly damaged. However in ischaemia, because of collateral blood supply, a surrounding area called a penumbra remains potentially viable for a limited time. This time period is usually about 3-4.5 hours, during which it will recover if the blood supply is restored. This is the target for the early treatment directed at decreasing thrombosis and improving blood supply. The swelling in the brain is caused by cytotoxic and vasogenic oedema as a result of infarction or haemorrhage.

This is frequently responsible for the clinical deterioration in the days immediately following on the acute stroke.

Vascular Risk Factors

The main risk factors for stroke are hypertension, atrial fibrillation, diabetes mellitus, smoking and lack of exercise (Table 5.1). Together, these account for over two thirds of all strokes and represent modifiable risk factors. The risk of stroke increases exponentially with age, with a much greater risk in the elderly population. Hypertension is the most important modifiable risk factor for both ischaemic and haemorrhagic stroke. The risk almost doubles with every 7.5 mm Hg rise in diastolic pressure even within the normal range of blood pressure. Established cardiovascular disease is an important risk factor for stroke, particularly a previous stroke or TIA, atrial fibrillation, rheumatic mitral valve disease and heart failure. Diabetes, high cholesterol and low density lipoproteins, sickle cell disease, the oral contraceptive pill, migraine and infections are all known risk factors for ischaemic stroke. The main modifiable life style risk factors include diet, salt intake, obesity, lack of exercise, cigarette smoking and increased alcohol consumption.

Table 5.1 Main risk factors for stroke

Risk factors	Relative degree of risk
ageing	highest
hypertension atrial fibrillation previous stroke or TIA	very high
ischaemic heart disease diabetes	high
life style: diet increased salt intake lack of exercise smoking alcohol	moderate
obesity	low

Key points

- age is the strongest non modifiable risk factor for stroke
- hypertension and AF are among the main modifiable risk factors in secondary prevention
- life style is the major modifiable risk factor in primary prevention

Main causes of stroke

- atheroma
- hypertension
- cardioembolism

CLINICAL PRESENTATION

The key features of a stroke are a sudden onset of a focal neurological deficit in a person who was previously well. Strokes occur more frequently at night and in the early morning. The clinical findings will depend on the type of stroke, the vascular site affected and the underlying cause. The most common presentations are a sudden, unilateral loss of power or sensation in an arm or leg or both, a loss of speech, vision or balance (Table 5.2). These help to localize the site of origin of the stroke. There are no features that can reliably distinguish between ischaemia and haemorrhage, although headache, vomiting, complete hemiparesis, reduced level of consciousness and severe hypertension are more common in haemorrhage. In subarachnoid haemorrhage (SAH), the onset is characterized by a new, sudden and severe headache with neck stiffness, usually without any focal neurological deficit, but alteration or loss of consciousness may be present. If the patient is unable to give a history, then the details should be obtained from a relative. The general examination should be directed at looking for the main underlying risk factors for stroke, including hypertension, atrial fibrillation, cardiac murmurs, carotid bruits and signs of systemic illness. CT imaging is usually necessary to distinguish between the two main types of stroke.

Table 5.2 Main clinical features of stroke

sudden onset either all at once or over minutes or hours
focal neurological symptoms and signs
loss of neurological function
motor loss: weakness of one side or part of one side of the body
sensory loss: decreased sensation on one side or part of one side of the body
aphasia: loss or impairment of speech, understanding, reading or writing
visual: loss of vision to one side, hemianopia (patient usually unaware)
other symptoms: altered consiousness, dysphagia, dysarthria, ataxia, diplopia, quadriparesis

Localization

Ischaemic strokes can be divided into anterior and posterior circulation strokes. Anteriorly the internal carotid artery (ICA) divides to form the anterior and middle cerebral arteries (ACA & MCA). Posteriorly the vertebral arteries join at the lower pons to form the basilar artery which in turn divides into two posterior cerebral arteries (PCA). The anterior and posterior circulations are joined in front by the anterior communicating artery and at the back by the posterior communicating artery to form the circle of Willis (Fig. 5.1). This ensures collateral circulation in the brain. The MCA supplies the anterior lateral two thirds of the brain and the ACA supplies the remaining medial two thirds. The PCA supplies the posterior one third or the occipital lobe. The brain stem and cerebellum are supplied in turn by the vertebral and basilar arteries. The most common sites affected are the MCA followed by the ACA, followed by lacunar and PCA (Table 5.3).

Table 5.3 Localization and strokes

Artery	Main clinical findings
Internal carotid artery	hemiplegia, (arm = face = leg)
	hemisensory deficit
	hemianopia
Anterior cerebral artery	hemiplegia, (leg > arm)
Middle cerebral artery	hemiplegia & numbness (face = arm > leg)
	aphasia *(if the dominant hemisphere involved)*
	hemianopia
	sensory inattention *(if the non dominant hemisphere involved)*
Posterior cerebral artery	hemianopia
Lacunar	hemiplegia, (face = arm = leg)
	hemisensory, (face = arm = leg)
Vertebro-basilar arteries (brain stem)	dysphagia, dysarthria,
	hemiplegia/quadriplegia
	cranial nerve palsies
	ataxia

* left hemisphere is dominant in most (>90%) right handed persons and in approx 70% of left handed persons

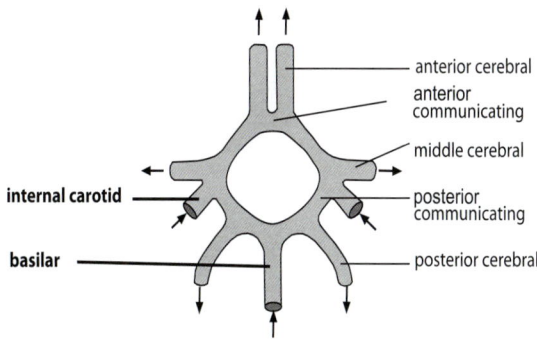

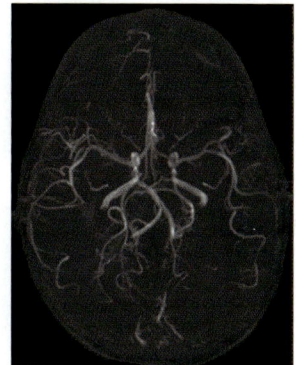

Figure 5.1 Circle of Willis. Angiogram of circle of Willis (COW). Normal (right).

Key points

- stroke is a sudden neurological deficit due to a vascular cause
- person is usually aware of a neurological deficit over minutes or less commonly hours
- hemiparesis is the most common finding
- neurological findings help to localize the site of the lesion
- most strokes occur in the anterior circulation

TRANSIENT ISCHAEMIC ATTACK (TIA)

A TIA is a sudden ischaemic focal neurological deficit that completely recovers in less than 24 hours. They typically last for minutes not hours. They are mostly caused by thromboemboli arising from the internal carotid arteries in the neck and their branches. Other sources of emboli are atrial fibrillation and heart disease. The vascular territory involved determines the

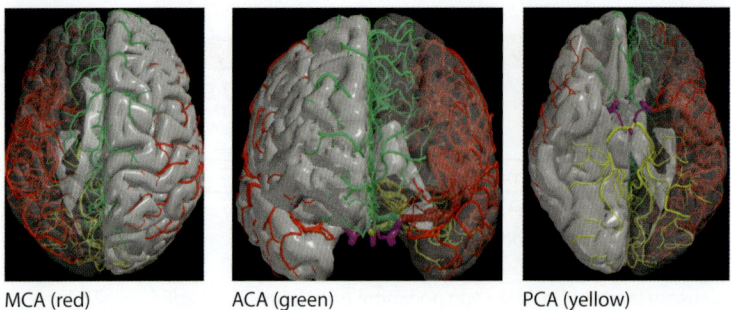

MCA (red)   ACA (green)   PCA (yellow)

Figure 5.2 Territories supplied by main cerebral arteries

CT scans showing infarcts

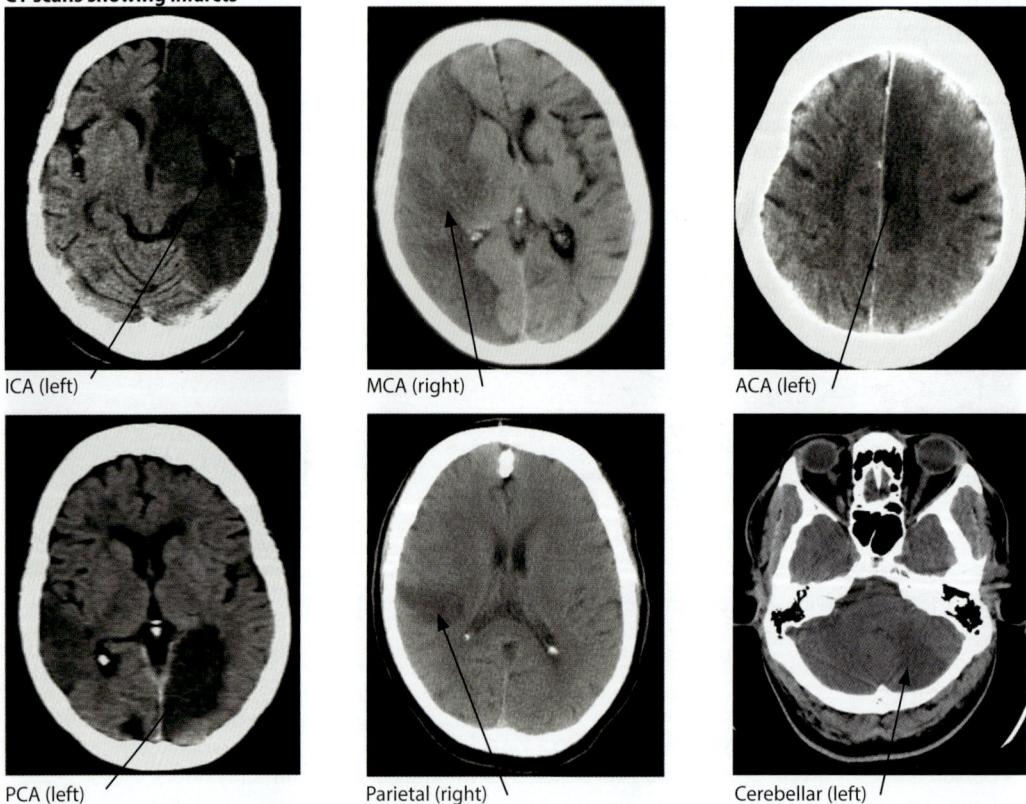

ICA (left)   MCA (right)   ACA (left)

PCA (left)   Parietal (right)   Cerebellar (left)

Figure 5.3 Infarction in territories of the main cerebral arteries

neurological findings and the presentations are similar to those already outlined for stroke but usually less severe. All TIAs should be investigated in a similar manner and with the same sense of urgency as stroke (Table 5.4). After a TIA the overall risk for stroke is about 10% per year, the greatest risk being in the days and weeks following the TIA. If the TIA lasts >90 mins in a person at risk, then the likelihood of a stroke is greatest (4-8%) within the next 48 hours and

CT scans showing ICH

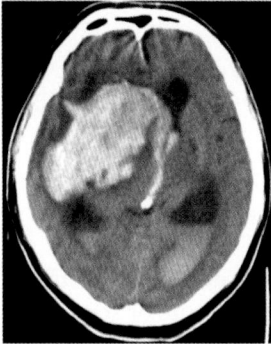

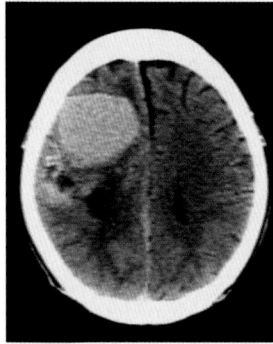

Frontal (right) & intraventricular   Frontal (right)   Internal capsule (right)

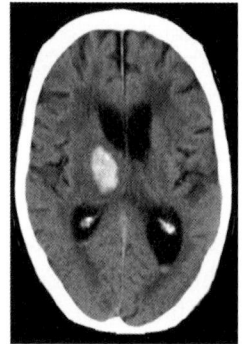

Figure 5.4 Intracerebral haemorrhage (ICH). CT scans showing ICH.

Carotid angiogram

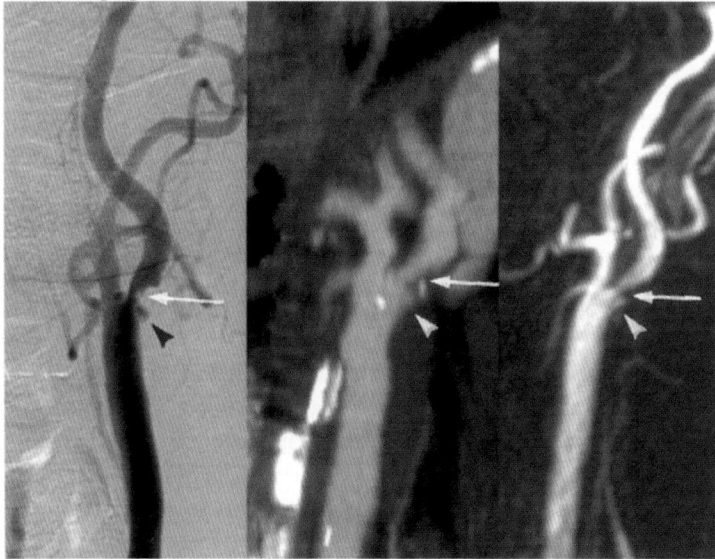

Stenosis ICA

Figure 5.5 Internal carotid artery stenosis

the patient requires urgent hospital admission. The aim of investigations and management is to identify and modify preventable risk factors such as smoking, exercise, diet and alcohol and aggressively treat underlying diseases such as carotid artery stenosis (Fig. 5.5), hypertension, diabetes and atrial fibrillation (Table 5.1). Antiplatelet drugs and anticoagulants are used as in the prevention of stroke (Table 5.6).

Key points

- most TIAs last for minutes not hours
- if TIA lasts >1-2 hours, the risk of stroke is greatest over next 48 hours
- annual risk for stroke after a TIA is around 10%
- don't wait for stroke to happen
- manage & treat TIA as if it were a stroke

Differential diagnosis

A history of a sudden onset of focal neurological deficit is almost always diagnostic of stroke. The differential diagnosis includes other disorders presenting with similar acute or semi acute neurological presentations. These include opportunistic processes in HIV disease, subdural haematoma, mass lesions, Todd's paralysis after an unwitnessed seizure, and other causes of acute encephalopathy. However in these cases the correct diagnosis should be suggested by a different clinical history, sub-acute onset and progressive nature of the neurological deficit. Venous sinus thrombosis may present with a stroke but this is uncommon. The clinical context, usually a pre-menopausal female with typical fundoscopy changes of venous engorgement with haemorrhages should suggest the correct diagnosis. A history of recent head injury or fall suggests the possibility of subdural haematoma (SDH), although a history of trauma may be absent (Chapter 19). CT scan of the brain may be necessary to make the correct diagnosis. There are a number of other medical conditions that can mimic a stroke or TIA at onset; these include focal seizures, migraine, hypoglycaemia, syncope, and hysteria. These are usually self-limiting often with a history of similar previous episodes and have a normal neurological examination.

INVESTIGATIONS AND DIAGNOSIS

Stroke is a clinical diagnosis and investigations are directed at establishing the cause and preventing recurrences. The main investigations for stroke are outlined in Table 5.4. Computerised tomography (CT) of the head is the investigation of choice in stroke. Ideally this should be done within 24-48 hours of onset of the stroke. Its primary role is to rapidly exclude haemorrhage, thereby allowing the administration of an antiplatelet drug, usually aspirin. In addition, it can determine the nature, size and site of stroke and exclude other disorders. In haemorrhagic stroke, CT shows haemorrhage as a white or hyperdense area almost as soon as it occurs. In small bleeds, the white area persists for around 48 hours while larger bleeds may persist for 1-2 weeks. After two weeks a bleed becomes indistinguishable from an infarct on a CT. CT shows ischaemia as an ill defined dark or hypodense area but this can take 24-48 hours to appear on the scan. Not all infarcts show up on a CT because of decreased sensitivity, small size and also poor imaging of the posterior fossa. If the initial CT is normal and a stroke is still suspected then a scan repeated after 3-7 days may show an infarct. If the clinical diagnosis of a stroke is certain, then a repeat scan may be unnecessary. In SAH the CT is highly sensitive during the first few days, after which it becomes negative and the diagnosis is then confirmed by lumbar puncture showing altered blood or xanthochromia. Magnetic resonance imaging (MRI) is more sensitive than CT for detecting early and small vessel strokes.

Table 5.4 Investigations for stroke

Department	Investigation	Risk factor
Haematology	FBC, ESR, sickle cell test	anaemia, polycythaemia, infection, vasculitis, sickle cell disease
Biochemistry	blood glucose, creatinine, electrolytes, liver function tests, lipids	diabetes, renal disease, hyperlipidaemia
Serology	HIV, VDRL	infections
Microbiology	malaria parasites, blood culture (if febrile)	infections
Cardiology	ECG	atrial fibrillation, myocardial infarction
Imaging	chest X-ray CT/MRI of head	cardiomegaly, hypertension ischaemia or haemorrhage
Ultrasound	echo heart (if cardiac origin suspected) carotid doppler (if carotid origin suspected)	mitral valve disease, thrombus, endocarditis large vessel atheroma

Key points

- CT head may be necessary in suspected stroke to make the correct diagnosis
- CT scan can detect over 90% of all strokes
- CT scan done during the first 24-48 hours after onset of stroke may miss ischaemia
- CT scan done during the first 1-2 weeks after onset of stroke usually confirms haemorrhage

SUBARACHNOID HAEMORRHAGE

SAH is the term usually reserved for spontaneous or non traumatic bleeding into the subarachnoid space which occurs as a result of a ruptured saccular (berry) aneurysm or an arteriovenous malformation (AVM) (Fig. 5.6). The majority (75-80%) occur as a result of bleeding from a ruptured saccular aneurysm. These aneurysms arise mainly at the junctions of the arteries that form the circle of Willis in the subarachnoid space at the base of the brain. In 5-10% of cases the SAH arises from an AVM and in a small percentage of cases no cause is found. SAH occurs in 5-10/100,000 persons per year in the UK. The frequency of SAH in SSA is not known but it may be more common there. A patient presenting with SAH is usually younger than in other types of haemorrhagic stroke (ICH) and first degree relatives are at an increased risk of stroke. Other risk factors for SAH include hypertension and a history of smoking.

Clinical presentation

The main clinical feature of SAH is a sudden explosive severe headache described as "like being hit on the back of the head with a hammer." There may be a prior history of sentinel or warning headaches for some weeks beforehand. The suddenness of onset helps to differentiate it from the pain of meningitis. The headache in SAH is usually accompanied by nausea, vomiting, fever, meningism and variable loss of consciousness. The loss of consciousness typically occurs at the moment of the bleed. The clinical findings vary from a fully alert patient with severe headache and meningism to a deeply comatose patient with decerebrate rigidity. Blood pressure is frequently elevated, mostly as a result of the SAH. Focal neurological signs and deficits may occur as a result of raised ICP, ICH or compression from the aneurysm. These include 3rd nerve palsy, 6th nerve palsy, hemiparesis, bilateral extensor plantar responses and papilloedema with or without subhyaloid haemorrhages (10-20%). Focal neurological deficits are more common in ruptured AVMs.

Investigations

CT of the head is highly sensitive for SAH with >90% of patients showing evidence of fresh blood in the subarachnoid space or ventricles (Fig 5.6). This lasts for 24-48 hours after which it becomes negative. CT may not show evidence of an aneurysm unless it is large but will usually show evidence of an AVM especially if contrast is given. In a patient with suspected SAH if a CT is normal or unavailable then it is necessary to do lumbar puncture (LP) and check for fresh uniformly mixed blood which fails to clear in all 3 consecutive CSF samples. The opening CSF pressure may be elevated in SAH. Xanthochromia occurs when the CSF is uniformly straw or yellow in colour. This is due to the presence of degraded blood in the CSF which is older than 24 hours and it persists for up to 2 weeks. The CSF may be entirely normal if examined within the first few hours or later than 2 weeks after the bleed.

Key points

- most common cause of SAH is a ruptured saccular aneurysm
- diagnostic feature of SAH is a sudden severe explosive headache
- meningism is a key feature of SAH
- level of consciousness in SAH ranges from being fully alert to deep coma
- diagnosis confirmed by finding evidence of blood either on CT or in CSF

Management

SAH carries a very high mortality during the first few days and if left untreated, there is a significant risk of rebleeding (20-30%) over the next 6 weeks. Management of acute SAH is therefore directed towards immediate treatment and the prevention of further bleeding. Patients should be nursed in bed with the head elevated 10-20 degrees, resting in quiet surroundings with adequate analgesia to avoid pain and surges in blood pressure. Aspirin should be avoided and constipation prevented. Intravenous hydration should be with approximately 3 litres per day of normal saline to avoid hypovolaemia. Antihypertensive medications should be avoided to prevent hypotension. In order to reduce arterial vasospasm and cerebral infarction secondary to the irritative effect of blood on vascular smooth muscle, the calcium channel blocker nimodipine 60 mg 4 hourly is prescribed for 3 weeks. Seizures occur in approximately10% of patients and usually respond to phenytoin 300 mg daily after a loading dose of 900 mg.

Neurosurgical

Neurosurgical intervention is indicated for SAH patients who are fully conscious or mildly confused with minimal or no neurological deficits. Patients with altered level of consciousness, coma or focal neurological signs less often benefit from neurosurgical intervention. The overall aim of neurosurgical intervention aim is to occlude the ruptured aneurysm. This can be achieved by either a neurosurgeon placing a clip over the neck of the aneurysm or by the neuroradiologist endovascularly embolising the aneurysm by packing it with metal coils. The latter is now the preferred method for the occlusion of most aneurysms. The optimum time for neurosurgical management is within the first 3 days after the initial bleed although the aneurysm can be operated on or coiled later.

CT (without contrast)

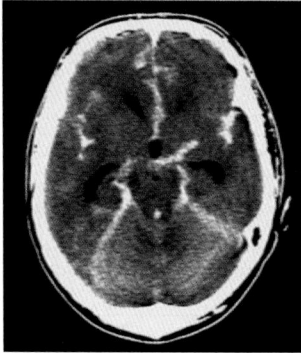

Blood in the subarachnoid space

Magnetic resonance angiogram COW

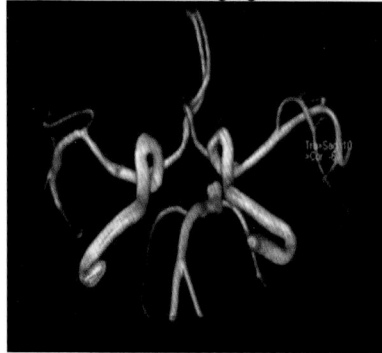

Aneurysm in left posterior cerebral artery

Figure 5.6 Subarachnoid haemorrhage & aneurysm

Prognosis

The case fatality rate for patients presenting with SAH due to aneurysms is high with >10% mortality within the first few days either as a result of the initial haemorrhage or its early complications. Of all those patients that do survive the initial bleed and do not have neurosurgical intervention, one third die within 3 months, one third go on to make a good recovery and one third are left with permanent neurological disability. Case fatality rates for patients presenting with SAH secondary to AVM are lower at around 10%.

Key points

- main aim of treatment is to prevent another bleed
- nimodipine helps to reduce vasospasm which may worsen the neurological deficit
- definitive surgical management is by either coiling or clipping the aneurysm
- overall mortality in SAH is high

MANAGEMENT

The overall aim of stroke care is to decrease morbidity and mortality, to optimise recovery of function and to prevent further strokes. This can be achieved by good nursing care, specific stroke treatment, maintenance of fluid and electrolytes, nutrition, avoiding systemic complications and early rehabilitation. The outcome improves when stroke care guidelines are followed and care takes place in a defined area in hospital by a dedicated team. In Africa hospital care starts usually with admission to a general medical ward. Management includes general (Table 5.5) and specific measures (Table 5.6).

Table 5.5 General measures in caring for acute stroke patient

1. Start neurological observations hourly and change to 4 hourly if stable
• level of consciousness using GCS • vital signs • oxygen saturation
2. Monitor blood glucose (if >11 mmol/L start insulin sliding scale)   intravenous fluids in dehydrated patients, unable to swallow

4. Evaluate swallowing after 24 hours
• observe the patient attempting to swallow sips of water in upright position
• check for coughing or gagging
• if swallowing impaired keep nil per oral (NPO)
• continue iv fluids for 48 hours then start nasogastric tube feeding if still unable to swallow
5. Urinary catheterization if incontinent or in retention
6. Prevent constipation by adequate hydration and laxatives
7. Prevent pressure sores by supervising 2 hourly turning*
8. Decrease the risk of deep vein thrombosis (DVT) by using compression stockings in addition to oral aspirin if ICH excluded

* this is done best by a relative or carer permanently at the bedside

Specific measures

Antiplatelet drugs

All ischaemic strokes should have aspirin immediately or as soon as possible after onset followed by long term treatment (Table 5.6). Ideally, haemorrhage should be first excluded on CT. If a CT scan is unavailable, then aspirin should be used cautiously in the first two weeks and then only in cases strongly suspected of having ischaemic stroke. Aspirin when given effectively prevents 15 deaths or major disability for about every 1000 patients treated during the first few weeks and prevents about a fifth of recurrent strokes when used longer term. There is a slight increased risk of gastro-intestinal haemorrhage. The dose is 300 mg po daily for the first 2 weeks followed by 75-150 mg po daily thereafter. Patients that are intolerant of aspirin should be treated with either clopidogrel or dipyridamole. Combination therapy with both aspirin and clopidogrel is increasingly used in acute stroke patients.

Blood pressure

Blood pressure (BP) rises after an acute stroke and tends to fall spontaneously after that. The modern management is to avoid lowering blood pressure during the first 24-48 hours as an acute drop in BP can reduce perfusion to an already ischaemic brain. Consider treatment only if BP is persistently elevated (Table 5.6). The upper limit of persistently elevated blood pressure in ischaemic stroke is systolic 210 mm Hg and diastolic 110 mm Hg. The aim is a daily reduction of 10-20 mm Hg. Lower levels should not be treated in the first 48 hours unless complicated by hypertensive encephalopathy, left ventricular failure or myocardial infarction. In ICH, the threshold for starting treatment is lower (>160/100, Table 5.6). If BP needs to be treated in the acute phase, consider using nifedipine sublingually for acute reduction and then orally twice daily. Other options include captopril for a more gradual reduction or atenolol and/or hydralazine.

Anticoagulation

Patients with a proven ischaemic stroke and a cardiac embolic source or atrial fibrillation should be anticoagulated to prevent further strokes (Table 5.6). Patients should be first treated with aspirin and anticoagulation be delayed for 2 weeks after the stroke because of the risk of intracerebral haemorrhage. Warfarin is then the drug of choice in a loading dose, usually 10 mg daily for 2 days followed by daily dose, depending on the prothrombin time or international normalized ratio (INR). The aim is to have and maintain an INR of 2-3 or a prothrombin time of twice the normal range. In patients with mechanical valve prosthesis the target INR is 2.5-3.5.

Thrombolysis

This is a recent development in stroke management and dramatically improves the outcome in some ischaemic stroke patients. Thrombolytic therapy is with alteplase, an iv tissue recombinant plasminogen activator (rtPA), a thrombolytic agent. This is beneficial in some patients with ischaemic strokes who have no early CT evidence of completed infarction or bleed. It has to be given as soon as possible after the onset of the stroke usually within 3 hours or 4.5 hours at maximum. Any later treatment has increased risk of bleeding and a lack of efficacy. However implementation requires a trained medical team on call and emergency CT scanning facilities. Currently <5% of all stroke patients with access in high income countries are treated with thrombolysis.

Table 5.6 Drug treatments in stroke

Measures	Treatment	Dose	Side effects
Blood Pressure (Indication for Rx in 1st 48 hours) >210/110 in infarction >160/100 in haemorrhage	nifedipine	10 mg/sublingually stat 10/20 mg/po/bd	hypotension headache
	captopril	6.25/12.5 mg/po/bd	cough, allergy
	hydralazine	25/50 mg/im/po/tid	rash
	atenolol	50/100 mg/iv/po/od	asthma, depression, hypoglycaemia
Antiplatelet drugs Indication: ischaemia	aspirin	300 mg/po/stat 75-150 mg/po/od	indigestion, nausea, GI bleeding
	clopidogrel	75 mg/po/od	indigestion diarrhoea
	dipyridamole	200 mg/po/bd	headache, indigestion
Anticoagulation Indication: risk of cardiac embolism	warfarin	10 mg/po/od/for 2 days 1-5 mg/po/od (according to INR)	bleeding

Key points

- acute ischaemic strokes should have aspirin immediately
- avoid aggressively lowering blood pressure during the first 48 hours of acute ischaemic stroke
- after first 48 hours, all persistently elevated blood pressures should be lowered
- embolic strokes should be anticoagulated, but not for two weeks after onset of stroke

COMPLICATIONS

Stroke patients are at risk for complications which may lead to death. Neurological worsening is common in the first 48 hours of stroke as a result of brain swelling, extension of the original stroke and complications. Patients with coma, extensive stroke and large haemorrhage have a poor prognosis.

Acute

The main acute complications are aspiration pneumonia, pulmonary embolism (PE), pressure sores and urinary tract infections. These occur in over half of hospitalized stroke patients and are associated with a poor prognosis. Pneumonia is the main cause of death in stroke in hospitalized patients. This occurs as a result of aspiration and is more frequent in patients with extensive strokes and coma. Management includes avoiding oral intake, chest physiotherapy and early antibiotics. Patients with stroke are at significant risk for DVT and PE. The use of prophylactic low dose aspirin and compression stockings decreases this risk. Heparin is contraindicated in the first 2 weeks after stroke as it increases intracerebral bleeding. Pressure sores, spasticity and contractures are common after a stroke and are reduced by early patient positioning, 2 hourly turning, passive exercises and limb splinting.

Chronic

Long term complications include spasticity, contractures, pain, depression, dementia and late onset seizures. Post stroke depression is common occurring in over half the patients. It is important to recognize it and if necessary offer treatment with tricyclics or selective serotonin reuptake inhibitors. Dementia as a result of stroke is common and is a major long term cause of dependency, particularly in the elderly. Seizures occur in about 2% of acute stroke patients but usually resolve in a few weeks and don't require long term treatment with anticonvulsants. Late onset seizures (6–12 months after stroke) occur in around 5% of stroke patients and are persistent, but they respond well to phenytoin.

Rehabilitation

Rehabilitation is one of the most important aspects in the care of stroke patients. Early mobilization and rehabilitation have been shown to help and improve outcome. This should take place on a daily basis in the general medical ward or in a specialized stroke area. Physiotherapy maximises functional recovery, occupational therapy is necessary for functional assessment and the provision of practical aids and speech and language therapy helps with aphasia, dysarthria and dysphagia.

Palliative care

Many stroke patients have no hope of recovery, and the best management is to ensure their comfort and avoid any unnecessary investigations and further suffering. It can be very distressing for family to witness a dying patient with noisy and laboured breathing because of retained airway secretions. Care is best achieved by good nursing and adequate palliative analgesia. It is important to explain to family and carers what is happening and many will at this stage choose to care for the patient at home.

Key points

- main acute complications are aspiration pneumonia & pressure sores
- pneumonia is a leading cause of death in stroke
- early mobilization and rehabilitation are critical to recovery
- long-term complications are disability, pain, depression, dementia & seizures
- palliative care is important where recovery is unlikely

PREVENTION

Antiplatelet drugs

Low dose daily aspirin 75-150 mg decreases the risk of another stroke by about one fifth in ischaemic strokes. About 10% of patients don't tolerate aspirin because of gastrointestinal side effects, mainly indigestion, nausea and rarely bleeding. This can be decreased by the concomitant use of a proton pump inhibitor and by using alternative antiplatelet drugs. Clopidogrel 75 mg daily is the drug of first choice in patients with aspirin intolerance but is more expensive. The combination of clopidogrel and aspirin is considered more effective than aspirin alone but has an increased risk of bleeding. Dipyridamole may also be used. Antiplatelet therapy has to be continued indefinitely.

Anticoagulants

The annual risk of embolism with either valvular heart disease or atrial fibrillation is around 10% per year without anticoagulation. Anticoagulation with warfarin decreases this risk very significantly by >50% per year. All ischaemic stroke patients presenting with atrial fibrillation or mitral valve disease should be anticoagulated indefinitely unless there is a contraindication.

Blood pressure

Treatment of hypertension significantly reduces the risk of strokes. There is strong evidence that lowering blood pressure, irrespective of the previous baseline level down to 130/70 reduces the risk of stroke. A mean drop of 9 mm Hg systolic and 4 mm Hg diastolic reduces the relative risk of stroke by about a quarter. Blood pressure treatment should be started in hypertensive stroke patients 48 hours after onset of the stroke and continued and monitored on discharge from hospital.

Carotid Stenosis

Athero-thromboembolism arising from the carotid and vertebral arteries is the main cause of ischaemic stroke in high income countries. Symptomatic carotid stenosis of >70% is an indication for carotid surgery wherever this is available (Fig. 5.5). Asymptomatic carotid stenosis of >70% and symptomatic stenosis of <70% are managed medically. However atheroma arising specifically from the carotids appears to be an uncommon source of ischaemic stroke in Africa.

Other factors

Life style measures such as salt reduction, low animal fat diet, decreasing alcohol consumption, stopping smoking and increasing exercise are all very important in both primary prevention of stroke at community level and secondary prevention when the stroke/TIA has occurred. Education is vital to the successful implementation of these measures. The use of cholesterol lowering drugs, simvastatin 20-40 mg po daily or another statin has been shown to decrease coronary events and recurrent strokes and these should be prescribed if possible after an ischaemic event. The expected relative risk reduction is in the order of 20%. However, the statins are expensive and have side effects including myalgia, myositis and liver dysfunction, which can lead to them being discontinued in about 10% of patients. An elevation of creatine kinase (CK) occurs in many individuals on statins and values up to 1000 IU can be tolerated. Adequate long term control of diabetes is important.

Prognosis

The outcome for stroke patients is poor. The mortality within the first year is over 30%, with a further one third disabled and about one third regaining independent living. The majority of deaths occur during the first week and month after the stroke and continue throughout the first year. The risk of recurrence continues over time. Over half of all stroke survivors are dead within 5 years. The long term prognosis for stroke is probably worse in Africa because of the lack of secondary and tertiary care.

Prognosis of stroke after one year

- one third die
- one third are disabled and dependent
- one third are independent

The future

The majority of strokes occur in low and middle income countries where most of the world's population live. With increasing urbanization, this burden is set to continue and increase over time. In low income countries especially, the majority of people have limited or no access to facilities for the prevention and management of stroke. These limitations extend from a lack of awareness to lack of treatment, rehabilitation and prevention. These in turn are related to a lack of trained specialists, education, resources and research. Clearly there is a need for more research and intervention particularly in the area of primary and secondary prevention of strokes in low and middle income countries, not forgetting the very important link between patient care and primary prevention of stroke in the community.

Key points

- prevention of stroke is now a top priority in Africa
- primary prevention must include public education concerning necessary lifestyle changes
- includes decreasing total salt intake, stopping smoking, dietary changes & increasing exercise
- secondary prevention includes targeting known diseases & risk factors for stroke
- tertiary measures are important to cope with increasing burden of death & disability

Selected references

Connor M, Rheeder P, Bryer A, Meredith M, Beukes M, Dubb A, et al. *The South African stroke risk in general practice study.* S Afr Med J. 2005 May;95(5):334-9.

Connor MD, Modi G, Warlow CP. *Differences in the nature of stroke in a multiethnic urban South African population: the Johannesburg hospital stroke register.* Stroke. 2009 Feb;40(2):355-62.

Connor MD, Walker R, Modi G, Warlow CP. *Burden of stroke in black populations in sub-Saharan Africa.* Lancet Neurol. 2007 Mar;6(3):269-78.

Feigin VL. *Stroke epidemiology in the developing world.* Lancet. 2005 Jun 25-Jul 1;365(9478):2160-1.

Giovannoni G, Fritz VU. *Transient ischaemic attacks in younger and older patients. A comparative study of 798 patients in South Africa.* Stroke. 1993 Jul;24(7):947-53.

Jusabani A, Gray WK, Swai M, Walker R. *Post-stroke carotid ultrasound findings from an incident Tanzanian population.* Neuroepidemiology. 2011;37(3-4):245-8.

Kumwenda JJ, Mateyu G, Kampondeni S, van Dam AP, van Lieshout L, Zijlstra EE. *Differential diagnosis of stroke in a setting of high HIV prevalence in Blantyre, Malawi.* Stroke. 2005 May;36(5):960-4.

Lemogoum D, Degaute JP, Bovet P. *Stroke prevention, treatment, and rehabilitation in sub-Saharan Africa.* Am J Prev Med. 2005 Dec;29(5 Suppl 1):95-101.

Mensah GA. *Epidemiology of stroke and high blood pressure in Africa.* Heart. 2008 Jun;94(6):697-705.

Mochan A, Modi M, Modi G. *Stroke in black South African HIV-positive patients: a prospective analysis.* Stroke. 2003 Jan;34(1):10-5.

Patel VB, Sacoor Z, Francis P, Bill PL, Bhigjee AI, Connolly C. *Ischemic stroke in young HIV-positive patients in Kwazulu-Natal, South Africa.* Neurology. 2005 Sep 13;65(5):759-61.

Poungvarin N. *Stroke in the developing world.* Lancet. 1998 Oct;352 Suppl 3:SIII19-22.

Qureshi AI, Mendelow AD, Hanley DF. *Intracerebral haemorrhage.* Lancet. 2009 May 9;373(9675):1632-44.

Swain S, Turner C, Tyrrell P, Rudd A. *Diagnosis and initial management of acute stroke and transient ischaemic attack: summary of NICE guidance.* BMJ. 2008;337:a786.

Tipping B, de Villiers L, Wainwright H, Candy S, Bryer A. *Stroke in patients with human immunodeficiency virus infection.* J Neurol Neurosurg Psychiatry. 2007 Dec;78(12):1320-4.

Wahab KW. *The burden of stroke in Nigeria.* Int J Stroke. 2008 Nov;3(4):290-2.

Walker RW, Jusabani A, Aris E, Gray WK, Mitra D, Swai M. *A prospective study of stroke sub-type from within an incident population in Tanzania.* S Afr Med J. 2011 May;101(5):338-44

Walker RW, McLarty DG, Kitange HM, Whiting D, Masuki G, Mtasiwa DM, et al. *Stroke mortality in urban and rural Tanzania. Adult Morbidity and Mortality Project.* Lancet. 2000 May 13;355(9216):1684-7.

Walker RW, Whiting D, Unwin N, Mugusi F, Swai M, Aris E, et al. *Stroke incidence in rural and urban Tanzania: a prospective, community-based study.* Lancet Neurol. 2010 Aug;9(8):786-92.

PART II – NEUROLOGICAL DISORDERS

CHAPTER 6
NEUROLOGICAL INFECTIONS

CONTENTS

CHAPTER 6

NEUROLOGICAL INFECTIONS

Introduction

Infections of the nervous system are common in Africa and account for a significant percentage of all deaths. The causes of these infections are viral, bacterial, fungal and parasitic, protozoa and helminths. Their estimated frequency and mortality is presented in Table 6.1. These infections result in CNS illnesses characterized mainly by meningitis, focal neurological disorders and coma. Since the onset of the human immunodeficiency virus (HIV) epidemic in Africa three decades ago there has been a dramatic change in the overall pattern of CNS infections in Africa. CNS opportunistic infections related to HIV have now become commonplace and are the leading cause of death in adults in many countries. The main causes are cryptococcal meningitis (CM), cerebral toxoplasmosis (CT) and tuberculous meningitis (TBM). At the same time cerebral malaria, acute bacterial meningitis (ABM), tetanus, trypanosomiasis, neurocysticercosis and brain abscess remain as major causes of neurological illnesses. This chapter presents an overview of the main bacterial, fungal and viral infections including clinical features, diagnosis and management. After reading this chapter the student should aim to be able to diagnose, treat and prevent meningitis and know the other main CNS infections.

Table 6.1 Estimated frequency & treated mortality of main neurological infectious disease in Sub Saharan Africa

Disease	Estimated frequency per year for whole population	Mortality rates (treated patients)
Acute Bacterial Meningitis	24/100,000 (children)	5-40% (children)
	12/100,000 (adults)	10-70% (adults)
Opportunistic infections in HIV	5-700,000	
cryptococcus		50%
toxoplasmosis		10-20%
TB		>50%
CNS TB (non HIV)	30,000	20-30%
Cerebral malaria	>0.5 million	10-20%
Human African trypanosomiasis	40,000-300,000	20-30%
Tetanus	100,000	40-60%
Rabies	10-20,000	100%
Leprosy	40,000	low

Meningitis

Meningitis is defined as inflammation of the pia and arachnoid meninges and the cerebrospinal fluid (CSF) that surrounds the brain and spinal cord. The main infectious causes are viral, bacterial and fungal. Meningitis is classified clinically as either acute or chronic. Acute meningitis occurs within hours or days, whereas chronic meningitis evolves over weeks. Acute meningitis is classified as aseptic which is mostly viral in origin or septic or pyogenic which is caused by bacteria.

The term **acute bacterial meningitis (ABM)** refers to acute infections caused by pyogenic bacteria. The main causes of pyogenic meningitis in Africa are *Streptococcus pneumoniae* **(pneumococcus)**, *Neisseria meningitidis* **(meningococcus)** *and Haemophilus influenzae* type b **(Hib).** Chronic meningitis by definition persists for weeks (four or more). The main causes in Africa are *cryptococcal infection* and *tuberculosis.* The overall pattern of meningitis in adults has changed in Africa, whereas ABM used to be the leading cause of meningitis, cryptococcus is now the most common cause followed by tuberculous meningitis (TBM) and ABM. Their exact order depends on the geographic location, the extent of HIV epidemic and the age group affected.

ACUTE BACTERIAL MENINGITIS (ABM)

EPIDEMIOLOGY

ABM causes over a quarter of a million deaths globally each year with a large proportion of these occurring in Africa. ABM occurs mostly in young children, particularly in those <2 years but affects all age groups including adults. Africa has some of the highest rates of ABM in the world affecting as many as 1/250 of children <5 yrs, in mainly urban parts of West Africa. However as many as 1-2% of whole populations in the "meningitic belt" may be affected during cyclical meningococcal epidemics which occur every 5-10 years. It is estimated that ABM in Africa is 5-10 times more common in children (24/100,000/yr) as compared to high income countries. Risk factors for ABM in Africa are crowded living conditions, extremes of age, organism virulence and antibiotic resistance, and host predisposition. Individual host factors include HIV infection, malnutrition, sickle cell disease, splenectomy, a non functioning spleen, recent head injury with fracture or, post neurosurgery with CSF leak, middle ear infection and pneumonia. The overall frequency of ABM in adults (10-12/100,000/yr) in Africa appears to have remained relatively constant despite the current HIV epidemic there.

Aetiology

In children in Africa the main causative organisms of ABM are *Hib, pneumococcus* and *meningococcus.* In those countries where *Hib* vaccination has been instituted, *Hib* has now been replaced as the main cause by *pneumococcus* and *meningococcus.* Recently a new pneumococcal conjugate vaccine is being used in children in some countries, including South Africa, Gambia and Kenya. In adults the main causative organisms are *pneumococcus* and *meningococcus.* Other less common causes include *group B streptococcus, nontyphoidal salmonella, (NTS), staphylococci,* and *Escherichia coli* in neonates. *Listeria monocytogenes* may cause ABM in pregnancy and in HIV. *Gram negative bacilli* and *salmonella* may cause ABM in HIV and in the elderly.

Streptococcus pneumoniae

Pneumococcus is a gram positive coccus which exists in pairs (Fig 6.1) with many subtypes. It affects mostly infants aged <12 months, young children and adults, but all age groups may be affected. It may occasionally occur as epidemics. The main source of meningeal infection is haematogenous spread arising from the respiratory tract (pneumonia) and from otitis media, although individual host factors are also important. Sporadic invasive pneumococcal disease has increased significantly since the arrival of the HIV epidemic and is a significant cause of bacteraemia, pneumonia and death in HIV disease. It accounts for >90% of cases of ABM in adults in the main HIV affected areas in Africa. The main risk factors for ABM have already been outlined above. The case fatality rate (CFR) in Africa in treated pneumococcal meningitis is high, ranging from 30-40% in children to 50-70% in adults.

Neisseria meningitidis

Meningococcus is a gram-negative diplococcus and infection results in meningococcal disease (fig. 6.2). It is classified into serogroups with A, B, C, Y, **W**-135 and X predominating. The most common serogroup in Africa is A but there have been recent outbreaks there with serogroups W-135 and X. Epidemic strains are sometimes introduced by Hajj pilgrims returning from Mecca, where similar epidemics have occurred. Protective vaccines exist for serogroups A and C and more recently a quadrivalent vaccine for A, C, Y, and **W**-135 (meningococcal A-conjugate vaccine) but not for group B or X. The usual incubation period for meningococcal disease is 2-7 days. The peak incidence is in children with a second peak in teenagers and young adults. The main risk factor for infection is close household contact with an infected person, when the risk of contracting the disease is increased a thousand fold. While most cases are sporadic, meningococcal disease also occurs as epidemics in Africa.

Large scale epidemics occur in sub-Saharan Africa during the dry season in approximately 10 year cycles. These epidemics occur in a large *"meningitis belt"* which stretches from the Gambia and Senegal in the West to Sudan and Ethiopia in the north and as far south as Kenya and Tanzania in the east and Nigeria and Ghana in the west. The reason for epidemics is unclear but has been attributed to the loss of accumulated herd immunity and the presence of suitably dry conditions for transmission, usually from March to May. During meningococcal epidemics, outbreaks occur typically in areas of overcrowding such as towns, schools, barracks, and prisons.

The overall case fatality ratio (CFR) in adults is of around 10% but this can vary (5-20%). A lower overall CFR (5%) generally reported across parts of Africa is attributed to infection with the most common serogroup A and to meningococcal disease presenting with mostly meningitis without associated septicaemia. However a higher CFR of around 20% has been reported recently in patients infected with serogroups W-135 and X, and also with HIV infection in South Africa.

Haemophilus influenzae type b (Hib)

Hib is a small gram-negative coccobacillus. It primarily affects young children under the age of six years and is a major cause of respiratory tract infection and ABM. *Hib* related ABM primarily affects infants 1-24 months and rarely occurs in adults. The CFR in Africa in children is 20-30% and is higher in adults 30-40%.

Key points

- ABM is a major cause of mortality & morbidity in Africa
- occurs in any age group but mostly in infants & young children
- main causes are pneumococcus, meningococcus & Hib
- host risk factors are HIV, sickle cell disease, asplenia & head injury
- meningococcal infection occurs in both sporadic & epidemic forms
- CFR varies with the organism & the age group affected

Pathogenesis

All the three main bacterial causes of meningitis colonise the nasopharynx in asymptomatic carriers. Colonisation rates of around 10-20% are commonplace in schools, universities etc with higher seasonal rates in children, young adults and in case contacts. Spread is by droplets from close physical contact with asymptomatic carriers or occasionally direct from cases. The presence of a lipopolysaccharide capsule helps bacteria survive and they reach the meninges via the bloodstream or by direct invasion. Clinical disease is rare and only occurs when there is penetration across the blood-brain barrier with infection of the meninges and subarachnoid space (Fig. 6.1). This may occur in association with bacteraemia and septicaemia. The multiplication of bacteria in the sterile CSF triggers a massive host immune response with release of inflammatory cytokines, which result in activated macrophages and invasion with neutrophils, immunoglobulins and other markers of inflammation. This leads to a further breakdown in the blood brain barrier and can result in vasculitis, thrombosis, infarction, raised intracranial pressure, brain damage and death.

Pathology

CSF microscopy

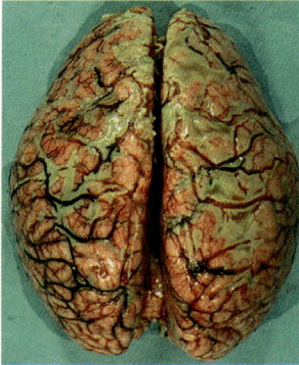

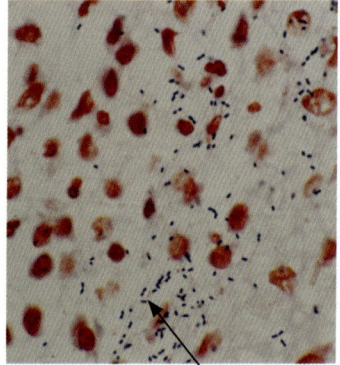

Purulent meninges

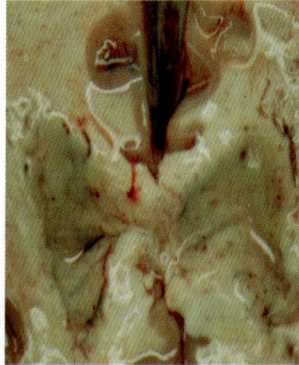

Purulent ventriculitis

Pneumococcus (Gm pos cocci)

Figure 6.1 Brain/csf in acute bacterial meningitis

Clinical diagnosis

The main clinical features of ABM are headache, fever and meningism. When this triad is accompanied by alteration in consciousness or seizures, the diagnosis is usually not in doubt. Other symptoms include photophobia, nausea, vomiting, backache and lethargy. The finding of a haemorrhagic rash on the skin is strongly suggestive of meningococcal infection. Progression occurs rapidly over 1-3 days but a smaller number may have an acute fulminant course lasting hours. However patients with HIV infection may present with only one or two of these main features.

Seizures occur in about one third of patients, typically in children and may be the presenting complaint. Focal neurological abnormalities, status epilepticus and coma occur mainly as complications. There may also be evidence of infection outside the CNS or an underlying condition predisposing to meningitis e.g. pneumonia, HIV, middle ear infection and head injury. The differential diagnosis for ABM in adults in Africa includes the other main causes of meningitis (cryptococcus, TBM and viral), opportunistic infections in HIV, cerebral malaria, viral encephalitis, typhoid fever and other CNS infections.

Signs of meningitis

The cardinal signs of meningitis are *neck stiffness* and *Kernig's sign* (Chapter 1). **Neck stiffness** is the most important sign and is present when the neck resists passive flexion to bring the chin on to the chest. It is found in most adults and over three quarters of children with ABM. **Kernig's sign** is elicited by passively attempting to straighten the leg with the hip and knee flexed to >90 degrees. In cases of meningitis this is met with resistance and pain, caused by spasm in the hamstrings as a result of stretching inflamed nerve roots. A forward flexing of the neck elicits involuntary hip and knee flexion or *Brudzinski's sign*. **Brudzinski's sign** is found mainly in infants and young children but not in adults.

These signs of meningitis are present in most cases of established meningitis but are less likely to be present early on in the disease and in the young and the elderly. In older children and adults, in addition to the classic features, there may be back pain and myalgia and seizures in around 20%. In infants, the combination of fever, respiratory distress, irritability, crying, vomiting, drowsiness and failure to feed may be the only findings. In babies, the association of bulging fontanel, neck retraction and seizures should prompt the correct diagnosis. In the elderly, alteration in the level of consciousness and fever may be the only clinical findings. It is important to remember that whenever in doubt about the diagnosis of meningitis, to return to re-examine the patient for signs of meningitis, in particular for neck stiffness.

Pneumococcal meningitis

Patients with pneumococcal meningitis present with marked meningism. Signs of an underlying pneumonia and septicaemia may be present particularly in children. Patients tend to progress rapidly in 24-48 hours to drowsiness, confusion, seizures and coma.

Meningococcal disease

The main clinical features of meningococcal disease are those of either septicaemia with or without meningitis or meningitis alone. The proportion of patients presenting with meningitis alone appears to be greater in tropical countries. Meningococcal meningitis without septicaemia has a favourable recovery rate (95%). The clinical features of meningococcal septicaemia may vary from mildly symptomatic patients to acute fulminant infection. The onset is typically abrupt over 24-48 hours. However, symptoms can progress rapidly from drowsiness and rash to circulatory failure, coma and death within hours of onset.

The diagnostic feature of meningococcal disease is the typical haemorrhagic rash, which is non-blanching and present in the majority of patients (Fig 6.2). However it may be absent, particularly in uncomplicated meningitis in children. The rash may begin as a maculopapular rash and develops in a matter of hours into a petechial and purpuric rash all over. The conjunctiva, palate, soles of the feet and palms of the hands should be carefully examined as the rash may be easily missed on the limbs and trunk in dark skin. The lesions do not blanch under pressure and this can be confirmed by pressure with a glass when the rash can be seen to persist. This is called the **"tumbler test"** (Fig 6.2). Petechiae may later progress to larger confluent purpuric areas called purpura fulminans. Complications of meningococcal disease include skin necrosis, arthritis, gangrene and Waterhouse-Friderichsen syndrome of adrenal failure.

Skin   **CSF microscopy**

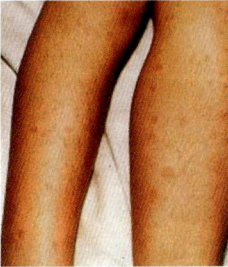 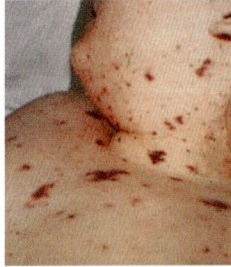 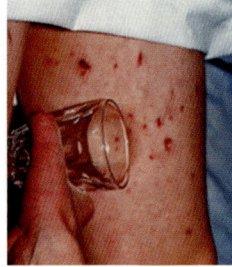 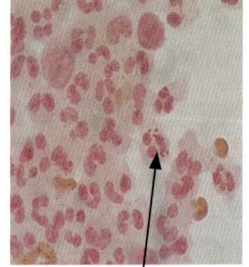

Macular rash   Petechial purpuric rash   The tumbler test   Gm neg cocci

Figure 6.2 Meningococcal meningitis

Hib meningitis
This has a characteristic slow onset over several days often starting with fever or respiratory tract infection. The onset of drowsiness, vomiting and convulsions in an infant in this setting may suggest the diagnosis.

Key points

- headache, fever & meningism are the cardinal clinical features of ABM
- neck stiffness is the most sensitive clinical sign
- signs are less sensitive in the young, old & in HIV infection
- meningism & bleeding into skin suggests meningococcal disease
- When in doubt about the diagnosis return & re-examine the patient

Diagnosis
The diagnosis of ABM is based on clinical and laboratory findings (Table 6.2). Laboratory tests include a full blood count, blood glucose, malaria slide, blood culture and an HIV test. A lumbar puncture (LP) is the key investigation and is an overall simple and very safe test (see appendix). It is always indicated in suspected ABM, unless there is a clear contraindication. A LP is contraindicated in the presence of suspected raised intracranial pressure (ICP). The clinical features suggestive of raised ICP in ABM are altered level of consciousness, coma, focal neurological deficit and papilloedema. These are all indications to avoid a LP and also for doing a CT scan of the head if it is available. The CT with contrast may show meningeal enhancement in ABM. If the CT of the head shows no mass lesion and there is no other evidence of raised intracranial pressure e.g. papilloedema then it is reasonable to proceed with the lumbar puncture. However it is important to note that even a normal CT may not necessarily rule out raised ICP, particularly if carried out early on in ABM.

CSF in ABM

The opening CSF pressure is typically elevated >20 cm and the colour is cloudy (Table 6.2). On analysis there is a characteristic high white cell count (>60% neutrophils), a very low glucose and an elevated protein. In HIV patients who are unable to mount a full inflammatory response, a much lower cell count is used as a cut off (>10 cells/mm^3) for diagnosis of ABM and any protein elevation is also less. A similar pattern may be seen with the other causes of meningitis in HIV disease. A gram stain should always be performed on the CSF and a specimen sent for bacterial culture. Suspected cases of chronic meningitis patients should have their CSF screened for cryptococcus by India ink and cryptococcal antigen (CRAg) if available and also for tuberculosis by Ziehl-Neelsen (ZN) stain and culture.

Table 6.2 Summary CSF findings in meningitis*

	acute bacterial meningitis	tuberculous	cryptococcal	viral
opening pressure (n = <20 cm in adults)	increased	increased	increased	normal/increased
appearance (n = clear)	cloudy, purulent	yellow/cloudy	clear/cloudy	clear (cloudy)
cells/mm³* n = <5/mm³ **main type**	high >2,000/mm³ neutrophils	increased 50-500 lymphocytes	normal/increased 0-100 lymphocytes	normal/increased 0-500 lymphocytes
glucose (n = >50% plasma)	very low/absent <1 mmol/L	low	normal/low	normal
protein (n=<0.5gm/L)	elevated 1-2	high/very high 1-5	normal/elevated 0.5-2	normal/elevated 0.5-1.0
diagnosis confirmed	Gm stain & culture	ZN stain & culture	India ink stain, CRAg/culture	PCR/culture

see appendix for exceptions

Management

The mainstay of management of ABM is prompt diagnosis and early treatment with antimicrobials (Table 6.3). It is important that antimicrobials should be given straight away (within 20-30 mins of first seeing the patient) and not to delay treatment because of ongoing investigations including a LP or CT. The early treatment is based on a presumed diagnosis of ABM and the patient is usually covered with antibiotics for the main possible bacterial causes (Table 6.3). In adults ceftriaxone or another extended-spectrum cephalosporin, cefotaxime are now the drugs of first choice. If unavailable then it is recommended to give soluble penicillin in combination with chloramphenicol. A history of anaphylaxis is a contraindication for penicillin but a history of a rash is not.

Patients at the extremes of life or with a particular risk factor may need additional antibiotic cover e.g. flucloxacillin for staphylococcal infection in neonates or gentamycin for some gram negatives in neonates and in old age. Additions or changes in antimicrobials are guided by laboratory based bacteriology stains and cultures. The use of steroids in the treatment of ABM in adults is currently not recommended in Africa as evidenced by recent prospective ABM studies in Malawi, showing no additional benefit. Supportive measures include oxygen, careful rehydration at less than 1-2 litres in the first 24 hours, maintenance of normal blood pressure, urinary output, electrolyte balance and control of pain and fever.

Table 6.3 Antimicrobial treatment of adult ABM

Drug	Dose/ route	Frequency	Duration*
ceftriaxone	2 gm/iv	12 hourly	10-14 days
or			
cefotaxime	2 gm/iv	4 hourly	10-14 days
or			
penicillin	2.4 gm or 4 million units/iv	4 hourly	10-14 days
&			
chloramphenicol	1 gm/iv	6 hourly	10-14 days

children with ABM & meningococcal disease may have shorter courses of antibiotics (5-7 days)

Outcome

Death is inevitable in untreated ABM. Mortality in treated ABM varies with the age group affected, the organism causing it and in particular how early on the appropriate antimicrobial was given. The case fatality ratio (CFR) in ABM is highest in neonates and adults (50-70%). In adults in Africa, CFR is highest in pneumococcus (70%) and lowest in meningococcus (10-20%). The lowest CFR in ABM is in children with uncomplicated meningococcal meningitis (5%). The presence of underlying HIV infection significantly increases the CFR in ABM. Resistance to penicillin (20%), chloramphenicol (20%) or both (10%) and a decreased susceptibility to cephalosporins (5%) is an increasing problem particularly in Africa because of their widespread usage. Permanent neurologic deficits persist in over a quarter of all surviving ABM patients. This also varies by age group and organism. Over 50% of neonates and 40% of those who survive pneumococcal meningitis have permanent neurological deficits, in contrast to about 5-7% of those with meningococcus. The main neurological deficits after ABM are hearing loss (>25%), motor loss (12%), cognitive impairment (9%) visual disturbance (6%) and seizures.

Key points

- death is inevitable in untreated ABM
- early antibiotics is the most important treatment affecting outcome
- cephalosporins are the drugs of first choice
- over a quarter of all surviving patients have permanent neurological disabilities
- disabilities includes deafness, motor loss, cognitive impairment, mental retardation, visual disturbance & seizures

Prevention

In sporadic meningococcal infection, chemoprophylaxis should be provided for all household and close contacts of the patient within the previous 24 hours. The risk of developing meningitis in close contacts is estimated to be about 1 in 300. Adults and children over 12 yrs should receive rifampicin 600 mg orally twice daily for 2 days or ciprofloxacin or azithromycin 500 mg orally as a single dose. Rifampicin should not be given in pregnancy. For children up to the age of 12 years, use rifampicin10 mg/kg twice daily for two days or ceftriaxone 125 mg im as a single dose. Chemoprophylaxis is not indicated for close contacts of pneumococcal or Hib meningitis. Early recognition is the key to management when epidemic meningococcal meningitis is suspected. If the number of cases exceeds 15/100,000 per week or 5-10 cases per week if the population <30,000, then emergency preventative measures include alerting the appropriate authorities, identifying the organism and use of mass chemoprophylaxis and vaccination. All three main causes of ABM are now largely preventable by vaccination.

Key points

- prevention of individual cases meningococcal infection is based on prophylaxis of close contacts
- epidemic prevention is based on early recognition, mass chemoprophylaxis & vaccination
- vaccines are available to prevent Hib & for some strains of meningococcus & pneumococcus
- ABM in SSA is largely preventable by vaccination

TUBERCULOUS MENINGITIS (TBM)

Each year there arc around 10 million new cases of tuberculosis worldwide, approximately one third of which occur in Africa. TBM now accounts for 8-44% of all cases of meningitis in SSA depending on the local HIV and TB prevalence. TB of the CNS is estimated to account for <1% of all new cases of TB, but this figure is significantly higher, when there is coexisting HIV infection. Tuberculous meningitis (TBM) is the most common CNS presentation. Other CNS presentations of TB infection include focal neurological disorders in intracranial tuberculoma and paraplegia in spinal cord involvement. In Africa, non HIV associated TBM affects mostly children, in particular the age group <5 years but can affect all age groups. In contrast TBM in HIV disease mostly affects adults. TB is clinically classified as pulmonary type (85%) and extra pulmonary type (15%). Only the pulmonary type is infectious to others. TBM can arise in two main ways: either as a complication of pulmonary e.g. disseminated or miliary, or less commonly as a result of reactivation of extra pulmonary TB.

Pathogenesis

Mycobacterium tuberculosis is the main cause of TB but other members of the *M. tuberculosis* complex such as *M. bovis* and *M. africanum* may also cause human disease. TB of the CNS arises indirectly from primary infection in the lungs, from where it spreads via the blood stream to other organs including the brain and spinal cord. In the brain or spinal cord, it has a predilection for the subpial sites, where it may present either acutely as TBM or lie dormant for years and later reactivate. Under different conditions, notably immunosuppression in HIV or sometimes pregnancy these tubercles which are known as Rich foci reactivate and rupture. If they rupture into the subarachnoid space they result in TBM, into the brain a tuberculoma, or into the spinal cord a myeloarachnoiditis. The immune reaction generated is mainly inflammatory with exudates particularly around the base of the brain and in the ventricles (Fig. 6.3). This may lead to multiple cranial nerve palsies, arteritis with strokes and obstruction to CSF flow and absorption resulting in hydrocephalus.

Clinical features

TBM is a difficult condition to diagnose and confirm clinically. The clinical features are those of slowly progressive chronic meningitis frequently with associated encephalopathy. Symptoms develop gradually, usually over 1-3 weeks but can be more acute in children. Constitutional TB symptoms including fever, night sweats, weight loss and malaise may be present for a week or more early on but these may also be absent or are not specific for TB. The main neurological symptoms suggestive of TBM are headache, nausea, vomiting, irritability, behaviour change and meningism of gradual onset usually for a period of one week or usually longer in adults.

Pathology

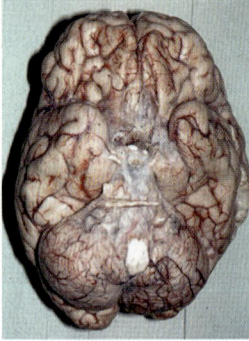

Basal meningitis

Histopathology

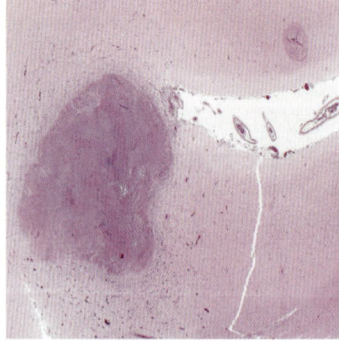

Rich focus

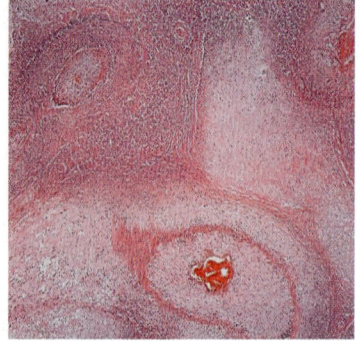

Endarteritis obliterans

Fundoscopy

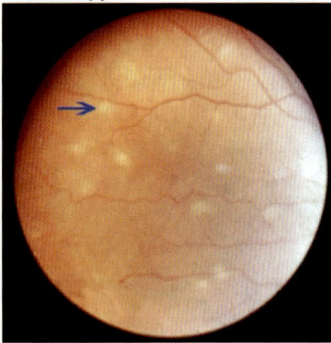

Retinal TB

Microscopy

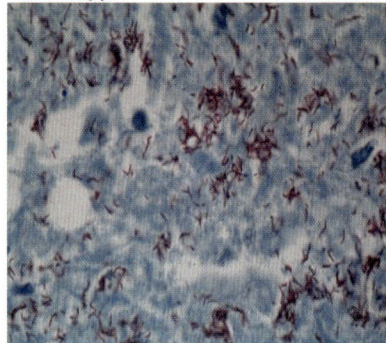

AFB on ZN stain

Figure 6.3 Brain/csf in tuberculous meningitis

However, headaches may be less prominent in children, fever may be absent in 10-20% of adults and the signs of meningitis are generally less prominent as compared to ABM. The main neurological signs are those of meningism including neck stiffness coupled with combinations of cranial nerve palsies (3rd, 4th, 6 th ,7th & 8th). The presence of focal neurological deficits, visual loss, papilloedema, altered level of consciousness, seizures and coma all suggest either parenchymal brain involvement or hydrocephalus. Fundoscopy may occasionally reveal typical TB retinopathy (characteristic white spots e.g. Fig 6.3). Hydrocephalus may be present early on or develop later during the course of the illness.

Other neurological presentations of TB involving the CNS are tuberculoma in the brain and spinal cord TB. Tuberculoma may be solitary or multiple presenting mainly as focal neurological deficits, seizures and occasionally raised intracranial pressure. Tuberculoma may sometimes complicate TBM and the most common site in adults is above the tentorium (supratentorium), whereas in children it is below the tentorium (infratentorium). Spinal cord TB presents as paraplegia and the site may sometimes be the source of TBM (Chapter 10). A WHO staging based on the main neurological features of TBM is outlined below (Table 6.4).

Table 6.4 WHO Staging of TBM

Disease Stage	Neurological features
Stage I	no disturbance of consciousness no *FND
Stage II	alteration in consciousness but not in coma or delirium, no FNDs, cranial nerve palsies may be present
Stage III	coma &/or FNDs

FND focal neurological disorder

Key points

- TBM occurs either as an acute complication of pulmonary TB or as a reactivation of extra pulmonary TB
- TBM affects mostly young children whereas TBM in HIV affects mostly adults
- HIV significantly increases the risk of TBM
- symptoms of TBM include headache, fever, vomiting, & meningism for >1 week
- signs include neck stiffness, seizures & multiple cranial nerve palsies

Differential diagnosis

The differential diagnosis includes cryptococcal meningitis, partially treated ABM, cerebral malaria, brain abscess and other infectious causes of meningoencephalopathies.

Diagnosis

The diagnosis of TBM is based on clinical suspicion and characteristic CSF findings (Table 6.2). Routine laboratory investigations are of limited value in the diagnosis of TBM. The tuberculin skin test is of little diagnostic benefit in adult populations with high levels of TB infection or previous BCG exposure and may also be negative in disseminated TB and HIV disease. The diagnosis of TBM is supported if there is evidence of concomitant TB elsewhere, most frequently pulmonary as evidenced by chest radiograph. Lumbar puncture is safe if there are no contraindications e.g., alteration in consciousness, lateralising clinical signs or signs of raised intracranial pressure (see appendix).

In TBM the opening pressure is often raised and the CSF clear in colour but may be slightly yellow in established disease. If a sample is left standing overnight in a test tube, the development of an appearance of a cobweb or lattice is supportive of TBM. The CSF white cell count in TBM is usually elevated, 50-500 cell/mm^3 mostly lymphocytes, but notably these may be absent in HIV disease or are polymorphs in early infection, particularly in young children. The CSF protein level is usually quite elevated and the glucose is low (<50% plasma glucose) but these can be normal in early disease and also in HIV infection. The organism is identified by acid-fast staining and culture. In TBM, the sensitivity of routine unconcentrated CSF staining with Ziehl-Neelsen stain is very low (<5%), but this yield can be improved markedly with increased quantity of CSF (10-20 ml in adult), by concentrating the CSF by centrifugation and by careful examination or the residue (for at least 20 mins) and by repeated CSF examinations. Polymerase chain reaction (PCR) has better sensitivity depending on bacillary load and good specificity (90-95%) but the test is not widely available in Africa and the result is no better than culture. A new automated PCR test on sputum is now available which gives a result in 4 hours but running cost is approx 20 US dollars per test which makes it relatively prohibitive in most parts of Africa. Also it has yet to be validated on CSF. Culture is the gold standard but limitations include the fact that the result takes 4-6 weeks which is too slow to be of value clinically and this facility is again not widely available. The CRAg test in TBM is negative.

Imaging with CT/MRI (Fig. 6.4) can be very helpful. In TBM it may show evidence of hydrocephalus and after contrast generalised meningeal enhancement with irregular basilar/cisternal involvement. It may also reveal infarction or tuberculoma. A tuberculoma shows as a rounded lesion with ring enhancement with irregular walls, nodular enhancement, oedema and mass effect. They are most commonly situated near the cortex, may be multiple and accompany TBM.

MRI with contrast

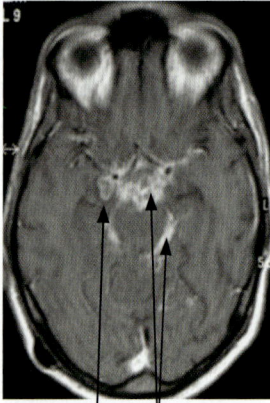

CT head

Tuberculoma & basal cistern & meningeal enhancement

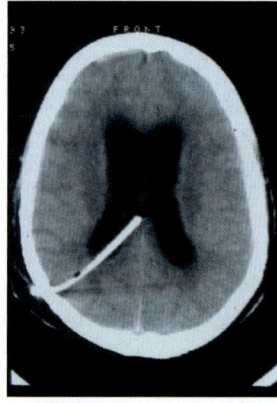

Hydrocephalus with shunt in TBM

Figure 6.4 Neuroimaging in TB CNS

Key points

- diagnosis of TBM requires a high index of clinical suspicion
- laboratory confirmation is by finding evidence of TB in CSF by ZN stain or culture
- routine CSF screening sensitivity for AFB is very low
- typical CSF findings in TBM are increased lymphocytes, elevated protein & low glucose
- CT findings in TBM include basilar meningeal enhancement & hydrocephalus

Management of TB

Treatment for CNS TB should start as early as possible with 4 drugs as any delay in treatment greatly increases mortality. These include isoniazid, rifampicin, pyrazinamide and a fourth drug ethambutol (Table 6.5). Streptomycin is also available but is a second line drug used when there is drug resistance or toxicity. The four drugs are continued for the first 2 months after which isoniazid and rifampicin are continued usually for another 10 months. In practice the standard total period of treatment is 12 months for TBM and longer for tuberculoma (18 months). A shorter period of treatment for TBM (total 9-10 months) has been proposed but is not common practice in Africa. The main side effects are hepatitis with isoniazid and rifampicin, neuropathy with isoniazid and deafness with streptomycin, and rarely optic neuritis with ethambutol (Table 6.5). Pyridoxine 20-50 mg daily should be prescribed with isoniazid to prevent neuropathy. All HIV uninfected patients with CNS TB in WHO Stages II and III of the disease should be given steroids for the first 6 weeks of chemotherapy. The dose can be decreased gradually after the first two weeks. Hydrocephalus is a major complication of TBM occurring in >50% cases and may require ventricular peritoneal shunting or drainage as early as is clinically indicated.

Table 6.5 Treatment of CNS tuberculosis, TBM

Chemotherapy	Dose/route/frequency/duration*	Main side effects
Isoniazid *(H)*	5-10 mg/kg/po/daily/12 months (300-600 mg daily) & **pyridoxine 20-50 mg** daily to prevent neuropathy	hepatitis, neuropathy
Rifampicin *(R)*	10-12 mg/kg/po/daily/12 months (600 mg daily)	hepatitis
Pyrazinamide *(Z)*	30 mg/kg/po/daily for 2 months 1.5-2.0 gm daily	nausea & vomiting & arthralgia, hepatitis
Ethambutol *(E)* *or* **Streptomycin** *(S)***	15 mg/kg/day/po/daily for 2 months (800 mg daily) 20 mg/kg/im/daily for 2 months (1 gm daily)	optic neuritis (rare) nerve deafness, nephrotoxicity
Dexamethasone *or* **Prednisolone**	0.4 mg/kg/iv/po/daily (24 mg od) for 2 weeks and tapering over next 4 weeks 60 mg/po/daily for 2 weeks and tapering over next 4 weeks	hyperglycaemia, peptic ulcer, hypertension & psychosis

* a longer course of treatment (18/12) is recommended in tuberculoma
** second line drug

TBM in HIV

The clinical, neuroimaging and laboratory features of TBM are very similar in both HIV positive and HIV negative persons apart from decreased or no evidence of inflammation in the CSF (15-20%) and more extra meningeal TB in HIV infection. Starting ART is recommended after the first 2 weeks of TB treatment. In general steroids are not contraindicated and the indications for their use are the same as in non HIV TBM with steroid cover for the first 6 weeks of TBM treatment. However the clinical course may be complicated by drug resistant TB, co-infection, bacteraemia, immune reconstitution inflammatory syndrome (IRIS) and decreased drug compliance.

Outcome

The outcome of TBM in Africa even with treatment is poor with published CFRs varying from 13-90%. In adults TBM has a mortality rate of >50%. This is mainly related to late clinical presentation and advanced stage of disease (WHO stages II & III) or to underlying HIV infection. WHO stage I disease is associated with a good outcome. Permanent deficits occur in at least 30-40% of survivors. These include deafness, blindness, paralysis, seizures and retardation.

Prevention

Prevention of TB is based on case or patient finding and treatment. Prophylactic treatment with isoniazid is used to prevent reactivation of TB in selected patients in particular with HIV infection. The use of BCG vaccination of neonates has been shown to decrease the overall risk of TBM in children in Africa.

Key points

- delay in diagnosis greatly increases mortality in TBM
- duration of treatment in TBM is 9-12 months
- steroids are indicated in TBM for the first 6 weeks in most patients
- CFR rates and morbidity rates are very high
- prevention is by BCG & prophylaxis & active case treatment

CRYPTOCOCCAL MENINGITIS

Introduction

Cryptococcal disease is caused by *Cryptococcus neoformans,* a yeast fungus found worldwide in soil and bird excrement. It is usually acquired asymptomatically by humans via inhalation of encapsulated yeast cells, mostly during the first 5 years of life. Cryptococcal disease in immunosuppressed persons occurs mostly as a result of reactivation of latent infection. It typically presents as a chronic meningitis in patients during the later stages of HIV disease occurring with CD4 counts of <100 cells/mm^3. Since the onset of the HIV epidemic, it has become the leading cause of meningitis in large parts of Africa accounting for 33-63% of all cases depending on the individual country. After TB it is the main cause of death in HIV disease in Africa, accounting annually for over half a million deaths or around 25% of all HIV related deaths.

Clinical findings

Cryptococcal disease may present clinically as cryptococcal meningitis (CM), pulmonary infection, or uncommonly disseminated disease with skin involvement. Pneumonia is the main pulmonary presentation. While occasionally severe, pulmonary involvement is relatively uncommon and usually self limiting. Pulmonary symptoms include cough, chest pain dyspnoea and fever. CM is the main clinical disease, presenting with a sub acute or chronic illness evolving usually over 1-2 weeks or occasionally longer, 3-4 weeks. The main symptoms are headache (80-100%), fever (70%) and alteration in mental status (25-30%).

Clinical features suggestive of CM include headaches which are usually severe and associated with nausea and vomiting, and the relative absence of meningism (25-50%). Notably confusion or behaviour change with or without fever may be the only clinical feature suggestive of underlying CM. Neurological findings include isolated cranial nerve palsies (mainly 6th nerves), decreased visual acuity and papilloedema. Neck stiffness is uncommon being present in only around 25% of patients. The presence of altered level of consciousness and coma are explained by raised intracranial pressure (ICP) secondary to decreased absorption of CSF in CM by the arachnoid granulations. Raised ICP is present in about 50% of patients at diagnosis and if not properly managed is associated with a worse prognosis. Clinically CM may be indistinguishable from TBM.

Diagnosis

The diagnosis of CM requires a high index of clinical suspicion. However, the presentation of a patient with an unexplained sub acute illness with headache, fever, altered mental status and evidence of underlying HIV infection (CD4 <100 mm^3) usually suggests the diagnosis. The CSF is abnormal in >80% of CM cases but CSF chemistry remains normal in about

20%, despite the presence of the disease, usually in early CM or in advanced HIV (Table 6.2). Typical abnormal CSF findings include increased opening pressure and increased WBCs. These include mostly lymphocytes (median 10-20/mm³) but can be <5/mm³, a normal or increased protein and normal or slightly low glucose levels in around 50% of cases.

The diagnosis is confirmed by demonstrating the presence of encapsulated yeast cells in the CSF by direct staining of a centrifuged sample with Gram's or India ink staining (Fig. 6.5). It is also demonstrated by the presence of cryptococcal antigen (CRAg) in CSF or blood. While the India ink staining method is relatively easy to perform i.e., adding a few drops to CSF, and is cheap, it is less sensitive (60-80%) than CRAg which is highly sensitive (>95%). In particular all adults in Africa presenting with meningitis and India negative CSF should ideally have a CRAg test. CRAg is mostly unavailable in hospitals in Africa because of cost. However a newer rapid lateral flow assay or dipstix test for the presence of cryptococcal antigen in blood, serum or urine, costing approx 1 dollar per test offers the hope of a more affordable, rapid and accurate diagnostic test in Africa. Fungal culture is more sensitive than India ink but takes 2-5 days for results, is also more complex to perform and is available only in some specialized laboratories. CT imaging of brain is less helpful in diagnosis, being normal in over half the cases. It may show meningeal enhancement or abscess formation with contrast but its main role is to exclude other opportunistic processes. The main differential diagnosis in HIV is with TBM and toxoplasmosis.

Pathology

Csf microscopy

India ink stain

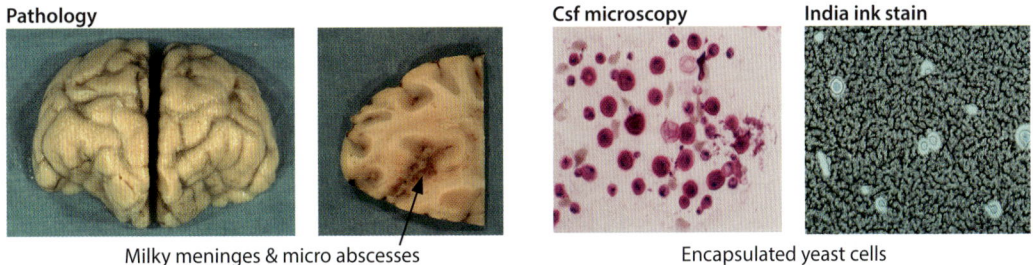

Milky meninges & micro abscesses

Encapsulated yeast cells

Figure 6.5 Brain/csf in cryptococcal meningitis

Key points

- CM is the leading cause of meningitis in adults in Africa
- accounts for >25% of all AIDS related deaths in Africa
- occurs mostly in patients with CD4 counts <100 cells/mm³
- symptoms include severe headache, fever and altered mental status for 1-2 weeks
- signs of meningism are frequently absent but papilloedema is common
- clinically it is often indistinguishable from TBM

Treatment

The treatment of CM in Africa is mostly based on fluconazole alone (Table 6.6). There are three phases, the induction phase lasts 2 weeks using fluconazole 1200 mg daily and the consolidation phase lasts the next 8 weeks using fluconazole 800 mg daily. The maintenance or prophylaxis phase uses fluconazole 200 mg daily until the CD4 count is >200/mm³ for >6 months. The higher treatment phase dosage of fluconazole "1200 mg daily" which is recommended here has been shown to be superior to "800 mg daily" in the induction phase in Africa but is not yet widely adopted. The recommended first line induction treatment for CM is amphotericin B (AmB) 0.7-1mg/kg/day in saline used in combination with flucytosine 100 mg/kg/day, for the first two weeks of infection followed by the consolidation phase of fluconazole, 400 mg po daily for 8-10 weeks followed by the 200 mg daily maintenance phase. This is the most effective regime and has been shown to have highest early fungicidal activity in the CSF. However the use of AmB and flucytosine in Africa is restricted mainly because of availability, cost and the need to monitor renal function every couple of days and check for any evidence of bone marrow suppression. Combining fluconazole with either AmB or flucytosine has also been shown to be superior to fluconazole alone.

Table 6.6 Fluconazole treatment for cryptococcal meningitis in Africa

Drug	Dose/route	Duration	Side effects
Fluconazole			
treatment phase	1200 mg/po/daily	2 weeks	headache, dizziness
consolidation phase	800 mg/po/daily	8 weeks	hepatitis
prophylaxis phase	200 mg/po/daily	until CD4 >200/mm³ for 6/12	

Lumbar puncture in treatment

Patients with symptomatic raised ICP, papilloedema or opening CSF pressures >25 cm (normal OP is <20 cm) benefit from frequent, daily or alternate day lumbar punctures with drainage of approx 10-15 ml (max 30 ml) at each LP until symptoms clear or the CSF pressure decreases consistently to below 20 cm. Serial lumbar punctures (day 1, 3, 7, & 14) have been shown to reduce CM mortality in Africa.

CM and ART

In CM the very early initiation of ART is associated with a higher case fatality rate. A delay in initiation of ART until at least 4 weeks after the start of the treatment phase appears to have a better outcome in fluconazole treated patients. In amphotericin treated patients starting at 2 weeks is better than at 6 weeks. Further studies are underway to determine the exact optimum time to start ART. Meanwhile best practice is to follow WHO and national guidelines. Adequate secondary prophylaxis with fluconazole is essential to long term survival. Although studies from South East Asia suggest that primary prophylaxis (treating all HIV patients with fluconazole 200 mg daily) decreases CM this may not be either feasible or practical in Africa. However there is strong evidence in Africa that in HIV patients with CD4 count <100/mm³ the presence of cryptococcal antigenaemia accurately predicts the onset of an attack of CM over the following 12 months. This highlights the need for a more targeted approach to screening of at risk HIV infected persons e.g. those starting ARTs and the treatment and chemoprophylaxis of the CRAg positives.

Prognosis

CM is fatal without treatment and has a high mortality even with treatment. In Africa the two week post treatment mortality is 20-40% and the six month mortality rate even with ART therapy is >50%. The overall high mortality rates seen in CM in Africa are ascribed to late clinical presentation, ongoing immunosuppression, concurrent infections e.g. TB, immune reconstitution syndrome (IRIS) which usually occurs within 3 months of initiating ART and high rates of relapse. The following clinical features at presentation are associated with poor prognosis, abnormal mental status, high fungal burden, increased CSF opening pressure and poor inflammatory response (<20 cells /mm^3). Relapse is common (approx 30%) and IRIS can occur months after initiating ART in patients with successfully treated CM. Management of IRIS includes excluding or treating possible CM relapse, decreasing intracranial pressure (by repeated LPs), excluding other possible opportunistic infections e.g. TBM and finally steroids if necessary.

Key points

- diagnosis is confirmed by CSF microscopy (India ink) and/or CRAg serology
- repeated lumbar punctures is critical in the management of ↑ICP in CM
- treatment is with fluconazole 1200 mg/po for 2/52 followed by 800 mg po for 8/52
- secondary prophylaxis is necessary until the CD4 count >200/mm^3 for 6/12
- initiating ART for CM patients should be delayed for 4 weeks after treatment
- long-term mortality in CM is high (>50%) even with ART

VIRAL MENINGITIS

Viruses are the commonest cause of meningitis worldwide. Viral meningitis is usually a benign disease that does not require hospitalization. It is commonest in the age groups 0-1yrs and 4-15 yrs but can affect all age groups. Human enteroviruses account for >90% of cases and are classified into polioviruses, coxsackie viruses and echoviruses. Other viruses that cause meningitis include the arboviruses and adenoviruses. Young children are the usual source with spread mostly via the faecal oral route within families. It occurs throughout the year with seasonal peaks in the hotter weather. Outbreaks can occur in hospitals and schools.

Clinical features

Clinically there may be a history of a viral like illness with fever, vomiting and rash. The onset can be acute or sub acute with fever and headache occurring in most patients. Neck stiffness is mild and present in half the cases. Neurologic abnormalities are rare but febrile convulsions may occur in young children. The illness can last over a week in children and longer in adults. Clinically at onset viral meningitis may be indistinguishable from bacterial meningitis and often requires emergency antibiotics until the diagnosis is confirmed by exclusion of other causes. A lumbar puncture may be normal or show mild abnormalities including polymorphs early on and later lymphocytes (Table 6.2). Treatment is mainly symptomatic and the prognosis is generally excellent.

VIRAL ENCEPHALITIS

Encephalitis is inflammation of the brain parenchyma caused by a viral infection. It is predominantly a disease of children. The causative virus is not known in >50% of cases. The most frequent known forms are caused by an unusual manifestation of common, mainly childhood viral infections including measles, chickenpox and mumps. Herpes simplex (HSV) is the most common cause of fatal sporadic encephalitis in adults worldwide but it appears to be uncommon in Africa. Other well known viruses causing encephalitis include HIV, cytomegalovirus (CMV), Epstein-Barr virus (EBV) and rabies. There are great geographic variations in the causes of viral meningo-encephalitis worldwide. Viruses specific to the African subcontinent including Ebola virus, Lassa fever, Marburg disease and Rift Valley fever are briefly reviewed on page 146.

The main arthropod borne infections causing viral encephalitis are Japanese B encephalitis virus in the Far East, West Nile virus in mainly West Africa and Rift Valley Fever in East Africa. The vectors are mosquitoes and the hosts may be humans, animals or birds depending on the location and virus. Viruses enter the CNS by two distinct routes, haematogenous which is the most common route as occurs in the arthropod borne group and by local replication at the site of infection and retrograde spread to the brain via peripheral nerves as occurs in herpes and rabies. Other main ways of acquiring CNS viral infection include enteric e.g. polio and by inhalation e.g. Ebola and sexually e.g. HIV.

Clinical features

Viruses cause a variety of CNS disease including aseptic meningitis, encephalomyelitis, myelitis and myeloradiculitis. The signs and symptoms of encephalitis include fever, headache, confusion, stupor, coma, seizures, upper motor neurone signs and less commonly focal neurological deficits. Virus infections may also infrequently result in a form of autoimmune encephalitis called **acute demyelinating encephalomyelitis (ADEM)** occurring mainly in older childhood/early teens which is very responsive to high dose parenteral steroids. The clinical presentation of ADEM is that of monophasic illness and can be very similar to encephalitis. However, it is difficult to diagnose and confirm in Africa without MRI scanning.

The diagnosis of viral encephalitis is made by immunological tests, neuroimaging and EEG but the viral cause is not usually identified. Effective antiviral therapy (such as the acyclic purine nucleoside analogue, aciclovir) is available only for the herpes virus group. The mortality is variable and depends on the virus. Preventive measures include control of vectors and vaccination when available.

Key points

- viruses are leading cause of meningitis/encephalitis worldwide & mainly affect children
- enteroviruses are main causes of viral meningitis in children
- transmission is by close physical contact: inhalation, ingestion, insect bites & sexual contact
- diagnosis is clinical in combination with CSF & serology findings
- outcome is excellent in viral meningitis but variable in encephalitis depending on the virus

HERPES ENCEPHALITIS

This is the most common form of fatal sporadic encephalitis worldwide and is important because it is treatable if diagnosed early. The frequency is not known in Africa but may be less there possibly because of early exposure in childhood. There are two main types, HSV-1 and HSV-2. Humans are the reservoir for both types; HSV-1 is more common and affects mainly older adults, whereas HSV-2 affects neonates. HSV-I is spread by close physical contact and causes predominantly encephalitis, whereas HSV-2 is considered a sexually transmitted disease and predominantly causes meningitis. The source of encephalitis is mostly reactivation of latent ganglionic infection or less commonly a primary infection. It spreads in a retrograde way either via the trigeminal or olfactory nerves to the temporal and frontal areas of the brain

Clinical findings

Clinically, HSV encephalitis begins as an acute or sub acute non-specific febrile illness characterised by headache, fever, irritability, and altered mental status. Most patients go on to experience confusion, personality change, dysphasia, focal neurological findings, memory loss and seizures affecting the temporal lobe. Herpetic skin lesions are rare. Symptoms typically evolve over several days and may take 2 to 3 weeks to reach their maximum severity. The differential diagnosis includes HIV related CNS infections, TB meningitis, partially treated acute bacterial meningitis, cerebral malaria and brain abscess.

Diagnosis

Diagnosis of HSV encephalitis is based on clinical findings and a characteristic CSF with lymphocytes, red blood cells and elevated protein. Infection in the CSF may be demonstrated by PCR, serologically and viral culture. PCR has a specificity of up to 100% and a sensitivity of 95% on CSF taken between day 2 and 10 after the onset of the illness, however serological tests are of no help in acute diagnosis of HSE, only in retrospect and then after 2 weeks. An EEG can be helpful with diagnosis, (triphasic complexes). CT/MRI of the head typically shows oedema and haemorrhage in the temporal/frontal lobe (Fig. 6.6).

Pathology

MRI T1

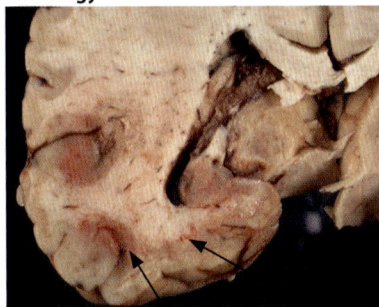

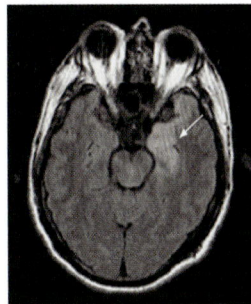

Temporal lobe oedema & multiple micro haemorrhages

Temporal lobe oedema

Figure 6.6 Brain in herpes encephalitis

Management

The antiviral drug aciclovir 10-15 mg/kg/iv 8 hourly is given for 14 days as soon as possible after the onset of symptoms if HSE is thought to be at all likely and for 21 days if HIV positive. Aciclovir is well absorbed orally if the parenteral form is unavailable. Seizures are treated as in status epilepticus. Rehabilitation includes physiotherapy, speech therapy, occupational therapy and later neuropsychological testing and support. Treated cases have a mortality of 10-20% and untreated 50-70%. Morbidity is high and includes memory loss, cognitive impairment and persistent seizures. The role of steroids is controversial but should be given at present if there is evidence of raised or increasing intracranial pressure.

RABIES

Rabies is mainly a disease of dogs, cats, jackals, mongoose and bats that is transmitted to humans. Transmission to humans in Africa is almost inevitably by the bite and saliva of a rabid dog or other animal. The severity and site of the bite from the rabid animal determines the risk of infection and 35-67% go on to develop rabies. Very rarely transmission is human to human e.g., by corneal graft. Rare cases have occurred by inhalation of bat urine in caves. There are over 50,000 deaths worldwide each year from rabies mainly in Asia but many also occur in

Africa. Post exposure prophylaxis can be 100% effective (Table 6.7) if it is given on the day of exposure or bite and the treatment precautions are rigorously adhered to.

Pathogenesis

Rabies starts with viral replication at the bite site. Then there is flow of the virus via the peripheral nerves towards the brain with replication in the brain nerve cells which gives rise to the characteristic neuronal inclusions called Negri bodies. Then there is flow back from the brain to the rest of the nervous system, in particular to the salivary glands and the clinical disease starts. Involvement of the limbic system in the brain results in furious rabies and involvement of the spinal cord results in paralytic rabies.

Clinical features

Rabies should be suspected if there are unexplained neurological, psychiatric or laryngo-pharyngeal symptoms in a patient with a history of an exposure. The usual incubation period is between 2-8 weeks but can vary from 9 days to 12 months or rarely more. The disease starts with a prodromal illness which lasts a few days, until either furious or paralytic rabies appears. The first symptom is itching, pain or paraesthesiae at the now healed bite site. Other prodromal symptoms include myalgia, fever, chills, irritability, anxiety, photophobia and headache.

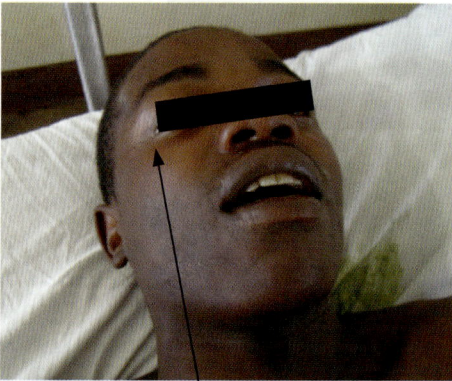

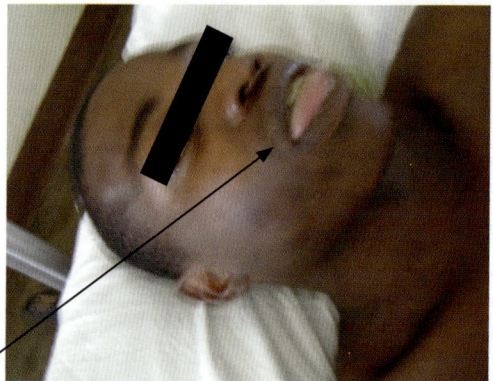

Furious rabies with tearing from the eyes, tongue protrusion & frothing

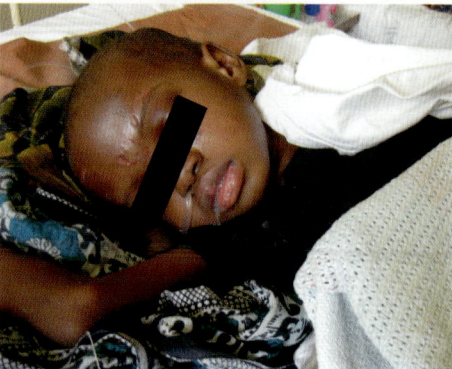

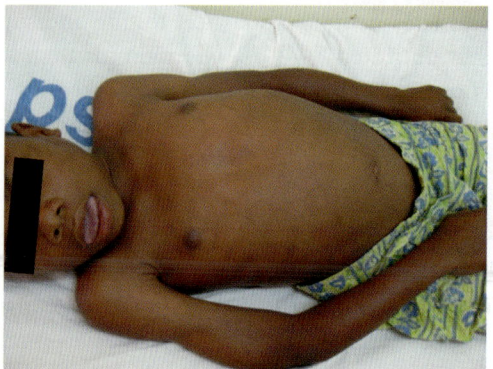

Paralytic rabies with facial scars (dog bite), hyper salivation & tongue protrusion

Figure 6.7 Rabies

The clinical features of furious rabies occur in 80% of cases and include hydrophobia, terror, pain, convulsions, hallucinations, aggression, cranial nerve palsies, paralysis and autonomic disturbance e.g. hyper salivation or frothing from the mouth, sweating and lacrimation (Fig 6.7). Periods of manic confusion may alternate with periods of calm and quiet. Rabies is characterised by terrifying hydrophobic spasms. These are typically provoked early on by sipping water, swallowing saliva or by blowing air onto the skin and later on by merely the sight, sound or mention of water. These are characteristically violent jerky spasms during which the neck and back are extended and the arms thrown upward. They can be very severe and end in seizures and death.

Paralytic or algid rabies occurs in about 20% of patients (Fig. 6.7). During this the patient begins with the usual prodromal symptoms followed by paralysis in the bitten limb, which eventually ascends to involve the remaining limbs and breathing. Death in rabies usually follows the onset of prodromal symptoms within 1-2 weeks and following the onset of spasms, coma and paralysis within days. The differential diagnosis includes causes of spasms including tetanus, tetany, dystonic drug reactions, poisoning and paralysis including Guillain-Barre syndrome, and CNS infections including cerebral malaria and encephalitis.

Laboratory diagnosis

The diagnosis is a clinical one based on a history of exposure and clinical findings. There are no routine laboratory or rapid tests for the diagnosis of rabies and the ante mortem diagnosis requires a reference laboratory as several tests are necessary. Antibodies are detectable in the unvaccinated patient during the second week of illness and the virus may be isolated from saliva and CSF although it may take 1-3 weeks for a result. Saliva can be tested by virus isolation or reverse transcription followed by polymerase chain reaction (RT-PCR). Skin biopsies at the nape of the neck can be examined for the presence of rabies antigen (IFA) in the cutaneous nerves. The brain of the biting animal and the patient can be examined microscopically for the presence of Negri bodies and immunofluorescent antibodies (Fig. 6.8).

Histopathology

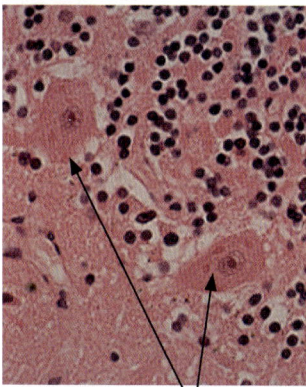

Negri bodies (small red inclusions)

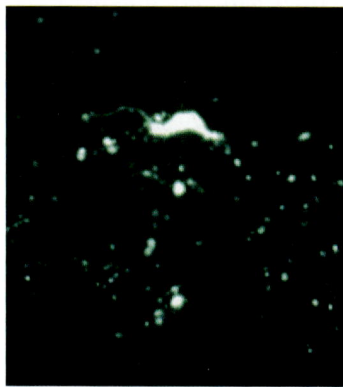

Immunofluorescence staining

Figure 6.8 Brain in rabies

Key points

- rabies is transmitted to humans mostly by the bite and saliva of a rabid dog
- diagnosis is by a history of exposure & unexplained neurological or psychiatric symptoms
- hydrophobia, terror, pain, convulsions & hallucinations occur in the majority of patients
- there are no routine clinical laboratory diagnostic tests for rabies

Treatment

Rabies patients should be nursed in a single room in isolation because the patient's saliva is potentially infective. Ideally there should be barrier nursing. Treatment is symptomatic as the disease is considered to be universally fatal once symptoms appear apart from a few isolated reports of survival with prolonged ICU care in high-income settings. Symptomatic treatment involves large doses of sedation using phenothiazines and phenobarbitone and adequate analgesia using morphine to relieve the fear and pain.

Prevention

Rabies is preventable by pre and post exposure vaccination (Table 6.7). Post exposure prophylaxis of rabies is based on using available rabies vaccines which are all equally safe and effective. These include human diploid cell vaccines (HDCV), purified vero cell vaccine (PVRV), purified chick embryo vaccine, (PCECV) and purified duck embryo vaccine (PDEV). The indications for prophylaxis are licks on skin or mucosa, scratches, abrasions and **bites** from animals in rabies endemic areas. Post exposure treatment consists of **1) vigorous wound debridement** and **cleaning with alcohol** or **iodine compounds, 2) starting the vaccine immediately** and **3) using rabies immunoglobulin,** if a major exposure (bites) has occurred. These measures, if carried out optimally, can reduce the risk of developing rabies to almost zero.

The vaccine should always be started as early as possible and be given regardless of the time lapse since exposure. Costs are reduced by using the intradermal route of administration. The WHO recommended vaccination schedules are presented below. *Vaccination may be discontinued if the animal, usually a dog or a cat remains healthy after 15 days of observation or if it is certain that the animal brain biopsy is negative for rabies.* The management and control of rabies in endemic areas depends on the control and immunization of dogs and the notification of the disease.

Table 6.7 WHO recommended immunization schedule for Rabies

Post exposure prophylaxis (all vaccines)	1.0 ml im (deltoid) never the buttock on day 0, 3, 7, 14, 28
Alternative regimes (where vaccine in short supply)	
8 site intradermal (HDCV & PCECV)	0.1 ml id @ eight sites* on day 0 0.1 ml id @ four sites** on day 7 0.1 ml id @ one site (deltoid) on day 28 & 90
2 site intradermal (PVRV, PCECV & PDEV)	0.2 ml id @ two sites (deltoid) on day 0, 3 & 7 & 0.2 ml id @ one site (deltoid) on day 28 & 90
Previously vaccinated (all vaccines)	1.0 ml im (deltoid) on day 0,3, &7

id = intradermal
* *deltoids, suprascapular, abdominal wall (lower quadrant) & lateral thighs*
** *deltoids & thighs*

POLIOMYELITIS

Poliomyelitis is a disease caused by the poliovirus which is characterized by an acute onset of flaccid paralysis. Poliovirus is a highly infectious enterovirus comprising of wild subtypes 1, 2 and 3. Transmission is by the faecal-oral, oral-oral route and occasionally by a shared common source e.g. water and milk. The main risk factors for outbreaks are high population density, poverty, poor faecal hygiene and low immunization rates. The majority of new infections are endemic with 75% occurring in the <3 year age group. It is rare after the age of 15 years but in epidemics however, a wider older non vaccinated age group may be affected. The incidence of polio has decreased dramatically from >250,000 cases 25 years ago to complete elimination countrywide, except for Nigeria, Pakistan and Afghanistan. There has however, been a resurgence of polio particularly in SSA. In 2013, 324/416 new cases reported to WHO were from Somalia, Kenya, Ethiopia, Nigeria and Cameroon. Transported wild type 1 and circulating vaccine derived poliovirus were responsible for the cases.

Clinical Features

The incubation period for poliomyelitis is 7-14 days (range 3-35). Out of infected cases, 70% are asymptomatic, 25% may have a minor febrile illness with sore throat or gastroenteritis and 4% have non paralytic poliomyelitis. Initial symptoms include fever, headache, vomiting, meningism, constipation or less commonly diarrhoea, myalgia and limb pain. A much smaller proportion (0.1-1.0%) develop paralytic poliomyelitis. Risk factors for acquiring the paralytic form include older age, male, recent injections, infections, surgery, trauma, stress and pregnancy. The main clinical features of paralytic poliomyelitis are fever, followed within 24-48 hours by asymmetrical limb paralysis affecting proximal more than distal muscle groups. There is no sensory loss or autonomic dysfunction. The legs (most commonly one limb) are most frequently involved but arms, breathing (diaphragm and intercostal muscles), swallowing, neck and face may be affected. The sites of pathology are the anterior horn cells in cord and brain with permanent loss of function in muscles supplied by the affected lower motor neurons. Paralysis with areflexia reaches its maximum within 2-4 days of onset. The CSF may initially contain a few polymorphs later changing to lymphocytes, whilst protein is elevated but sugar is normal. While there may be partial recovery of function paralysis remains permanent (>60 days) in >75% of cases. The case fatality rate is 5-10% and increases with age with most deaths due to bulbar and respiratory failure. A post-polio syndrome or a new onset motor weakness may occur 20-40 years later.

Differential Diagnosis

The differential diagnosis in SSA includes Guillain-Barre syndrome, post diphtheria paralysis, algid rabies, enterovirus polio-like paralysis, transverse myelitis, viral meningoencephalitis, sciatic nerve injury (post injection) and acute neuromuscular weakness.

Management

There is no antiviral treatment and therapy is aimed at preventing complications and starting rehabilitation. In the acute phase injections are avoided and paralyzed limbs are supported in a neutral position. Respiratory function is carefully monitored and supported with assisted ventilation if necessary. As soon as pain has disappeared rehabilitation exercises are started. The long term aim is to assist mobilization and rehabilitation back into society.

Prevention

Poliomyelitis is preventable as a disease and global threat. This can be achieved by education, vaccination, vigilant surveillance, case notification and virus isolation

Viral Haemorrhagic Fevers

The main causes, epidemiological and clinical features of the viral haemorrhagic fevers (VHFs) in SSA are summarized below in Table 6.8. These are caused by highly infectious viruses typically with a reservoir and source in either animals or humans. They are transmitted mostly by close physical contact (contagion) with or rarely inhalation from an infected patient or by a biting vector *i.e.* mosquito or tick. Parenteral, laboratory and workplace transmission is a particularly high risk. The disease occurs mostly as epidemics although Lassa Fever, Dengue, Yellow fever and C-CHF also occur in an endemic form. The clinical presentations are characterized by very high fever at onset usually coupled with severe pain/myalgia. This is frequently complicated over the following days by varying degrees of shock, bleeding, encephalitis and organ failure depending on which virus is involved and the severity and route of exposure. Management is largely symptomatic and supportive. Careful fluid replacement is a key measure coupled with the use of blood products *i.e.* whole blood, plasma and platelets. Ribavirin is used in cases of suspected Lassa and Rift Valley fever. Immediate infection control measures include strict barrier care precautions, index case identification and reporting to local health authorities. Public health measures include education, high risk contact identification, isolation and surveillance. The very high CFRs underscore the urgent need for prevention.

Table 6.8 Summary of Main Viral Haemorrhagic Fevers in SSA

Virus	Geographic Distribution	Main Reservoirs & Transmission Mode	ICP (R) days	Main Clinical Features	Prevention	CFR %
Ebola	**West**, East & Central Africa *(DRC, Guinea, SL, Liberia, Congo, Gabon, IC, Sudan, Uganda)*	**Fruit bats**, Primates, **Humans** *Contact:* **DC, PC, (Ingt)**	5–10 *(2–21)*	High Fever, Rash Vomiting, Diarrhea, HF: 50%, Shock, Encephalitis	IC, PHM	50–90
Marburg	**Central & East** Africa *(DRC, Angola, Kenya, Zimbabwe, Uganda)*	**Bats**, Primates **Humans.** *Contact:* **DC, PC (Ingt)**	5–10 *(2–21)*	High Fever, Rash, HF/conjunct/haem, Encephalitis, Shock	IC, PHM	20–80
Lassa	**West** Africa *(Nigeria, Liberia, SL, Guinea, Mali, Senegal)*	**Rodents** (urine/faeces) **Humans.** *Contact:* **Inhl/Ingt, DC, PC**	7–12 *(2–18)*	Fever, pharyngitis lymphadenopathy Encephalitis, HF	IC, PHM	15–20
Rift Valley Fever	**East, Central, West** & Sth. Africa *(Kenya, Tz, Sudan, Somalia, Senegal, Nigeria, CAR, SA)*	**Domestic animals** Contact: **Mosq bite:** *(A. aegypti)* **PC**, (DC, Inhl from animals)	2–7	Fever, Arthralgia, Jaundice, *(HF & Encephalitis 1–5%)*	IC, MC, PHM	1
Dengue	**East Central &** **West** Africa	**Humans**, Primates *Contact:* **Mosq bite:** *(A. aegypti, & albopictus)* **PC**	3–10	Fever, Myalgia, Rash, Shock, HF *(Encephalitis 1–2%)*	IC, MC, PHM	1–5
Yellow Fever	**West** Central & East Africa *(Nigeria Guinea, Ghana, Gabon, Liberia, Gabon, Senegal, Cameroon, DRC, Kenya)*	**Primates, Humans** Contact: **Mosq bite:** *(A. aegypti)* **PC**	3–6	Fever, Shock, Jaundice, HF, Renal failure, Encephalitis	IC, MC, PHM, Vaccination	20
C-CHF	**West, Central, East** & **SA** *(DRC, Congo BF, Senegal, Uganda, Tz, SA, Kenya, Mauritania)*	**Domestic & wild animals.** *Contact:* **Tick bite, PC (DC)**	3–7 *(2–13)*	High Fever, HF++, Encephalitis, *(Liver & Renal failure)*	IC, PHM	30–70

Contact/Contagion **PC:** *percutaneous: needle/mosquito/tick,* **DC:** *direct contact: skin/mucosa,* **Inhl:** *inhalation* **Ingt:** *ingestion.* **C-CHF:** *Crimean-Congo* **HF:** *Haemorrhagic Fever,* **ICP:** *Incubation period,* **HF:** *Haemorrhagic Fever,* **IC:** *Infection control,* **PHM:** *Public Health Measures,* **MC:** *Mosquito Control.* Countries in SSA: DRC, Democratic Republic of Congo, SL Sierra Leone, IC Ivory Coast, Tz Tanzania, BF Burkina Faso, SA South Africa.

TETANUS

Tetanus is caused by exposure to spores of *Clostridium tetani*, a gram positive anaerobic rod which is commonly found in soil. Tetanus follows contamination of a wound by tetanus spores. Most cases of adult tetanus follow an acute and sometimes relatively trivial injury to feet or legs. Most cases of neonatal tetanus occur as a result of contamination of the umbilical cord after birth. The disease is still prevalent in Africa despite the widespread introduction of immunization programs for neonates and pregnant women. Tetanus is estimated to cause almost a quarter of a million deaths worldwide annually, many of whom live in Africa. It is predominantly (90%) a disease of children under five years mainly affecting neonates but also affects adults, and in particular males.

Pathogenesis

The tetanus spores incubate in the wound under anaerobic conditions and mature into vegetative bacteria. They in turn produce potent neurotoxins, tetanolysin and tetanospasmin. Tetanospasmin spreads via nerves by retrograde axonal flow to the spinal cord and brain. In the spinal cord and brain, tetanospasmin binds the presynaptic terminal and produces presynaptic inhibition of gamma amino butyric acid (GABA) release. This denies the anterior horn cells and the alpha motor units of inhibition, resulting in uncontrollable spasms by both agonist and antagonist muscles. In addition a lack of neural control of the adrenal glands results in release of catecholamines, thus producing a hyper sympathetic state and widespread autonomic instability. Recovery only occurs when new terminal synapses are sprouted after 3-4 weeks.

Clinical features

The incubation period for tetanus is between 3-21 days with a median of 7 days. The clinical disease progresses over the course of the first 1-2 weeks and then continues for a total of 3-4 weeks in all. The clinical characteristic of tetanus is increased muscle tone at rest and continuing muscle spasms. On examination, there is rigidity of the muscles involving the face, neck, back and abdomen. The face may show risus sardonicus (lock jaw) and the body may be held arched in the opisthotonos like position (Fig 6.9). Reflex muscle spasms arise spontaneously and are provoked by noise, touch, and light and last from seconds to a minute. Their frequency and duration is variable from every few seconds to hours and they typically continue for most of the duration of the 3-4 week illness. Spasms are painful as full consciousness is retained. Prognosis is worse in those patients with wounds nearer the head and with a short incubation time. The main complications are pneumonia, asphyxia, hypoxia, arrhythmia and rarely fractures. Death usually occurs because of prolonged spasms provoking anoxia, pneumonia or autonomic involvement.

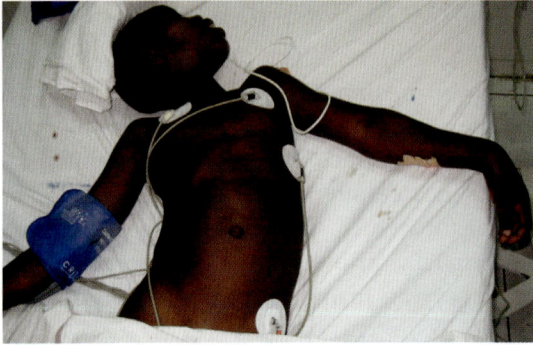

Figure 6.9 Tetanus. Opisthotonos, extensor spasms with arching of the back

Diagnosis

The diagnosis is made clinically as there are no confirmatory laboratory findings. The differential diagnosis includes dystonia, tetany, rabies, meningitis and poisoning (strychnine).

Management

The patient is nursed in a quiet and darkened area or room to avoid stimuli provoking spasms. The acute management involves wound debridement and exploration for foreign bodies, passive immunization with human antitetanus serum, human immunoglobulin 150 IU/kg (3-6000 iu) im, and penicillin with metronidazole to treat the infection. Diazepam is the most commonly used drug to treat muscle spasms. It may be necessary to use 10-20 mg/po or iv, initially 6 hourly increasing the frequency of administration to 4 or 2 hourly as necessary in cases of severe muscle spasms. Chlorpromazine, 50 to 100 mg/im, initially 12 hourly and increasing the frequency of administration to 6 hourly may be used in combination with diazepam. Phenobarbitone is also sometimes used in combination with diazepam. The use of regular iv magnesium sulphate has been shown to improve prognosis by decreasing the need for antispasmodics and antiarrhythmics. The choice of antispasmodic and their order, dose, frequency and duration should be according to the severity of the spasms and local treatment protocols. It is good practice to start with lower doses and over sedation should be avoided.

Beta blockers in the form of atenolol or labetolol or verapamil may be necessary to treat and prevent cardiac arrhythmias or hypertension. If there is failure to control the spasms or there is respiratory depression or pneumonia, then a tracheostomy or/and mechanical ventilation may be necessary. As the required period of intubation is usually prolonged (>7-10 days), early tracheostomy is common practice. Active immunization by tetanus toxoid is necessary when the disease has resolved as tetanus infection does not confer lasting immunity.

Prognosis

The case fatality rate with treated tetanus varies between 40-60%, more commonly the latter. Those who recover rarely have a neurological deficit.

Prevention

Primary prevention is by vaccination in early childhood as part of the routine, diphtheria, tetanus and pertussis (DTP) immunization and by booster at 4-7 years, in adolescence and once again in adulthood. For others who are non immune including pregnancy, these should receive primary immunization followed by 10 yearly booster doses for a total of 5 doses. If a person has not been vaccinated during the last 5 years and they receive a tetanus prone injury then a booster dose should be given.

Key points

- tetanus arises from wounds contaminated by soil containing spores of *C. tetani*
- management is by passive immunoglobulin, wound debridement & antibiotics
- spasms are controlled by diazepam, chlorpromazine & magnesium sulphate
- complications are pneumonia, asphyxia, hypoxia, arrhythmia & rarely fractures
- tracheostomy and mechanical ventilation may be necessary,
- CFR is frequently >50%

SYPHILIS

Syphilis is caused by the spirochete *Treponema pallidum*. It is a sexually transmitted disease and this route of transmission accounts for most adult cases. However syphilis can be transmitted vertically *in utero* resulting in congenital syphilis or also by blood transfusion. The natural history of syphilis is divided into three stages, primary, secondary and tertiary. Primary syphilis occurs 1-6 weeks after exposure, secondary syphilis 6-8 weeks post primary and tertiary syphilis 1-45 years afterwards. It is infective during all stages and transmission rates vary from 10–60%.

Epidemiology

There are over 12 million new cases of primary syphilis worldwide annually approximately one third of which occur in Africa. The prevalence rates for syphilis serology indicating previous exposure varies from less than one in ten in pregnancy to one in two in some sex workers. Over the last decades, there has been a marked decline in neurosyphilis worldwide. This has been attributed to the widespread use of antibiotics accidentally treating syphilis. The annual incidence of neurosyphilis is low (<0.5/100,000) in high income countries. Data on the incidence of neurosyphilis is not available for Africa. There is some clinical evidence that the incidence may be higher in HIV infected adults in Africa but there is no clear epidemiological data to support that.

Pathogenesis of Neurosyphilis

The treponeme invades the CNS within 3-24 months of untreated primary infection in about 25% of cases. The pathology of neurosyphilis is made up of two main stages: a vascular stage causing endarteritis and thrombosis and a granulomatous stage causing gumma formation.

Neurological findings

Neurosyphilis is divided into two main phases, *asymptomatic* and *symptomatic*. Symptomatic neurosyphilis is divided into four distinct clinical entities. These include **acute syphilitic meningitis** which occurs in about 25% of untreated cases of primary syphilis and **meningovascular syphilis**, **tabes dorsalis** and **generalised paralysis of the insane** which occurs in <10% of untreated primary cases.

Asymptomatic

The asymptomatic phase occurs in the period 1-10 yrs after primary infection. During this phase the infection is active but there are no symptoms and the only finding is an abnormal

CSF showing lymphocytosis, elevation in protein, low glucose and positive serological tests for syphilis.

Symptomatic

Meningitis

This occurs within 2 years of primary infection. The clinical presentation ranges from an isolated aseptic meningitis with fever and rash, to an acute basal meningitis presenting with cranial nerve palsies and hydrocephalus.

Meningovascular syphilis

This occurs 5-10 years after primary infection as a result of an obliterative endarteritis affecting the small or medium sized arteries supplying the internal capsule. It presents mainly as stroke in a younger person.

Tabes Dorsalis (TD)

TD is a late manifestation of tertiary syphilis occurring 15-20 years after primary infection. It arises as result of degeneration in the posterior columns in the spinal cord and in the brain stem. It presents with unexplained lightning and abdominal pains in combination with an ataxic gait disorder. There are characteristic neurological findings including an ataxic stamping gait, positive Romberg's sign, Argyll Robertson pupils and Charcot's joints, late in the disease.

General paralysis insane (GPI)

GPI is a late manifestation occurring 10-25 years after primary infection. This is characterised by a progressive dementia with delusions of grandeur and mania, coupled with varying degrees of paralysis.

Diagnosis of neurosyphilis

The diagnosis of neurosyphilis requires a high index of clinical suspicion combined with CSF findings and serological evidence of syphilis in blood and CSF. Laboratory CSF examination shows increased lymphocytes, increased protein and a normal or reduced glucose level. Diagnosis is by specific treponemal tests; flocculation treponemal antibody (FTA) and Treponema pallidum haemagglutination assay (TPHA) and non-treponemal tests including venereal disease reference laboratory (VDRL) and rapid reagin tests (RPR). Both RPR and VDRL are used as a screening test for syphilis in Africa. VDRL is positive in the blood in nearly all cases of syphilis but false positives occur with endemic treponematoses and in other diseases e.g. tuberculosis and malaria. However VDRL is positive in the CSF in only <80% of cases of neurosyphilis, therefore a negative VDRL in CSF does not exclude the diagnosis. False negatives may occur in primary and late syphilis and also in HIV infection. A more specific antibody test is the TPHA test. A negative TPHA in the CSF excludes neurosyphilis.

HIV and Neurosyphilis

The natural history of neurosyphilis may be altered in HIV disease. There may be an accelerated progression to neurosyphilis, atypical clinical presentation, negative antibody tests and response to penicillin may be less effective. Treatment may require a longer and repeated course of penicillin.

Treatment of neurosyphilis

The treatment of neurosyphilis is with soluble penicillin 20-24 million units (4 million units 4 hourly) daily iv for 14-21 days (>17 days). Persons who are allergic to penicillin should have erythromycin 0.5 gm 6 hourly or doxycycline 200 mg bid for 28 days. Steroids are given with the first few doses of penicillin because of the rare occurrence of the Jarich-Herxheimer reaction. The prognosis depends on the stage. Treatment of asymptomatic and meningitis stages are curative. Treatment of the other tertiary stages results in an improvement in about one third and stabilization in the rest. A follow up CSF examination should be done every 6 months for 2 yrs and every year if HIV positive. If the CSF shows signs of activity (lymphocytes +++) then the patient should be retreated with penicillin. The VDRL may remain positive in CSF and become negative in serum. The principles of prevention and control include public education, screening, partner notification and treatment.

Key points

- syphilis is one of the most common STDs globally with 1/3 of new cases in Africa
- neurosyphilis occurs in <10% of untreated primary syphilis
- neurosyphilis is uncommon & is altered in HIV disease
- confirmation relies on positive serological test in the CSF
- treatment is with high dose penicillin iv for 14-21 days

BRAIN ABSCESS

A brain abscess is caused by infection, the main causative organism being either bacteria or protozoa. An abscess may be clinically classified as pyogenic and non pyogenic depending on the organism. Toxoplasmosis and tuberculosis are the main non pyogenic causes. The main causative organisms in pyogenic brain abscess are ***Streptococcus viridans, Staphylococcus aureus*** and ***Bacteroides fragilus***. Intracranial pyogenic abscess is a focal infection within the brain, subdural or epidural space. They are uncommon and can affect any age group. The majority arise within the brain from a purulent infection elsewhere in the body so it is important to try to find the primary source. The source of infection is either local or haematogenous. Local spread arises directly from otitis media, mastoiditis, sinusitis, dental abscess or recent head injury in particular skull fracture. Haematogenous spread arises from the heart (e.g. endocarditis), the lungs (e.g. bronchiectasis), or from any other infected source (e.g. skin abscess).

Clinical features

Most patients present with headache, fever and focal neurological disorders (FND). Headache is the most frequent initial symptom. FNDs include seizures, focal motor sensory or speech disorders or confusion or alteration in consciousness. The fever is usually low grade or absent depending on the duration being usually absent in a mature abscess. Seizures occur in about a quarter of patients. Any neurological deficit will depend on the origin, site and extent of the abscess. The time from onset to complications usually takes a couple of weeks but may occasionally occur in days. Signs of the probable source of the brain abscess may be present.

Differential diagnosis

The differential diagnosis includes any other cause of a space occupying lesion resulting in a focal CNS disorder. These include non pyogenic brain abscess e.g. toxoplasmosis or TB, parasitic cyst, intracerebral haemorrhage, subdural haematoma and brain neoplasm.

Diagnosis

The diagnosis if not already suspected clinically is made by a CT scan of the head. A CT with contrast typically shows a ring enhancing mass lesion in the brain with a central area of low density surrounded by oedema with mass effect or a subdural/epidural collection (Fig 6.10). LP is contraindicated in any suspected intracranial mass lesion.

CT scan (with contrast)   **Pathology**

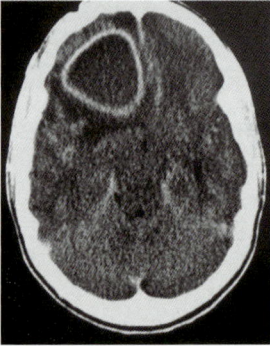

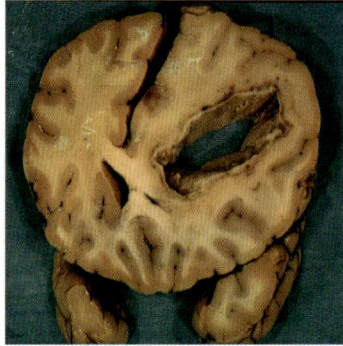

Frontal lobe (right)   Frontal lobe (left)

Figure 6.10 Brain abscess

Management

Management is based on antibiotics and surgical drainage. The choice of antibiotics should be based on the likelihood of the primary source of infection. This includes a combined daily dose of penicillin 20-24 million units iv in divided doses 4-6 hourly, chloramphenicol 1 gm iv 6 hourly and metronidazole 500 mg iv 8 hourly. Alternately an extended-spectrum cephalosporin e.g. ceftriaxone 2 gm iv twice daily with metronidazole can also be used depending on availability and cost. Where *Staphylococcus* or gm negatives are suspected flucloxacillin or gentamycin, respectively, should be added. Ciprofloxacin intravenously is also an alternative. Surgical drainage is indicated in large abscesses or collections of pus (>3cm). This is usually done by Burr hole aspiration or by craniotomy.

All antibiotics should be given intravenously and continued for a total of not less than a period of 4-6 weeks. A follow up CT of the head is recommended to assess response to treatment. Anticonvulsants may be necessary if there are seizures. The case fatality rate in the high-income countries varies from 10% in uncomplicated cases to >50% in patients with coma. Morbidity is about 30% and includes epilepsy and focal neurological deficits.

Key points

- pyogenic brain abscesses arise from either direct or haematogenous spread
- local sources are mastoiditis, sinusitis, dental & skin infections
- haematogenous sources are skin, heart & lungs
- clinical features are headache, seizures & focal neurological deficits
- antibiotics are iv for 4-6/52 & surgical drainage is necessary for large abscesses

APPENDIX LUMBAR PUNCTURE

Indications

A lumbar puncture is indicated in the following clinical situations:

1) diagnosis of suspected CNS infections, haemorrhage and encephalopathies

2) to reduce CSF pressure e.g. in cryptococcal meningitis and benign intracranial hypertension

3) administration of intrathecal medications e.g. radio-opaque media

Contraindications

LP is a safe procedure but there is a risk of brain herniation when CSF pressure is high. A fundoscopy to exclude papilloedema should always be carried out prior to an LP. An LP is contraindicated in the following clinical situations.

1) raised intracranial pressure
2) suspected CNS mass lesion
3) bleeding disorder e.g. anticoagulation, low platelets
4) local infection at the LP site

Positioning

An LP should start with an explanation, reassurance and a warning concerning possible complications. The procedure is performed on a bed with a firm or hard edge or alternatively on a table. Proper positioning is critical to successfully completing an LP. The patient lies horizontally facing away from the operator, usually in the left lateral decubitus position with the neck firmly flexed and the knees drawn up to the chin. The back should be in line with the edge of the bed with the shoulders and hips aligned in the same vertical plane and the patient's spine maximally flexed in order to open up the lower lumbar spaces. The head may be supported by a thin pillow (Fig 6.11). If it is necessary to perform an LP with the patient sitting upright this can be done with the patient either sitting astride a chair or on the side of a bed with the spine semi flexed and head supported by a pillow and table. The site of the LP should now be identified. The spinal cord ends at L1 (L2) in adults and a line drawn down from the top of the iliac crest bisects the L3-4 interspace which is safe and avoids the danger of damaging the spinal cord. After palpating and identifying the spines, either the L3-4 or L4-5 interspace should be marked with a pen or a scratch. The LP should now be done under full sterile technique using gloves. The steps in the procedure are outlined below

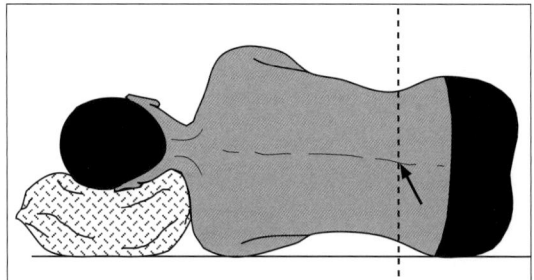

Figure 6.11 Lumbar puncture

Procedure

1) clean the L3-4 area including the iliac crest starting centrally and working outwards

2) infiltrate the skin overlying the L3-4/4-5 interspace with 2% lignocaine and wait a few minutes for it to work

3) insert the spinal 22 gauge needle in the L3-4 interspace horizontally aiming slightly towards the patient's head

4) the spinal needle is advanced slowly but firmly through the interspinous ligaments with the tip aiming for the umbilicus.

5) if the needle cannot be advanced it is likely that bone is encountered. Withdraw the needle partially and start advancing again with the needle parallel with the floor and the tip again pointing toward the umbilicus

6) the needle is advanced a short distance and continually checked until CSF obtained. Care must be taken not to advance the needle too far as it may enter the vertebral vein or disc space

7) if correctly positioned the advancing needle encounters resistance at the ligamentum flavum. After penetrating this ligament there is a sudden release as the needle enters the subarachnoid space

8) then remove the stylet from the needle to see if CSF drains, it usually does this slowly

9) CSF pressure is then measured by attaching a manometer to the needle. Ensure the patient is relaxed by slightly straightening the legs, when the column of CSF stops rising, its height is then measured (opening pressure)

10) CSF is drained from the manometer and from the spinal needle into 3 collection tubes. Approximately 2-3 ml CSF are collected into each tube and sent to the laboratory for cell count, protein, glucose concentrations and bacteriology

11) remove the LP needle and press on the LP site for about 1-2 mins and then apply a small dressing over the site

12) instruct the patient to lie flat for about 2-3 hours preferably prone to reduce the risk of post LP headache

Complications

herniation of brain or spinal cord: this is the most serious consequence of an LP. If during or after an LP the level of consciousness deteriorates or respiration alters or falls, the patient should be placed in the head down position and an infusion of 20% mannitol started. Emergency resuscitation measures should begin including possible surgical decompression.

dry or unsuccessful tap: this usually means that the technique was faulty or the disc space too narrow. In such cases another attempt should be done at either the disc space above or below. If the puncture is still unsuccessful then the LP should be attempted in the sitting position or consult a senior person with neurological or neurosurgical experience

bleeding: the spinal needle is likely to be in a vein so withdraw and try again at a different level

post LP headache: treat symptomatically with NSAIDs. Severe headaches may require a blood patch

infections: these include ABM and epidural abscess and are generally related to poor antisepsis

Interpretation of LP findings

CSF is evaluated under the following main headings *appearance, pressure, microscopy (cells mm³), protein (gms/litre) glucose (mmols/litre)* and *bacteriology* (Table 6.2).

Appearance

The normal CSF is clear and colourless. In meningitis the colour ranges from purulent or cloudy in ABM to mostly clear in viral meningitis. If in doubt the colour of CSF can be compared to water (which is the same as normal CSF) against a background of white sheet of paper when even the slightest opaqueness or yellowness (xanthochromia) in CSF is always abnormal.

Bloody CSF

It is important to distinguish between a traumatic tap and SAH. The following points are helpful. In SAH the CSF remains uniformly blood stained throughout the procedure and the opening pressure is usually elevated. In contrast in traumatic tap the bleeding into the CSF lessens as it flows and pressure is normal. This will have been evident as the CSF leaves the spinal needle and when comparing the 1st and 3rd collection tubes which show a clearing or lessening of blood. Blood in CSF can persist for up to one week but is gradually replaced by bilirubin (xanthochromia) which stays for >2 weeks. A bloody spinal tap will falsely elevate the CSF WCC and protein.

Xanthochromia (yellow discolouration)

This is seen from 24 hours to >2 weeks after a bleed, usually a SAH. It may also be seen in a subdural haematoma, high CSF protein, jaundice and rifampicin treatment.

Pressure

The normal CSF opening pressure in adults is 8-16 cm. The normal CSF pressure should never be over 20 cm water. CSF pressure is elevated in brain swelling in infections (e.g. meningitis), mass lesions, hydrocephalus and trauma. *Suspected elevation in intracranial pressure is the main contraindication to an LP.*

Cell count

The normal CSF contains up to five WBC/ml, either lymphocytes or monocytes. The count may be higher in children. Increased white cells in CSF usually indicate infection until proved otherwise. The presence of predominant neutrophils indicates pyogenic infection, in particular **ABM** and presence of lymphocytes indicates **TBM** or **CM** in HIV or viral infection. However neutrophils can predominate in early **TBM** and in some viral and fungal infections **(CM)** and lymphocytes can predominate in partially treated ABM, particularly in the very young. The presence of a small number of RBCs may be related to the trauma of the LP but if persisting in all 3 samples suggest a CNS source.

Protein

The normal CSF protein is <0.5gm/litre. Elevation in CSF protein is a common abnormality in neurological disorders. Moderate elevations 0.5-1gm/litre suggests infection e.g. meningitis, cerebral malaria, abscess, infarction and tumours whereas a more marked elevations in protein can be a feature of TBM, Guillain Barre Syndrome or spinal block.

Glucose

The normal CSF glucose is >50% blood glucose. *A concurrent blood glucose (ideally fasting) should be checked at the time of the LP.* CSF glucose can be reduced, very low or even absent in CNS infections. Very low or absent glucose is a characteristic of ABM and may also occur in TBM.

Microbiology

Normal CSF is sterile. Gram's stain for bacteria, acid fast stain for TB and India ink stain for cryptococcus are indicated in all suspected cases of meningitis. If India ink is negative then a cryptococcal antigen test (CRAg) should be carried out on all patients in whom the diagnosis of cryptococcal infection is possible. Microbiological screening includes appropriate cultures.

Selected references

Anyangu A, Gould L, Sharif S, Nguku P, Omolo J, Mutonga D et al: *Risk Factors for Severe Rift Valley Fever Infection in Kenya*, 2007. Am. J. Trop. Med. Hyg. 2010; 83:(Suppl2):14–21.

Bhigjee AI, Padayachee R, Paruk H, Hallwirth-Pillay KD, Marais S, Connoly C. *Diagnosis of tuberculous meningitis: clinical and laboratory parameters.* Int J Infect Dis. 2007 Jul;11(4):348-54.

Bicanic T, Harrison TS. *Cryptococcal meningitis.* Br Med Bull. 2004;72:99-118.

Bicanic T, Jarvis JN, Muzoora C, Harrison TS. *Should antiretroviral therapy be delayed for 10 weeks for patients treated with fluconazole for cryptococcal meningitis?* Clin Infect Dis. 2010 Oct 15;51(8):986-7.

Bisson GP, Lukes J, Thakur R, Mtoni I, MacGregor RR. *Cryptococcus and lymphocytic meningitis in Botswana.* S Afr Med J. 2008 Sep;98(9):724-5.

Caron M, Grard G, Paupy C, Mombo IM, Bi Nso B, Roland F et al: *First Evidence of Simultaneous Circulation of Three Different Dengue Virus Serotypes in Africa.* PLOS one: 2013 October; 8:10: e78030

Ergönül O. *Crimean-Congo haemorrhagic fever.* Lancet Infect Dis 2006; 6:203–14.

Farrar JJ, Yen LM, Cook T, Fairweather N, Binh N, Parry J, et al. *Tetanus.* J Neurol Neurosurg Psychiatry. 2000 Sep;69(3):292-301.

Fitch MT, van de Beek D. *Emergency diagnosis and treatment of adult meningitis.* Lancet Infect Dis. 2007 Mar;7(3):191-200.

Garg RK. *Tuberculous meningitis.* Acta Neurol Scand. 2010 Aug 1;122(2):75-90.

Gill G, Beeching N. *Lecture notes on tropical medicine* 6th edition. 2009 Wiley-Blackwell.

Greenberg David, Aminoff Michael & Roger Simon, *Clinical Neurology*, McGraw Hill Fifth edition 2002.

Godlwana L, Gounden P, Ngubo P, Nsibande T, Nyawo K, Puckree T. *Incidence and profile of spinal tuberculosis in patients at the only public hospital admitting such patients in KwaZulu-Natal.* Spinal Cord. 2008 May;46(5):372-4.

Greenwood B. *Pneumococcal meningitis epidemics in Africa.* Clin Infect Dis. 2006 Sep 15;43(6):701-3.

Greenwood BM. *Corticosteroids for acute bacterial meningitis.* N Engl J Med. 2007 Dec 13;357(24):2507-9.

Hemachudha T, Laothamatas J, Rupprecht CE. *Human rabies: a disease of complex neuropathogenetic mechanisms and diagnostic challenges.* Lancet Neurol. 2002 Jun;1(2):101-9.

Jackson A, Hosseinipour MC. *Management of cryptococcal meningitis in sub-saharan Africa.* Curr HIV/AIDS Rep. 2010 Aug;7(3):134-42.

Jarvis JN, Lawn SD, Vogt M, Bangani N, Wood R, Harrison TS. *Screening for cryptococcal antigenemia in patients accessing an antiretroviral treatment program in South Africa.* Clin Infect Dis. 2009 Apr 1;48(7):856-62.

Jarvis JN, Meintjes G, Harrison TS. *Outcomes of cryptococcal meningitis in antiretroviral naive and experienced patients in South Africa.* J Infect. 2010 Jun;60(6):496-8.

Kambugu A, Meya DB, Rhein J, O'Brien M, Janoff EN, Ronald AR, et al. *Outcomes of cryptococcal meningitis in Uganda before and after the availability of highly active antiretroviral therapy.* Clin Infect Dis. 2008 Jun 1;46(11):1694-701.

Kennedy PG. *Viral encephalitis: causes, differential diagnosis, and management.* J Neurol Neurosurg Psychiatry. 2004 Mar;75 Suppl 1: i10-5.

Longley N, Muzoora C, Taseera K, Mwesigye J, Rwebembera J, Chakera A, et al. *Dose response effect of high-dose fluconazole for HIV-associated cryptococcal meningitis in southwestern Uganda.* Clin Infect Dis. 2008 Dec 15;47(12):1556-61.

Makadzange AT, Ndhlovu CE, Takarinda K, Reid M, Kurangwa M, Gona P, et al. *Early versus delayed initiation of antiretroviral therapy for concurrent HIV infection and cryptococcal meningitis in sub-saharan Africa.* Clin Infect Dis. 2010 Jun 1;50(11):1532-8.

Mangal T, Aylward R, Mwanza M, Gasasira A, Abanida E, Pate M et al. *Key issues in the persistence of poliomyelitis in Nigeria: a case-control study.* Lancet Glob Health 2014;2: e90–97

Marais S, Pepper DJ, Schutz C, Wilkinson RJ, Meintjes G. *Presentation and outcome of tuberculous meningitis in a high HIV prevalence setting.* PLoS One. 2011;6(5):e20077.

Marais S, Thwaites G, Schoeman JF, Torok ME, Misra UK, Prasad K, et al. *Tuberculous meningitis: a uniform case definition for use in clinical research.* Lancet Infect Dis. 2010 Nov;10(11):803-12.

Monath TP. *Yellow fever: an update.* The Lancet Infectious Diseases 2001; Vol 1:11-20.

Muzoora CK, Kabanda T, Ortu G, Ssentamu J, Hearn P, Mwesigye J, et al. *Short course amphotericin B with high dose fluconazole for HIV-associated cryptococcal meningitis.* J Infect. 2012 Jan;64(1):76-81.

Nathoo N, Nadvi SS, Narotam PK, van Dellen JR. *Brain abscess: management and outcome analysis of a computed tomography era experience with 973 patients.* World Neurosurg. 2011 May-Jun;75(5-6):716-26; discussion 612-7.

Ogbua O, Ajuluchukwub E and Unekec C. *Lassa fever in West African sub-region: an overview.* J Vect Borne Dis. 2007; 44:1–11.

Sanya EO, Taiwo SS, Olarinoye JK, Aje A, Daramola OO, Ogunniyi A. *A 12-year review of cases of adult tetanus managed at the University College Hospital, Ibadan, Nigeria.* Trop Doct. 2007 Jul;37(3):170-3.

Scarborough M, Thwaites GE. *The diagnosis and management of acute bacterial meningitis in resource-poor settings.* Lancet Neurol. 2008 Jul;7(7):637-48.

Sichizya K, Fieggen G, Taylor A, Peter J. *Brain abscesses--the Groote Schuur experience, 1993-2003.* S Afr J Surg. 2005 Aug;43(3):79-82.

Sloan D, Dlamini S, Dedicoat M. *Management of cryptoccocal meningitis in resource-limited settings: a systematic review.* S Afr Med J. 2009 May;99(5):310-2.

Solomon T. *Exotic and emerging viral encephalitides.* Curr Opin Neurol. 2003 Jun;16(3):411-8.

Stephens DS, Greenwood B, Brandtzaeg P. *Epidemic meningitis, meningococcaemia, and Neisseria meningitidis.* Lancet. 2007 Jun 30;369(9580):2196-210.

Thwaites CL, Farrar JJ. *Preventing and treating tetanus.* BMJ. 2003 Jan 18;326(7381):117-8.

Thwaites CL, Yen LM, Loan HT, Thuy TT, Thwaites GE, Stepniewska K, et al. *Magnesium sulphate for treatment of severe tetanus: a randomised controlled trial.* Lancet. 2006 Oct 21;368(9545):1436-43.

Thwaites GE, Schoeman JF. *Update on tuberculosis of the central nervous system: pathogenesis, diagnosis, and treatment.* Clin Chest Med. 2009 Dec;30(4):745-54, ix.

Timmermans M, Carr J. *Neurosyphilis in the modern era.* J Neurol Neurosurg Psychiatry. 2004 Dec;75(12):1727-30.

Towner J, Sealy T, Khristova M, Albarin C, Conlan S, Reeder S, et al. Newly Discovered Ebola Virus Associated with Hemorrhagic Fever Outbreak in Uganda. Plos Pathogens: 2008; Nov: Vol 4:11: e1000212.

Wajanga BM, Kalluvya S, Downs JA, Johnson WD, Fitzgerald DW, Peck RN. *Universal screening of Tanzanian HIV-infected adult inpatients with the serum cryptococcal antigen to improve diagnosis and reduce mortality: an operational study.* J Int AIDS Soc. 2011 Oct 11;14:40.

Wall EC, Everett DB, Mukaka M, Bar-Zeev N, Feasey N, Jahn A, et al. *Bacterial meningitis in Malawian adults, adolescents, and children during the era of antiretroviral scale-up and haemophilus influenzae type b vaccination, 2000-2012.* Clin Infect Dis. 2014;58(10):137-145.

Whitley RJ, Gnann JW. *Viral encephalitis: familiar infections and emerging pathogens.* Lancet. 2002 Feb 9;359(9305):507-13.

Wilde H, Hemachudha T, Jackson AC. Viewpoint: *Management of human rabies.* Trans R Soc Trop Med Hyg. 2008 Oct;102(10):979-82.

CHAPTER 7
PROTOZOAL AND
HELMINTHIC INFECTIONS

CONTENTS

CHAPTER 7

PROTOZOAL AND HELMINTHIC INFECTIONS

This chapter is concerned with the main protozoal and helminthic infections affecting the nervous system in Africa. These include cerebral malaria, toxoplasmosis, and human African trypanosomiasis (HAT), neurocysticercosis, schistosomiasis and hydatid disease. The student should aim to be familiar with these, including life cycles, clinical presentations, diagnosis, management and prevention.

CEREBRAL MALARIA

Cerebral malaria is a severe neurological disease of the brain that is caused by *Plasmodium falciparum* and is characterized by fever, altered level of consciousness and laboratory evidence of malaria infection. The research definition of cerebral malaria is unrousable coma, (Glasgow coma scale ≤8 or Blantyre coma scale for young children ≤2 (Table 7.2) in the presence of a peripheral parasitaemia after other causes of coma have been excluded.

Epidemiology

Each year there are over 300 million new cases of malaria in Africa resulting in over 1 million deaths there, occurring mostly but not exclusively in children. Cerebral malaria is one of the most important complications. It is invariably fatal without treatment and each year there are over half a million new cases of cerebral malaria in Africa. Most cases occur in non immune children (<5 yrs) and the incidence declines progressively as children become older. Cerebral malaria also occurs in adults but much less frequently. The mortality rate in treated cerebral malaria in children is 15-20% and 10-15% in adults. Recent reports and clinical experience in Africa suggest that the overall burden of severe malaria is decreasing significantly there.

Pathophysiology of cerebral malaria

The mechanism of brain injury in cerebral malaria is not fully understood. The main theories involve parasite sequestration, endothelial dysfunction and injury with cytokine release and blood brain barrier dysfunction. The brain at post mortem in cerebral malaria is typically congested and darkened in colour (Fig 7.1). The histopathology shows many parasitized red blood cells (RBCs) sequestered in the capillaries and small blood vessels particularly in the grey matter and petechial perivascular ring haemorrhages in white matter (Fig 7.1). The sequestration is attributed to cytoadherence or the sticking of parasitized RBCs to vascular endothelium and to rosetting; the sticking of unparasitized RBCs around a parasitized RBC, which in turn may lead to congestion of the capillaries. These findings have led to the mechanical theory of decreased microcirculation or blocked capillaries being a main mechanism. An alternative theory is that sequestration and rupture of trapped parasitized RBCs release many mature malaria parasites, trophozoites and schizonts leading to increased local glucose consumption and massive local release of endotoxins and cytokines. These in turn result in breakdown in the blood brain barrier, increased cerebral blood flow, cerebral oedema and coma.

Pathology

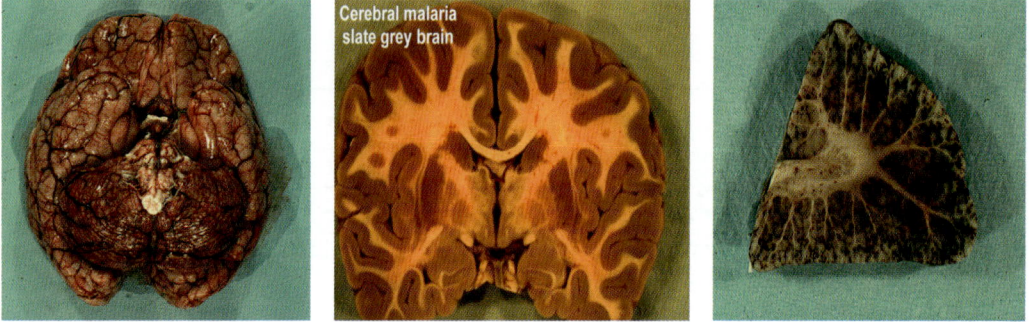

Darkened brain with congestion & haemorrhages

Histopathology   **Microscopy**

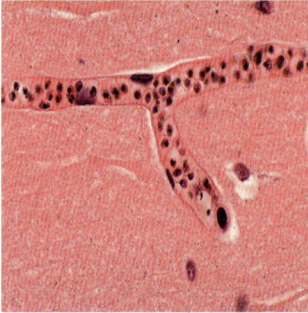 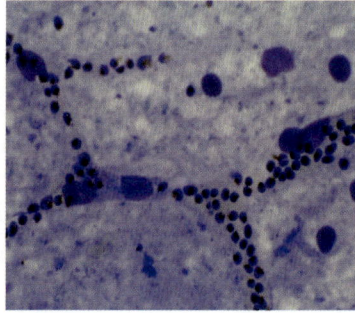 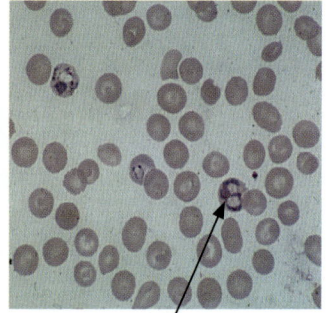

Parasitized red blood cells blocking capillaries   P. Falciparum

Figure 7.1 Brain in Cerebral Malaria (CM)

Clinical features

The first symptoms of cerebral malaria in adults include fever, headache, myalgia, malaise followed by progressive drowsiness, confusion, delirium, stupor and coma. These symptoms usually develop over 1-3 days but may occur in <24 hours. The onset can be relatively sudden with the patient presenting with a febrile illness over hours followed by a generalised seizure and or coma. This is a more common presentation in children and in non immune hosts. Seizures occur in >50% of children and about 20% of adults, either at onset or throughout the course of the illness. In adults the main neurological findings are those of an acute encephalopathy with symmetrical upper motor neurone signs. These include altered level of consciousness, divergent gaze, bruxism (teeth grinding), hypertonia and extensor plantar reflexes. The duration of coma after starting treatment is on average 1-3 days but may persist for longer in adults. Systemic complications include anaemia, acidosis, renal failure, respiratory distress syndrome and secondary bacterial sepsis.

A characteristic malaria retinopathy has recently been described in Malawi occurring in children and also in adults with cerebral malaria (Fig. 7.2). This retinopathy is characterized by areas of retinal whitening best seen immediately around the macula/fovea but sparing it, coupled with white or orange discolouration of some retinal vessels and capillaries. These features are now considered to be specific for cerebral malaria. They are best seen with the direct ophthalmoscope provided that the pupils have been dilated and the examiner is already familiar with them. The more classical fundoscopy findings in cerebral malaria include retinal haemorrhages (<10% of adults) and papilloedema (<1% of adults). Characteristic white centered retinal haemorrhages are found in most children and papilloedema in 10%. These however are not specific for cerebral malaria.

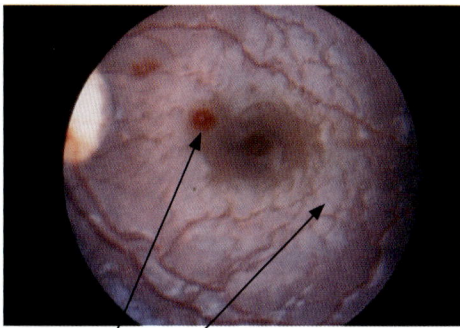

Haemorrhages & whitening around fovea

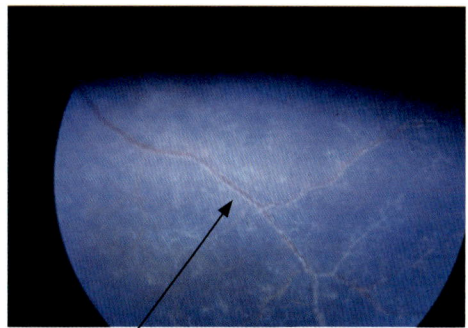

White discolouration of blood vessel wall

Figure 7.2 Retina in CM. *Photographs courtesy of Susan Lewallen Ophthalmology Dept, KCMC*

Differential diagnosis

The high prevalence of asymptomatic parasitaemia may make the diagnosis less certain and therefore other causes of encephalopathy need to be excluded. Infectious causes include acute bacterial meningitis (ABM), partially treated ABM, viral meningoencephalitis including rabies, semi acute presentations of the main HIV related CNS infections including cryptococcal and tuberculous meningitis and toxoplasmosis. Non-infectious causes include metabolic abnormalities, intoxication, epilepsy, stroke and other causes.

Diagnosis of malaria

The diagnosis of cerebral malaria is supported by laboratory evidence of infection. This is usually done by the demonstration of malaria parasites on a peripheral blood slide. A blood slide, usually a thick film is taken first on admission, after the first 24 hours and again at 48 hours. A negative blood slide on admission needs to be repeated if cerebral malaria is still suspected.

Newer methods of diagnosis include rapid diagnostic tests (RDT) which detect parasitic enzymes or antigen in whole blood. Most are sensitive and specific for *P. falciparum* and are very helpful particularly where skilled microscopy is unavailable. RDTs based on antibody detection are of less value clinically as they don't distinguish between old or recent infection and are non specific for falciparum.

A full blood count is frequently normal but may show anaemia especially in children. The presence of leucocytosis and thrombocytopenia usually indicates severe systemic malaria or coexistent sepsis. Hypoglycaemia is common in severe malaria particularly in children and blood glucose should always be regularly checked in cerebral malaria. Other investigations include renal, liver function, coagulation screen, arterial and blood gases. Urine in malaria may rarely be dark or black in colour and an analysis shows red blood cell casts. CSF examination is clear in colour with no increase in cells but may show a slightly elevated opening pressure with a mild elevation in protein. Neuroimaging is typically normal.

Key points

- cerebral malaria is a major cause of death in children <5 yrs
- clinical features include headache, fever, myalgia, altered consciousness & seizures
- symptoms typically progress over 1-3 days
- diagnosis is supported by evidence of malaria parasites in blood
- other causes of encephalopathies need to be excluded

Treatment of cerebral malaria

The treatment of a patient with cerebral malaria is based on specific drug treatment and the early recognition and management of complications. Management of complications includes urgent measures to treat hypoxia, hypoglycaemia, seizures, hypovolaemia, anaemia and acidosis. Because most deaths in cerebral malaria occur within 24 hours of onset, patients should if possible be admitted to a high dependency care area or an intensive care unit and have emergency management. Blood sugar should be checked every 4-6 hours particularly in children because of recurrent hypoglycaemia. Fluids need to be restricted in the first 48 hours, if raised intracranial pressure is suspected. Complicated cases may need intubation, ventilation, exchange transfusion and dialysis if available. A summary of the steps in emergency management of complications is outlined below.

Management of complications of cerebral malaria

- maintain airway with oxygen if hypoxaemic or in respiratory distress
- if high fever present reduce temperature with paracetamol
- correct hypovolaemia in children with NS, infusion @ 2-3 ml/kg/hr ↓
- treat hypoglycaemia with iv bolus one ml/kg of 50% dextrose
- give 5-10% dextrose infusion to all cerebral malaria patients to prevent hypoglycaemia
- control seizures using either diazepam or lorazepam or phenytoin/phenobarbitone
- offer blood transfusion if the haematocrit is <15% in children or <20% in adults
- give fresh whole blood, frozen plasma and vitamin K for spontaneous bleeding
- give first-line antibiotics for possible pyogenic meningitis and sepsis until excluded
- ventilate adults with respiratory distress syndrome and refer for dialysis if in renal failure

Specific drug treatment

The specific drug treatment of cerebral malaria includes the artemisinin compounds and quinine (Table 7.1). Recent studies in severe malaria show that parenteral artemisinin compounds are superior to quinine; they are easier to administer, better tolerated with no major side effects and have a better outcome. Intravenous artesunate was shown to be more potent than quinine (35% greater reduction in mortality rate) in treating cerebral malaria in adults in Vietnam. It is also more potent than artemether, possibly because of a more rapid effect. Parenteral artesunate is now the drug of first choice in the treatment of cerebral malaria in Africa.

Meanwhile quinine is still being used for the treatment of cerebral malaria in many countries in Africa and its use should never be delayed if artemisinins are unavailable. The main side effects of quinine are cinchonism (tinnitus, deafness, dizziness, nausea and vomiting), cardiac depression, hypotension, hypoglycaemia, blindness and very rarely blackwater fever. Quinine should also be used cautiously in patients with heart disease and in the elderly. In adults a loading dose of 20 mg/kg is given iv over 2-4 hours and then continued by iv infusion at 10 mg/kg/8 hourly for 5 days or until able to take orally. After 3 days of iv treatment the dose can be reduced from 8 to 12 hourly. Intramuscular quinine administered according to instructions can be used if iv route is not possible.

Table 7.1 Drug treatment of cerebral malaria

Drug	route	Dose loading	Dose maintenance	Duration
artesunate	iv	2.4 mg/kg	2.4 mg/kg/ @ 12 and 24 hours & then daily	7 days
or				
artemether	im	3.2 mg/kg	1.6 mg/kg/daily	5 days
or				
quinine dihydrochloride	iv	20 mg/kg (max 1400 mg) over 4 hours in 5% dextrose or dextrose/saline	10 mg/kg/8 hourly*	5 days

* infused over four hours in adults & changed to oral as soon as the patient can swallow

Prognosis in Cerebral Malaria (CM)

The mortality rate in quinine and artemisinin treated children with cerebral malaria in Africa is 15-20%. Mortality rates are lower <10%, in both artemisinin and quinine treated adult patients. However mortality rates in pregnancy are up to 50%. Risk factors for death in cerebral malaria in adults include anaemia, seizures, respiratory distress syndrome and renal failure. Prolonged and deep coma, elevated intracranial pressure and hypoglycaemia are risk factors in children. While the majority of patients make a full recovery from treated cerebral malaria, permanent neurological deficits still occur in >20% of children and <5% adults. Deficits including psychoses, ataxias are usually transient and clear within weeks or months. Gross neurological deficits occur in about 10% of children, these include, hemiparesis, quadriparesis, cerebellar ataxia, and severe brain damage. Neurocognitive and behavioural dysfunction are also more common occurring in >20% and epilepsy occurs in about 10%. Hemiparesis is the main deficit in adults.

Key points

- parenteral artemisinin is superior to quinine in treatment of cerebral malaria
- mortality in treated children is 15-20% and <10% in adults
- morbidity occurs in >20% of children and <5% adults
- morbidity (children), neurological & cognitive deficits, behavioural abnormalities & epilepsy
- hemiparesis is most frequent complication in adults

Table 7.2 Blantyre coma scale*

To obtain coma score add the scores from each section**	
Best motor response	
Localizes painful stimulus	2
Withdraws limb from painful stimulus	1
No or inappropriate response	0
Best verbal response	
Cries or speaks appropriately with painful or verbal stimuli	2
Moans or abnormal cry to painful stimulus	1
No vocal response to painful stimulus	0
Eye Movements	
Watches or follows e.g. mother's face	1
Fails to watch or follow	0

* for use in children
** Score ≤2 & a positive blood slide suggests cerebral malaria

TOXOPLASMOSIS

Introduction

Toxoplasmosis is caused by infection with *Toxoplasma gondii*. T. gondii is an intracellular protozoan parasite whose definitive host is the cat. Humans and other animals may become infected accidentally from infected cats via ingestion of food or water contaminated with cat faeces. Transmission in Africa is most probably from ingestion of undercooked meat of infected animals. Human infection occurs mostly during childhood and antibody seroprevalence rates are a measure of latent infection. Worldwide seroprevalence rates vary from 20% to 75% and a similar pattern occurs in Africa varying from 27% in Uganda to 75% in Nigeria. Nearly all toxoplasmosis illnesses in Africa are caused by reactivation of latent infection in HIV related immunosuppression. Cerebral toxoplasmosis or toxoplasma encephalitis (TE) is the main form of the disease resulting from reactivation. The frequency of cerebral toxoplasmosis in HIV varies within Africa, depending on the local pattern of latent infection. In one major HIV autopsy study in West Africa, evidence of cerebral toxoplasmosis was present in15% and was considered the main cause of death in 10%. Toxoplasmosis is considered to be the most common cause of a focal brain lesion in AIDS patients in most parts of Africa.

Clinical presentation

Clinically patients present sub acutely over days or more commonly 1 or 2 weeks with headache and fever often in combination with focal neurological signs. Focal neurological signs occur in around three quarters of patients and include hemiparesis, cranial nerve palsies, ataxia, confusion, altered consciousness and seizures. The pattern of neurologic signs will depend on the site of the focal lesion within the brain and its duration. There may be associated toxoplasma chorioretinitis in 5-10% of affected patients. Cerebral toxoplasmosis occurs mainly in patients with a CD4 count of <100 cells/mm³ and is frequently the first presenting complaint of HIV infection.

Diagnosis

Laboratory investigations are of limited value in the diagnosis. A positive serological screening test for toxoplasmosis usually indicates previous exposure rather than active disease. However a negative result does not exclude the disease. The CSF is also non diagnostic showing predominantly lymphocytes with an elevated protein and a modest decrease in glucose. CT scan of the head with contrast is very helpful for the diagnosis. In cerebral toxoplasmosis, it shows a single or more commonly multiple ring-enhancing lesions with surrounding oedema situated usually in the basal ganglia or/and at the junction of the grey white matter in the cortex (Fig 7.3).

CT (with contrast) **Pathology** **Histopathology**

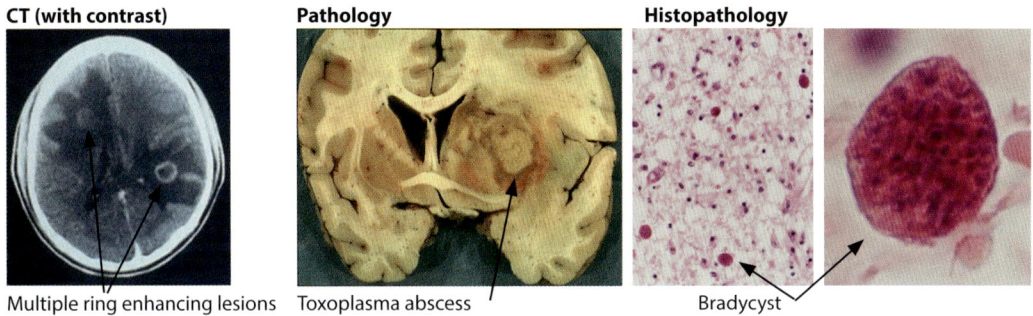

Multiple ring enhancing lesions   Toxoplasma abscess   Bradycyst

Figure 7.3 Brain in toxoplasmosis

Differential diagnosis

The differential diagnosis of cerebral toxoplasmosis includes other causes of focal neurological disorders in HIV disease, including tuberculoma, primary CNS lymphoma, and rarely progressive multifocal leucoencephalopathy (PML). Other HIV related infections including cryptococcal and TB meningitis may also need to be considered. The clinical presentation of tuberculoma can be very similar to that of cerebral toxoplasmosis, although the clinical course in tuberculoma is usually slower and there may be evidence of concomitant TB elsewhere e.g. chest X-ray. CT features of tuberculoma in adults are those of a single or multiple ring enhancing lesions, with irregular walls of varying thickness and surrounding oedema situated mainly in the cortex. Primary CNS lymphoma is relatively uncommon in HIV in Africa occurring in <1% of HIV patients. The CT in lymphoma may be similar to toxoplasmosis and shows ring enhancing lesions in the deep white matter near the corpus callosum or subependymal areas. In the absence of a CT scan empirical treatment for toxoplasmosis should be started in all HIV patients presenting with focal neurological signs and CD4 count <200 cells/mm³.

Key points

- toxoplasmosis is the most common cause of focal brain lesion in AIDS
- occurs mostly in patients with CD4<100 mm³
- clinical features include headache, fever & focal neurological signs over days or weeks
- diagnosis supported by ring enhancing lesions on CT brain scan
- differential diagnosis includes tuberculoma & lymphoma

Treatment

Treatment is based on drugs that interfere with the ability of *T. gondii* to synthesise folate and replicate. High dose trimethoprim/sulphamethoxazole (TMP-SMX) is the recommended first line treatment for cerebral toxoplasmosis in Africa (Table 7.3). The dose is one TMP-SMX tablet (80/400 mg) for each 8 kg body weight, taken in two or three divided doses per day. For the average adult this is usually 4 tablets, (1920 mg) twice daily for four weeks, followed by two tablets twice daily for another 8 weeks. Long term secondary prophylaxis with two tablets daily is indicated if the CD4 count is <200/cm^3 and should be considered for all patients with CD4 counts < 350 cells/cm^3. A clinical response to treatment is usually seen within 3-4 days of starting treatment and definite improvement after 2-3 weeks in over 80% of patients. If there is inadequate or no response to treatment, then other diagnoses other than toxoplasmosis should be considered including tuberculoma. Relapses should be retreated with full course (TMP-SMX). Patients who are intolerant of TMP-SMX because of drug rash or neutropenia can be treated with pyrimethamine 50-75 mg daily in combination with clindamycin 600 mg 8 hourly or azithromycin 1 gram daily. These are continued for a total of 6 weeks. Limiting side effects include drug rashes and bone marrow depression. Folinic acid 15 mg daily should be prescribed with pyrimethamine.

Prognosis

The mortality in Africa in treated cases of cerebral toxoplasmosis is 10-15% mainly because of late disease and co-morbidity in HIV disease. Relapse rates are considered to be in the order of 20%, occurring up to 6 months after successful treatment. Antiretroviral therapy (ART) should be started within two weeks of starting treatment for suspected or proven toxoplasmosis.

Key points

- treatment is with high dose TMP-SMX for 4/52 & maintenance dose for 8/52
- long term chemoprophylaxis should continue until CD4 is >350 cm3
- ART should start within two weeks of starting treatment
- case fatality rate in treated cases is 10-15%

Table 7.3 Drug treatment for toxoplasmosis

Drug	Dose/route	Duration	Side effects
trimethoprim/sulphamethoxazole (TMP-SMX)			
treatment phase	4 tab (1920 mg) /po/ twice daily	4 weeks	rash, neutropenia
maintenance phase	2 tab/po/twice daily	8 weeks	
chemoprophylaxis phase	2 tab/po/ daily	until CD4 >350/cm3	

HUMAN AFRICAN TRYPANOSOMIASIS (HAT)

This is a protozoan parasitic infection caused by parasites of the ***Trypanosoma brucei,*** which are transmitted to humans by the bite of the tsetse fly (*Glossina* spp) (Fig 7.4). Human African trypanosomiasis (HAT), better known as sleeping sickness, is restricted to the distribution of tsetse flies in a vast area throughout sub-Saharan Africa (Fig 7.4). It stretches from 14° north to 20° south latitude, putting a total of over 60 million people in 36 countries at risk. HAT occurs in both epidemic and endemic forms. There are two main types of HAT with differences in epidemiology, biology and clinical features: ***Trypanosoma brucei rhodesiense*** **(T.b.r.)** affects eastern and parts of southern Africa with savannah bush with game animals and cattle as its main reservoir. It accounts for fewer than **5%** of reported cases and causes an acute illness. ***Trypanosoma brucei gambiense*** (**T.b.g.**) affects Central and West African river and water hole areas with humans as its main reservoir; it accounts for over **95%** of all cases and causes a chronic illness. In Uganda both types of HAT occur, indicating local geographical overlap between **Tbr** and **Tbg** infections. The people most at risk live in rural areas and depend on agriculture, fishing, animal husbandry and hunting in African rivers and waterhole areas. HAT has re-emerged during the last decades as a threat to public health in those affected areas. Precise details of disease prevalence are difficult to ascertain. It is estimated that around 300,000 people in Africa are infected with most of those occurring in Southern Sudan and the Democratic Republic of Congo (DRC). Of those approximately 40,000 cases are reported annually to WHO.

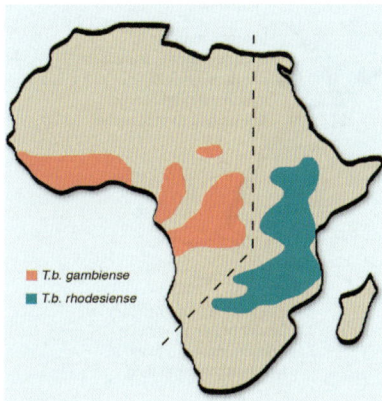

Main sleeping sickness areas in Africa   Tsetse fly

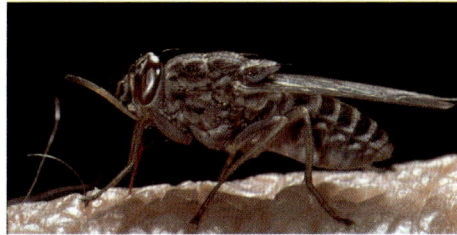

Figure 7.4 Map of trypanosomiasis distribution in Africa

Key points

- thousands cases of HAT or sleeping sickness occur annually in Africa
- HAT is transmitted by tsetse fly bites & people most at risk live in rural areas
- two main types, T. b. r in E. & S. Africa and T. b. g in C. & W. Africa
- wild animals and cattle are the main reservoirs of infection in E. & S. Africa
- infected humans are the main reservoir in C. & W. Africa

Clinical features

Tsetse flies acquire the infection by feeding on infected humans **(Tbg)**, wild animals or domestic cattle **(Tbr)**. The disease can also be transmitted vertically from mother-to-child and occasional accidental infections have occurred in the laboratory, mostly from needle stick injuries. The tsetse fly becomes infective approximately 3-5 weeks after biting an infected animal or human and later may transmit the trypanosomes to humans by biting. HAT may begin in humans at the site of the bite, as a painful indurated erythematous boil-like lesion or **primary chancre**. The primary chancre starts 3-15 days after the bite increasing to a couple of centimetres in size over the following 2-3 weeks. It usually does not suppurate and then slowly clears leaving a mark on the skin. Primary chancre formation occurs in less than half of cases of T.b.r. cases and is uncommon in T.b.g. The trypanosomes multiply at the chancre site, then invade the blood stream and lymph nodes and may eventually cross the blood–brain barrier and infect the brain. This invasion gives rise to two characteristic clinical stages, the early or **haemolymphatic stage** and the late, or **encephalitic stage**. T.b.g infection is characterised by distinct stages, a long asymptomatic phase followed by a sub acute illness and a chronic, late encephalitic stage, with the whole illness lasting up to 3 years or more before death in untreated cases. T.b.r infection presents with a more acute illness and less distinct stages with 80% of deaths occurring within 6 months of onset in untreated cases. The life cycle is outlined below in Figure 7.5.

Sleeping Sickness, African (African trypanosomiasis)
(Trypanosoma brucei gambiense)
(Trypanosoma brucei rhodesiense)

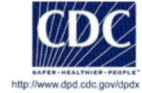

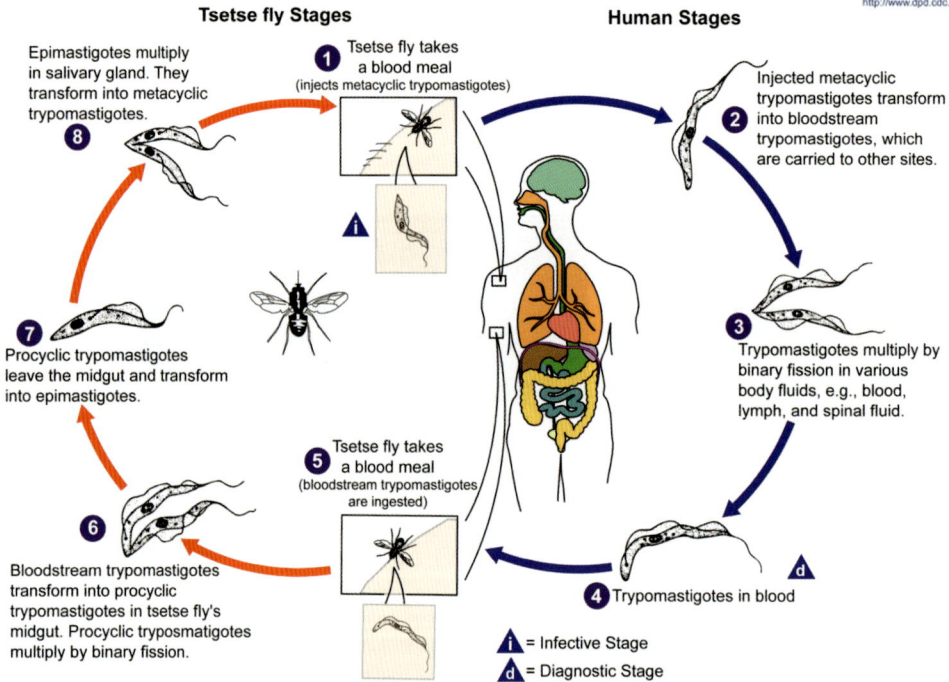

Tsetse fly Stages

Human Stages

8 Epimastigotes multiply in salivary gland. They transform into metacyclic trypomastigotes.

1 Tsetse fly takes a blood meal (injects metacyclic trypomastigotes)

i

2 Injected metacyclic trypomastigotes transform into bloodstream trypomastigotes, which are carried to other sites.

7 Procyclic trypomastigotes leave the midgut and transform into epimastigotes.

3 Trypomastigotes multiply by binary fission in various body fluids, e.g., blood, lymph, and spinal fluid.

5 Tsetse fly takes a blood meal (bloodstream trypomastigotes are ingested)

6 Bloodstream trypomastigotes transform into procyclic trypomastigotes in tsetse fly's midgut. Procyclic trypomastigotes multiply by binary fission.

4 Trypomastigotes in blood   d

i = Infective Stage
d = Diagnostic Stage

Figure 7.5 Life cycle for trypanosomiasis

Haemolymphatic stage

The onset is variable but usually occurs 1-3 weeks after the bite. Irregular episodes of fever lasting 1-7 days occur together with generalised lymphadenopathy. Palpable lymph nodes in the cervical triangle of the neck are called **Winterbottom's sign** (Fig. 7.6). Early associated symptoms include headache, joint pains, weakness and weight loss. Systemic involvement may then occur with multiple organs affected. In **T.b.r** this is characterised by fevers, pleural and pericardial effusions, myocarditis, hepatosplenomegaly, jaundice, anaemia and endocrine disorders. This stage in **T.b.r** can be fatal within weeks or more commonly progresses to the late encephalitic stage. In **T.b.g**, this early stage is usually less pronounced and more chronic and is characterised by hepatosplenomegaly and skin involvement. It may last many months to a couple of years before progressing on to the late or encephalitis stage.

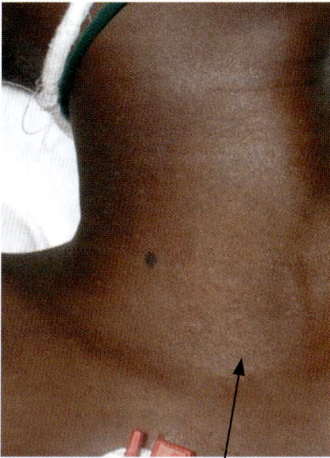

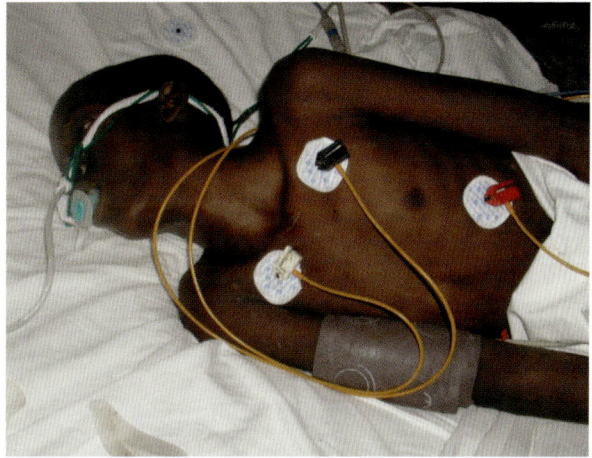

Winterbottom's sign (enlarged lymph glands)   Encephalitic stage (late)

Figure 7.6 Clinical findings in trypanosomiasis

Encephalitic stage

After the haemolymphatic stage, HAT may remain quiet until invasion of the CNS takes place. There is not always a clear recognisable transition from early to late stage disease. In **T.b.r**. disease this occurs within weeks or months of onset, whereas in **T.b.g** disease the late stage takes months or years to develop. The onset of encephalitis is often subtle and unnoticed and neurological presentations are variable. These can be generally grouped into behavioural and psychiatric symptoms, motor, sensory disorders and sleep disorders all of which may overlap. Behavioural and psychiatric presentations vary from irritability, headache, personality and habit change, to agitation, psychosis and mania with confusion and sleep. Accompanying motor signs include limb tremors, incoordination, dysarthria, involuntary movements, pyramidal and extra pyramidal findings. Sensory complaints include pruritus, painful hyperaesthesia and polyneuritis. The sleep disturbances include undue tiredness and an uncontrollable urge to sleep during the day time accompanied sometimes by insomnia at night. Untreated the disease eventually progresses to immobility, seizures, continuous sleep, coma and eventually death (Fig. 7.6). Late stage neurological features may not be seen in **T.b.r** as coma and death may intervene.

Diagnosis

HAT is diagnosed in Africa on the basis of characteristic clinical findings in a patient coming from an endemic area and confirmed by laboratory investigations. Other causes of febrile diseases especially malaria, HIV and TB need to be considered. Routine laboratory investigations may show a mild anaemia and elevated erythrocyte sedimentation rate (ESR). The laboratory diagnosis of HAT is dependent on showing evidence of infection either by direct visualization of trypanosomes by microscope or by serological detection of antibody to trypanosomes in blood and csf (Fig. 7.7). Direct visualization of trypanosomes in blood is usually successful in the haemolymphatic stage of **T.b.r** because of the continuous parasitaemia, whereas it is difficult in **T.b.g** because of low or intermittent parasitaemia. Chancre aspiration and lymph node aspirate may be helpful when these are negative. Concentration methods including centrifugation are used to detect low levels of parasitaemia. The methods of direct visualization involve examining the peripheral blood, the buffy coat, csf or rarely bone marrow for evidence of motile trypanosomes on a wet preparation or on Giemsa stain. In general the longer the duration of the illness the more difficult it is to find the organisms and the tests may have to be repeated in suspected cases more than once. The test of choice in suspected **T.b.g** infection is the antibody-detecting card agglutination trypanosomiasis test (CATT) which is easy to perform and widely available in endemic areas. Limitations include decreased sensitivity (87-98%) and specificity (93-95%).

CSF examination

It is critical to determine whether or not there is encephalitic involvement because to miss it and not to treat it results in the death of the patient. An LP is therefore indicated when encephalitis is clinically suspected and also in all cases of CATT positive tests as there are no reliable criteria for detecting exclusive early stage disease. It is performed only after one or two doses of suramin or pentamidine have been given in order to reduce the risk of parasites inadvertently entering the CSF from blood during the procedure. Direct evidence of encephalitis includes finding trypanosomes in centrifuged CSF either by direct visualization or by serology in the case of **T.b.g.** (Fig 7.7). Indirect evidence according to WHO includes lymphocytes >5 per ml and a raised protein in the CSF, although a cut off at a higher level of lymphocytes >20 per ml has been proposed to increase its diagnostic specificity. CT of brain is non diagnostic but may show non specific white matter changes and ventricular enlargement in long standing disease.

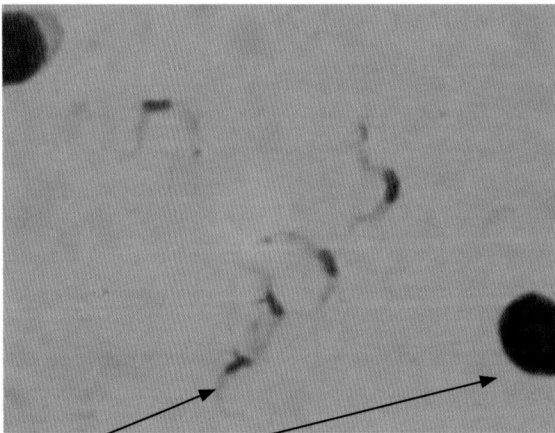

Trypanosomes and lymphocytes

Figure 7.7 CSF in trypanosomiasis

Key points

- HAT occurs in two stages, haemolymphatic & encephalitic
- diagnosis: finding typical clinical & lab findings in pts from endemic area
- HAT confirmed by microscopy in T.b.r & by serology & microscopy in T.b.g
- LP indicated if encephalitis is suspected & in all CATT positive persons
- LP is done only after 1-2 doses of suramin or pentamidine

Treatment

The treatment of HAT is complex and toxic and must be closely monitored (Table 7.4). It is determined by the stage of the disease and whether it is ***T.b.r*** or ***T.b.g***. The early haemolymphatic stage of ***T.b.r.*** is treated with ***iv suramin*** and of ***T.b.g.*** with ***im pentamidine***. Allergy with suramin is uncommon (<1%) but can be fatal and a test dose is always administered before using it for treatment. Associated nephrotoxicity is usually reversible. This treatment is usually successful if the disease is confined to this stage. The late encephalitic stage of ***T.b.r*** and ***T.b.g.*** is treated with ***iv melarsoprol***. This is usually preceded by 1-2 doses of suramin to clear peripheral trypanosomes. In ***T.b.r melarsoprol*** is usually administered as a series of 3-4 cycles of 3 consecutive daily injections (Table 7.4) with a 7 day rest period between each cycle. The main danger is an acute reactive encephalopathy which occurs in 5-10% of treated patients, a half of whom die because of the drug, therefore just giving melarsoprol therapy has an overall fatality rate of 2.5-5%. *A new shorter 10 day course of iv melarsaprol at 2.2 mg/kg/daily may be effective for* ***T.b.g.*** Resistance to melarsoprol has recently been reported from the DRC. The concomitant use of steroids is controversial but there is evidence that their use may decrease the chance of developing the post-treatment encephalopathy particularly in ***T.b.g***. One steroid regime is dexamethasone 30 mg iv stat, and 15 mg q 6 hourly or prednisolone 1mg/kg po daily starting before the first dose and continuing through the last dose. ***Eflornithine (DFMO,)*** is a safer therapy than melarsoprol for late stage HAT but is only effective for disease caused by ***T.b.g.***, being ineffective in the East African disease, ***T.b.r***. However eflornithine is expensive and requires 2 weeks of continuous iv drug treatment in hospital. A combination of ***eflornithine infusion,*** for 7 days and the drug ***nifurtimox*** orally, for 10 days has been recently introduced (2009) and now appears to be effective primary therapy for ***T.b.g***. It is not effective against ***T.b.r***.

Table 7.4 Drug treatment of human African trypanosomiasis

Drug	Type	Stage	Route	Dose/duration	Side effects
Suramin	T. b rhodesiense	Stage 1	iv	(5mg/kg test dose slowly iv on day 1). 20 mg/kg/iv (max 1 gm) on days 1,3, 5, 12, 19 & 26	allergy, anaphylaxis, renal failure, neurologic effects
Pentamidine	T. b gambiense	Stage 1	im	4 mg/kg im/od/ for 7–10 days	nephrotoxicity, hypoglycaemia low BP, site pain. nausea, leucopoenia
Melarsoprol (Mel B)	T. b rhodesiense & T. b gambiense	Stage 2	iv	3.6* mg/kg/od for 3 day cycles (series of 3-4 cycles)	acute reactive encephalopathy, neuropathy, diarrhoea and rash
Eflornithine	T. b gambiense	Stage 2	iv	100 mg/kg iv q 6hourly for 14 days in diluted normal saline/infused over 2 hours	leucopoenia, anaemia, diarrhoea and convulsions
Nifurtimox	T. b gambiense	Stage 1	po	15mg/kg /po/daily (5mg, 8 hourly) for 10 days	nausea, vomiting, abdominal pain, seizures, agitation tremor (neuropathy)

* different treatment schedules with doses ranging from 1.2 to 3.6 mg/kg/daily (in 3 divided doses) for consecutive 3 day cycles administered by slow iv injection, using a glass syringe and avoid leakage as it causes tissue necrosis. Total series of 3 to 4 cycles with a 7 day rest period between each cycle (see WHO recommendations),

Key points

- Rx of early stage in **T.b.r.** is with suramin & in **T.b.g** is with pentamidine
- Rx of encephalitic stage in **T.b.r.** & **T.b.g** is melarsoprol or **T.b.g** eflornithine
- Rx of early & late stage **T.b.g** is with eflornithine & nifurtimox
- encephalopathy occurs in 5-10% of patients treated with melarsaprol
- 50% of patients with melarsaprol encephalopathy die

Prognosis

HAT is invariably fatal if untreated. It has been estimated that 20-30% of affected persons in endemic areas in Africa may die even with treatment either because of late diagnosis or inadequate treatment. The rate of relapse after treatment for the encephalitic stage is up to 20%. LPs are necessary every 6 months to confirm cure which cannot be assumed until after a 2 year follow up.

Prevention

HAT in Central and West Africa is prevented by active case finding through systematic community screening and passive clinical case finding and the treatment of all infected persons. In East Africa HAT is controlled by avoiding being bitten and by vector control through fly trapping and the clearing of riverine tsetse habitat.

Key points

- overall mortality in trypanosomiasis is high
- follow up is necessary after treated encephalitic stage and relapse is common
- prevention in **T.b.g** is by active case screening & passive case treatment
- prevention in **T.b.r** is by avoiding tsetse bites & by vector control

Table 7.5 Summary

	Gambiense (T.b.g)	**Rhodesiense (T.b.r)**
location	Central & West Africa	East Africa
reservoir	humans	cattle & wild animals
clinical presentation	sub-acute/chronic	acute
diagnosis	CATT/lymph node/CSF	blood film/CSF
management	pentamidine/eflornithine & nifurtimox	suramin/melarsoprol
control/prevention	case finding & treatment	avoid tsetse bites/vector habitat control

NEUROCYSTICERCOSIS

Neurocysticercosis arises from the larvae of the pork tapeworm *Taenia solium*. This tape worm is endemic in large parts of the world including large parts of Africa (Fig 7.8). It is estimated that over 50 million people worldwide are infected with cysticerci and it accounts for over 50,000 deaths annually. As many as 20 million persons in Africa may be infected. Around 10-40% of infected persons develop seizures and it is responsible for up to 30% of late onset epilepsy in endemic areas. It is the most common parasitic infection causing disease of the nervous system.

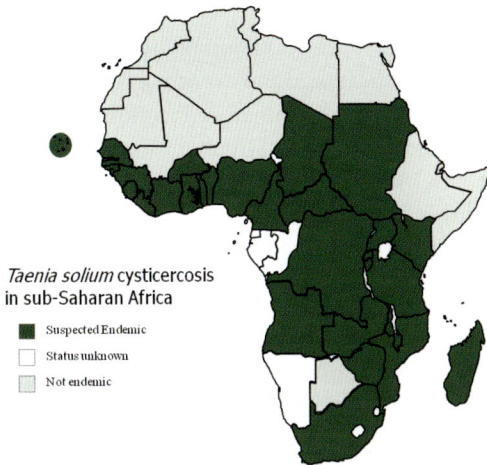

Figure 7.8 Map of cysticercosis distribution in Africa

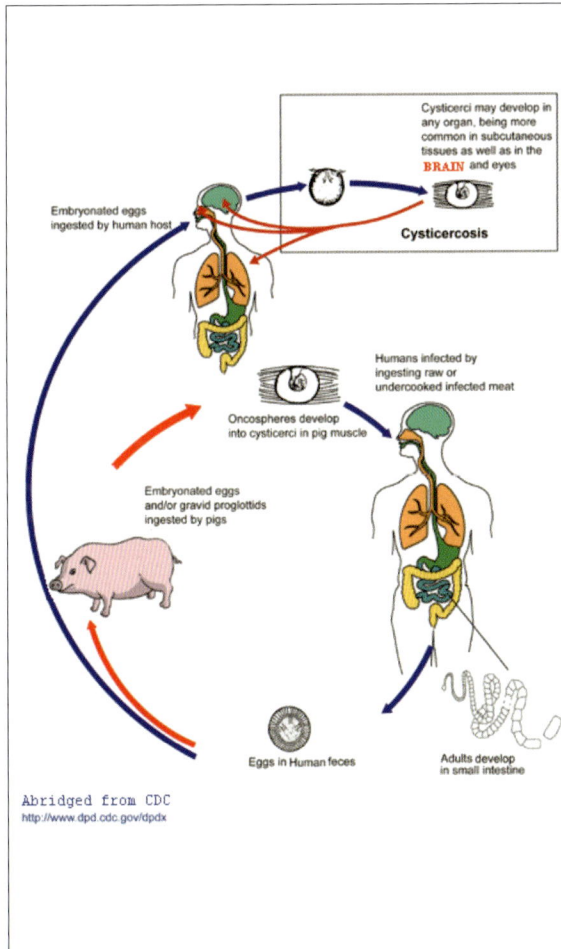

Life cycle

Humans are the definitive hosts of the 2-4 meters long tapeworm that excretes viable ova in the stool. The pig is the intermediate host. Following ingestion of human faeces by the pig, ova migrate mainly to the pig's muscles and become larvae or cysticerci. Humans eat undercooked and measly pork containing the viable larvae. The life cycle is then complete when the larvae develop into an adult tapeworm in the small intestine of humans (Fig 7.9). However when humans accidentally become the intermediate host by ingestion of the ova through faecal-oral contamination from someone else's faeces or their own, the larval form may migrate and develop into cysts either in human brain or other organs, mainly muscles skin and eye. The most frequent source of ova is a symptom free tapeworm carrier in the household. Vegetarians and non pork eaters may thus acquire cysticercosis. About 15-25% of patients with neurocysticercosis will either have a past history of tapeworm or harbour a live one.

Figure 7.9 Life cycle cysticercosis

Pathology

Once in the brain, the mature larvae live dormant for 2-6 yrs and occasionally for 10 years or longer. These are known as cysticerci. They expand to 1-2 cms in size and eventually die causing the wall of the cyst to break down resulting in an intense local inflammatory reaction and later calcification. This cycle of pathology is responsible for the main clinical presentations including seizures. The clinical findings will depend on the site, number and stage of cysticerci. They occur in many tissues in particular, skin, muscle and brain. Typical skeletal muscles involved are those of the limbs and back. The main sites within the brain are the cortex, ventricles and subarachnoid space and infrequently the spinal cord.

Clinical Features

The most common clinical feature of neurocysticercosis is single or repeated seizures. These occur in >90% of cases. In endemic countries, including large parts of rural Africa neurocysticercosis is the most common cause of acquired epilepsy in adults. The cysts may infrequently cause focal neurological disorders; these include hemiparesis, hydrocephalus due to intraventricular cysts and rarely paraplegia (5%) due to spinal cord disease. The finding of hydrocephalus and raised intracranial pressure are an indication for shunting. There may also be evidence of cysts outside the CNS mainly in skin, muscle and eye (1-3%).

Diagnosis

The diagnosis is made mainly by a high index of clinical suspicion in a patient suffering from epilepsy coming from an endemic area. The diagnosis is supported by the finding of radiological evidence of cysts in muscle or brain. A radiograph of shoulder or thigh muscles may reveal typical calcifications following the planes of muscle fibres (Fig 7.10). A CT of head shows evidence of neurocysticerci (Fig 7.10), in particular their number, location and activity. However MRI is necessary to show intraventricular cysts or the racemose variety. The racemose variety of neurocysticercosis is seen on MRI as multiple thin walled cysts with the same signal as CSF and no central scolex (Fig 7.10). On CT cysts appear as small isolated or multiple lesions at the grey white matter junction or widespread throughout the brain. During this dormant phase after contrast, they appear as hypo dense cysts with little enhancement and a visible dot like central scolex (Fig 7.10). This is diagnostic of neurocysticercosis. In the later mature or dying cyst phase, they appear as ring enhancing cysts surrounded by an area of oedema. Older cysts may calcify and there may be hydrocephalus (Fig 7.10). Serological testing should be used together with results from neuroimaging to help establish the diagnosis. These include ELISA and enzyme immunosorbent/blot/assay tests on both serum and CSF. The tests may be negative in isolated cysts, but are usually positive where there are multiple cysts. However newer antigen and antibody based serological tests appear more sensitive to detect both active and inactive disease. The CSF is abnormal in about half the cases with elevation in white cells and protein. There may be an associated eosinophilia early on and also evidence of tape worm infection with eggs in the patient's stool in <20% of patients.

Treatment

The main indication for treatment is active parenchymal CNS disease. The suggested treatment for cysts is albendazole 15 mg/kg po daily for 10-28 days, although a higher dose of 30 mg/kg po daily has been used in patients with subarachnoid cysts. An alternative but less effective treatment is praziquantel 25mg/kg/po three times daily for 14-21 days (Table 7.6). There is controversy over the benefits and duration of treatment which ranges from 7 days to 3 months

X-ray thigh

CT head

CT head (with contrast)

Cysts in muscle

Old calcified cysts

Dying cyst & surrounding oedema

CT head (with contrast)

MRI T1(with contrast

Multiple cysts with central scolex & hydrocephalus

Racemose cysts

Pathology

Cysticercosis
(Racemose)

Histopathology

Multiple cysts in brain

Inflammation around cysts

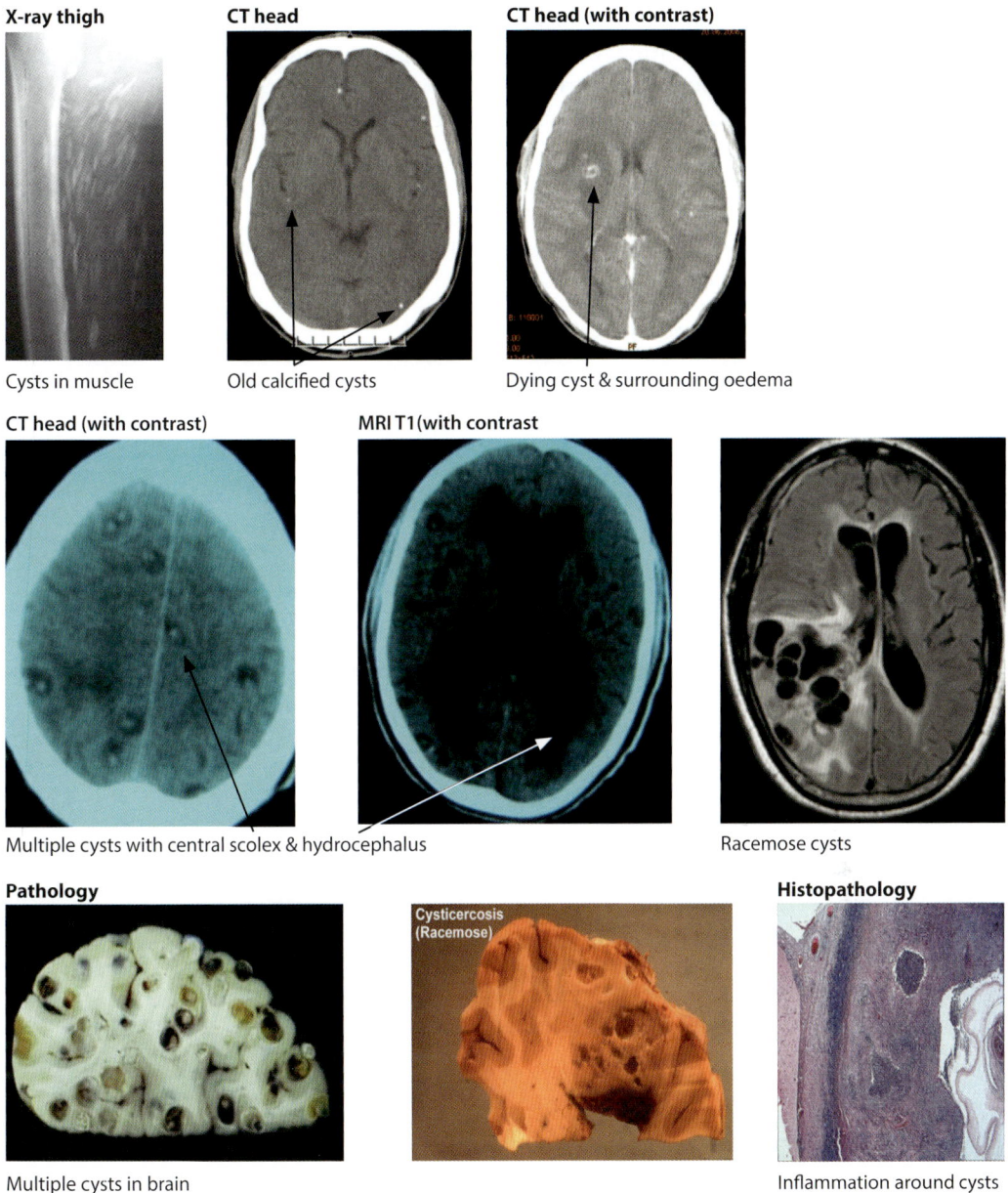

Figure 7.10 Muscle and brain in cysticercosis

or longer. In general the greater the cyst burden the longer the course of treatment. Cimetidine 400 mg tds given concurrently increases available blood levels of both anti parasitic drugs. Side effects of anti parasitic drug treatment include seizures, headaches and muscle enlargement. By starting treatment more cysts may die or die more quickly thereby causing more inflammation, oedema and consequently more headaches, seizures and sometimes encephalopathy.

This risk can be decreased by prescribing steroids. This is in the form of dexamethasone 0.4 mg/kg/po/daily (24 mg) or prednisolone 60 mg daily during active treatment. This is started either a few days before or at the start of antiparasitic drug treatment and continued for at least 7 days throughout the treatment course or as long as symptoms e.g. headache persists. The presence of subarachnoid, intraventricular and too many intracerebral cysts are a relative contraindication to antiparasitic drugs because of danger of fatal encephalopathy. Neurosurgery in particular a shunt may be indicated for obstructive hydrocephalus which is mostly due to intraventricular forms of cysts blocking the ventricles. Seizures can be controlled with standard antiepileptic medications. The outlook in a single symptomatic cyst is excellent. However, the more malignant forms presenting with neurological deficits and coma have a grave prognosis with CFR of >50%.

Table 7.6 Drug treatment of Neurocysticercosis

Drug	route	Dose
albendazole or	po	15 mg/kg/daily for 10-28 days
praziquantel	po	25 mg/kg/tds for 14-21days
&		
dexamethasone or	po	8 mg/tds for >7 days
prednisolone	po	60 mg/daily for >7 days

Prevention

Neurocysticercosis is a largely preventable infectious disease. The main strategies for prevention include hygiene measures to interrupt direct person to person transmission. This involves potentially mass human chemotherapy to eliminate the tapeworm stage, improved human sanitation i.e. safe faeces disposal, pig husbandry and meat inspection.

Key points

- man is the definitive host of Taenia solium & excretes ova in faeces
- neurocysticercosis develops when humans ingest ova from human faeces
- epilepsy is the most common clinical manifestation
- diagnosis supported by serology & X-rays showing cysts in muscle & brain
- treatment is with albendazole 2-4/52 & steroids 1-4/52
- prevention: personal hygiene & mass Rx & safe, faeces disposal, pig husbandry & meat inspection

HUMAN SCHISTOSOMIASIS

Epidemiology

Schistosomiasis is caused by trematode flatworms (flukes) transmitted by snails. The disease is endemic in the tropics with an estimated 200 million people worldwide infected, 80% of whom are in Africa. The main species in Africa are *Schistosoma mansoni* and *S. haematobium*. *S. japonicum* is the main species in southeast Asia and China. Infection of the CNS is unusual in Africa but occurs in 2-4% of patients with *S. japonicum* infection.

Life cycle

Humans are infected by contact with fresh water, usually when working, playing or swimming. Cercariae, the larval form released from infected snails, penetrate the skin. The larval forms then migrate and unite as pairs of mature worms with mansoni and japonicum living in the lower mesenteric veins (the intestinal form) and haematobium in vesical veins (the urinary form). They may live in the veins for up to 30 years but their usual life span is probably 3-5 years. Humans are the definitive host of the adult worms and excrete their eggs in either stool or urine depending on the type of infection. The snail is the intermediate host and miracidiae released from eggs coming from humans into water enter the snails and are later released as cercariae which in turn penetrate the skin and the life cycle is complete (Fig 7.11).

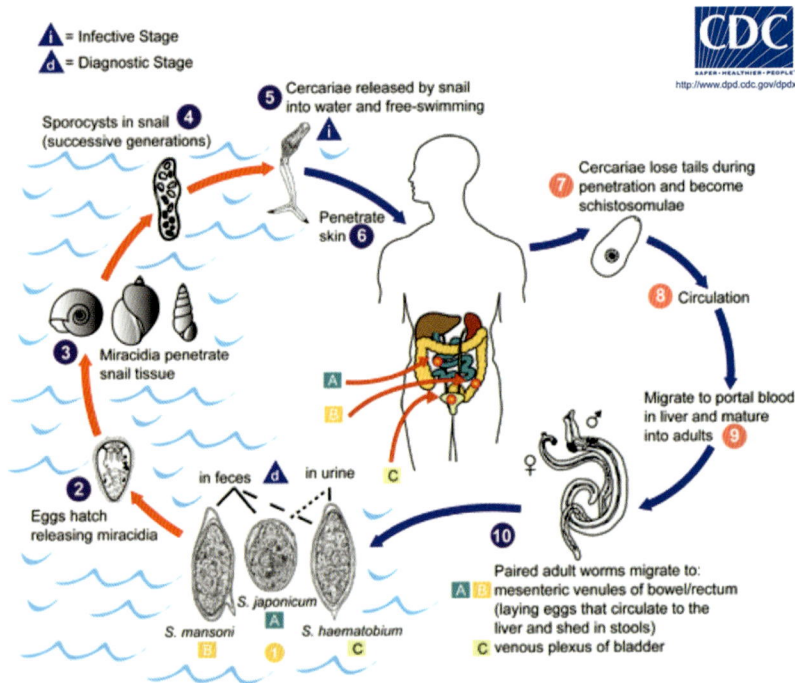

Figure 7.11 Life cycle schistosomiasis

Pathogenesis

The adult worms evade host immunity and some of their released eggs travel with the blood flow and get trapped in viscera and release antigens. This provokes a vigorous cell mediated inflammatory response particularly in early infection which forms intense granulomas around eggs, which gives rise to local pathology in the organ involved. The main sites for trapped *S. mansoni* and *S. japonicum* eggs are liver mainly causing portal hypertension and also the large intestine. *S. haematobium* eggs get deposited in the genitourinary tract causing bladder wall calcification, polyps, bladder stones and an increased risk of squamous cell cancer. The severity of systemic disease is proportional to the duration of worm infection and the egg load. When the eggs are deposited in the spinal cord or brain, this can lead to neurological disease. This can happen in two main ways, migration of egg laying worms to ectopic sites or embolization of eggs. Ectopic sites for worms include the inferior venacaval system with a right to left cardiac shunt or the paravertebral veins in the cord/cauda equina, or the cerebral cortical veins in the brain (Fig 7.12). Retrograde spread to the spinal cord from the inferior mesenteric veins through valveless pelvic veins is also a proposed mechanism for paraplegia. CNS involvement is unusual in both *S. mansoni* and *S. haematobium*. Spinal cord disease accounts for >95% of all CNS disease in Africa. It occurs particularly in early infection with mansoni in the non immune host and when there is a heavy worm and egg load.

MRI brain T1 (enhanced)

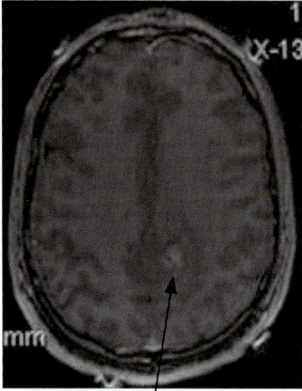

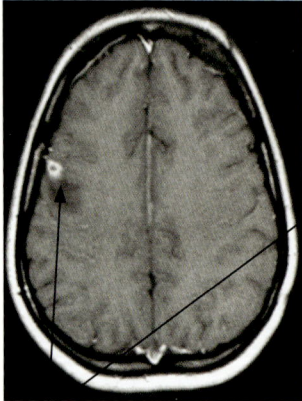

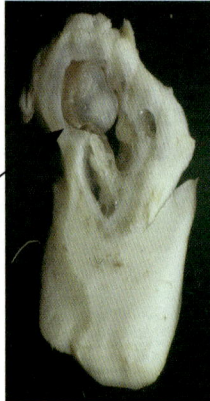

Histopathology

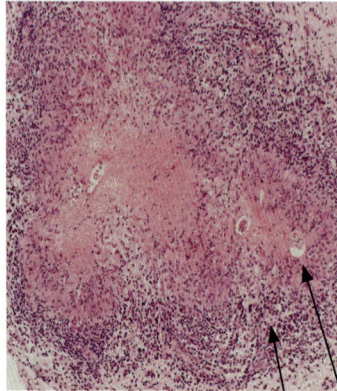

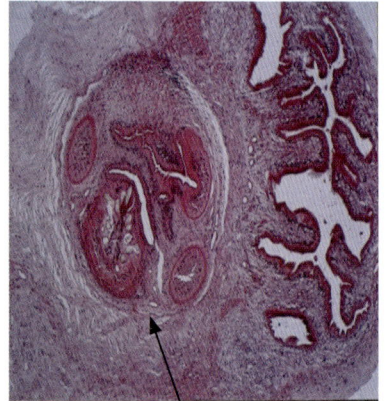

Eggs & surrounding oedema

Granuloma & eggs

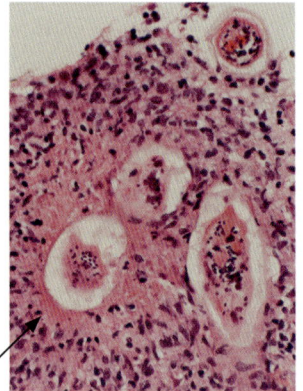

MRI brain T1 (enhanced)

Pathology

Histopathology

Eggs & granuloma in brain

Eggs & surrounding granuloma

Figure 7.12 Brain in schistosomiasis

Clinical Features

The neurological findings occur as a result of eggs deposited in the spinal cord (lower end) or rarely in the brain. In the spinal cord, they cause a myeloradiculopathy which may result in paraparesis, mostly flaccid in type. Clinical features include low back pain, lower limb weakness, paraesthesia, bladder and bowel dysfunction and impotence. This is the most common neurological presentation of mansoni. Eggs in the brain present as space occupying lesions with focal neurological deficits, seizures and encephalopathy.

Diagnosis

The diagnosis is suggested by a previous or recent history of water exposure in an endemic area and confirmed by ELISA antibody tests or the demonstration of eggs in the stool by faecal smear or urine by sedimentation or filtration. Although an ELISA antibody test is less useful in endemic areas, a positive CSF test result (sensitivity <60%, specificity >95%) supports the diagnosis. CSF may show a mild elevation of cells and protein and slight decrease in glucose. Eosinophilia may be present especially early on in the disease. Neuroimaging requires MRI as CT is not sensitive for spinal cord disease. MRI shows enlargement of the lower end of spinal cord below T6 level usually involving T11-L1 with thickening of the nerve roots and cauda equina

Treatment

Patients with neurological disorders should be treated with praziquantel and steroids (Table 7.7). There is no consensus on the dose or duration of treatment and doses of praziquantel range between 40-60 mg/kg/po/daily for 1-14 days, although in suspected and confirmed cases a longer course is frequently used. Steroids should be used in the first instance for 2-6 weeks and sometimes continued for 3-6 months.

Table 7.7 Drug treatment of neuroschistosomiasis

Drug	route	Dose/duration
praziquantel	po	40-60 mg/kg/po/od 1-14 days
and		
methyprednisolone	iv	15-20 mg*/kg/iv/od (max 1gm) 5-7 days
or		
prednisolone	po	1.5 mg/kg/po/od for 3-6/52 and a tapering dose

* followed by oral prednisolone 1.5 mg/kg daily for 2-6 weeks

Prognosis

The prognosis in treated spinal cord disease is good with 70% making a complete recovery. Recovery usually begins early within 1-2 days of starting treatment. The remaining patients are left with permanent deficits.

Prevention

The main methods of prevention involve regular intermittent mass drug treatment of exposed at risk populations usually school children with praziquantel, reduced contamination of water and a reduction or elimination of snails.

Key points

- neuroschistosomiasis is an uncommon complication of Schistosoma infection
- paraplegia is the most common neurological disorder & mostly occurs in the non immune host
- diagnosis is by serology & microscopic evidence of eggs & neuroimaging
- Rx is with praziquantel for 1-14/7 and steroids for 2-6 weeks
- secondary prevention: intermittent mass treatment of at risk populations with praziquantel
- primary prevention: reduced contamination of water & reduction or elimination of snails

HYDATID DISEASE

Echinococcosis in humans is mostly caused by the dog tapeworm *Echinococcus granulosus*. The dog is the definitive host and the adult tapeworm inhabits its intestine. Hydatid disease occurs, when humans come into contact with dog's faeces and the ingested ova develop into the cystic stage. The disease is estimated to affect 2-3 million people globally. It is endemic in large parts of Africa, mainly affecting the traditional cattle and sheep grazing communities. The prevalence in endemic areas ranges from 0.25 to 25%. Neurological involvement occurs in about 1-2% of cases.

Life cycle

The dog excretes the tapeworm eggs in its stool and these are accidentally ingested by grazing herbivores which then become intermediate hosts. These are mainly sheep, cattle and goats. The larval form penetrates the intestinal mucosa of the animal to lodge in the intestinal mesentery, liver and lungs, and develop into cysts. When the animal is killed the dog in turn ingests these organs which contain larval hydatid cysts. These larval cysts contain tapeworm heads or scolexes, which attach themselves to the intestinal wall of the dog and mature into the adult tapeworm and the life cycle is complete. Humans become accidentally infected by ingesting food or drink which has been contaminated by faeces containing ova from infected dogs. They then accidentally become the intermediate hosts (Fig 7.13).

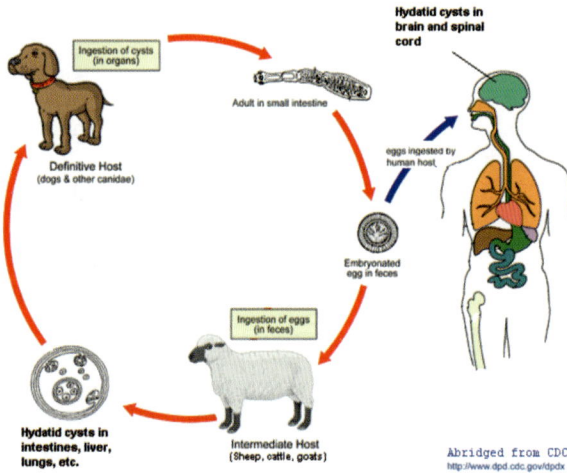

Figure 7.13 Life cycle Hydatid disease

Clinical features

Hydatid disease is characterized by slow growing cysts. It is a chronic disorder mainly of children and young persons but adults are also affected. The main sites are liver, lung but other organs may be involved. Neurological features depend on the site, age and maturity of the cysts. Cysts in the brain occur mostly in children and younger adults. They may be asymptomatic or present acutely with hydrocephalus, focal neurological deficits and seizures. Cysts in the spinal cord occur more in adults than children and present with paraparesis.

Diagnosis

The diagnosis is made by neuroimaging. CT reveals a striking large well defined rounded smooth thin walled unilocular, usually single cyst with mass effect. Calcification occurs in 20-40% of cases (Fig 7.14). Cysts may occasionally be multiple. The finding of a peripheral eosinophilia may be worrying as it may indicate that the hydatid cyst is leaking. Serology screening is not sensitive for extra hepatic involvement. The main differential diagnosis is between cystic brain tumours, an arachnoid cyst and abscesses.

CT head (without contrast)   **MRI T1cervical cord**

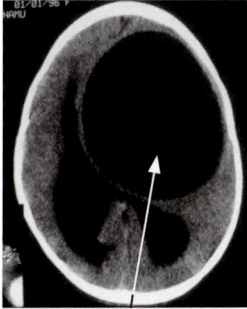

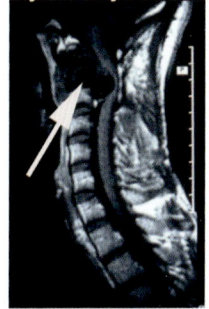

Hydatid cyst in child   Calcified cyst and hydrocephalus   Cyst pressing on cervical cord

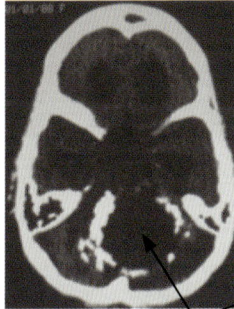

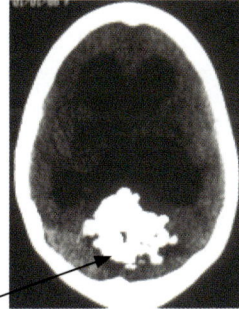

pathology   **histopathology**

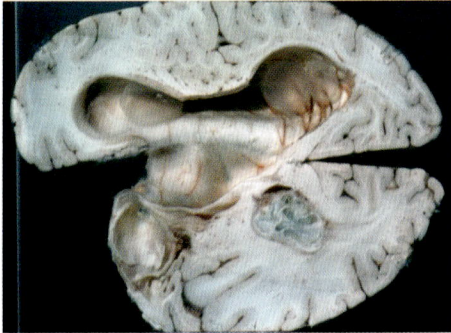

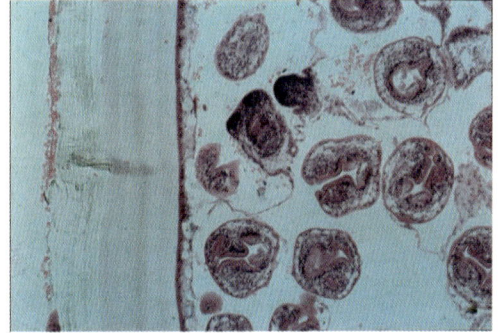

Multiple cysts in brain & ventricles   Hydatid daughter cysts

Figure 7.14 Brain and spinal cord in hydatid disease

Treatment

Management is both medical and surgical. Medical treatment is with albendazole alone or in combination with praziquantel. The recommended dosage of albendazole is 400 mg twice daily over a three or six month period. The optimum period of treatment remains uncertain. There is limited data on praziquantel but 40 mg/kg/week in combination with albendazole has been suggested and is the currently recommended treatment of choice. The advantage of two drugs is that while albendazole acts on the germinal membrane, praziquantel kills the proto-scolices or daughter cysts. The indications for medical treatment include multiple inoperable sites and to prevent secondary spread, and as an adjunct to surgery. Outcome with medical treatment is variable but clinical improvement and radiological resolution of cysts has been shown. Surgery is the management of choice for a lesion when there is symptomatic CNS involvement.

Prevention

Preventative measures in endemic areas include prophylactic dosing of dogs for tapeworm, avoiding feeding uncooked offal and raw meat to dogs and the regular inspection of meat for the presence of cysts.

Key points

- echinococcosis is caused by cystic stage of dog tapeworm
- humans infected when they accidentally ingest faeces from infected dogs.
- CNS disease occurs in 1-2% & includes hemiplegia, seizures & paraplegia
- diagnosis is by imaging showing cysts/Ca++ in the brain and spinal cord
- Rx: albendazole & praziquantel for >3/12 & surgery if symptomatic
- prevention: prophylaxis of dogs for tapeworm & inspection of meat for cysts

Selected references

Amogne W, Teshager G, Zenebe G. *Central nervous system toxoplasmosis in adult Ethiopians.* Ethiop Med J. 2006 Apr;44(2):113-20.

Beare NA, Taylor TE, Harding SP, Lewallen S, Molyneux ME. *Malarial retinopathy: a newly established diagnostic sign in severe malaria.* Am J Trop Med Hyg. 2006 Nov;75(5):790-7.

Beraud G, Pierre-Francois S, Foltzer A, Abel S, Liautaud B, Smadja D, et al. *Cotrimoxazole for treatment of cerebral toxoplasmosis: an observational cohort study during 1994-2006.* Am J Trop Med Hyg. 2009 Apr;80(4):583-7.

Bhigjee AI, Rosemberg S. *Optimizing therapy of seizures in patients with HIV and cysticercosis.* Neurology. 2006 Dec 26;67(12 Suppl 4):S19-22.

Blum J, Schmid C, Burri C. *Clinical aspects of 2541 patients with second stage human African trypanosomiasis.* Acta Trop. 2006 Jan;97(1):55-64.

Bygott JM, Chiodini PL. *Praziquantel: neglected drug? Ineffective treatment? Or therapeutic choice in cystic hydatid disease?* Acta Trop. 2009 Aug;111(2):95-101.

Carod-Artal FJ. *Neurological complications of Schistosoma infection.* Trans R Soc Trop Med Hyg. 2008 Feb;102(2):107-16.

Carpio A. *Neurocysticercosis: an update.* Lancet Infect Dis. 2002 Dec;2(12):751-62.

Dedicoat M, Livesley N. *Management of toxoplasmic encephalitis in HIV-infected adults (with an emphasis on resource-poor settings).* Cochrane Database Syst Rev. 2006;3:CD005420.

Dondorp AM, Fanello CI, Hendriksen IC, Gomes E, Seni A, Chhaganlal KD, et al. *Artesunate versus quinine in the treatment of severe falciparum malaria in African children (AQUAMAT): an open-label, randomised trial.* Lancet. 2010 Nov 13;376(9753):1647-57.

Ferrari TC, Moreira PR, Cunha AS. *Clinical characterization of neuroschistosomiasis due to Schistosoma mansoni and its treatment.* Acta Trop. 2008 Nov-Dec;108(2-3):89-97.

Fevre EM, Picozzi K, Jannin J, Welburn SC, Maudlin I. *Human African trypanosomiasis: Epidemiology and control.* Adv Parasitol. 2006;61:167-221.

Garcia HH, Del Brutto OH. *Neurocysticercosis: updated concepts about an old disease.* Lancet Neurol. 2005 Oct;4(10):653-61.

Garcia HH, Moro PL, Schantz PM. *Zoonotic helminth infections of humans: echinococcosis, cysticercosis and fascioliasis.* Curr Opin Infect Dis. 2007 Oct;20(5):489-94.

Gryseels B, Polman K, Clerinx J, Kestens L. *Human schistosomiasis.* Lancet. 2006 Sep 23;368(9541):1106-18.

Gwer S, Thuo N, Idro R, Ndiritu M, Boga M, Newton C, et al. *Changing trends in incidence and aetiology of childhood acute non-traumatic coma over a period of changing malaria transmission in rural coastal Kenya: a retrospective analysis.* BMJ Open. 2012 Apr 1;2(2):e000475.

Idro R, Jenkins NE, Newton CR. *Pathogenesis, clinical features, and neurological outcome of cerebral malaria.* Lancet Neurol. 2005 Dec;4(12):827-40.

Idro R, Marsh K, John CC, Newton CR. *Cerebral malaria: mechanisms of brain injury and strategies for improved neurocognitive outcome.* Pediatr Res. 2010 Oct;68(4):267-74.

Kariuki SM, Ikumi M, Ojal J, Sadarangani M, Idro R, Olotu A, et al. *Acute seizures attributable to falciparum malaria in an endemic area on the Kenyan coast.* Brain. 2011 May;134(Pt 5):1519-28.

Mafojane NA, Appleton CC, Krecek RC, Michael LM, Willingham AL, 3rd. *The current status of neurocysticercosis in Eastern and Southern Africa.* Acta Trop. 2003 Jun;87(1):25-33.

Maude RJ, Dondorp AM, Abu Sayeed A, Day NP, White NJ, Beare NA. *The eye in cerebral malaria: what can it teach us?* Trans R Soc Trop Med Hyg. 2009 Jul;103(7):661-4.

Milner DA, Jr. *Rethinking cerebral malaria pathology.* Curr Opin Infect Dis. 2010 Oct;23(5):456-63.

Mishra SK, Newton CR. *Diagnosis and management of the neurological complications of falciparum malaria.* Nat Rev Neurol. 2009 Apr;5(4):189-98.

Nok AJ. *Arsenicals (melarsoprol), pentamidine and suramin in the treatment of human African trypanosomiasis.* Parasitol Res. 2003 May;90(1):71-9.

Pal DK, Carpio A, Sander JW. *Neurocysticercosis and epilepsy in developing countries.* J Neurol Neurosurg Psychiatry. 2000 Feb;68(2):137-43.

Welburn SC, Odiit M. *Recent developments in human African trypanosomiasis.* Curr Opin Infect Dis. 2002 Oct;15(5):477-84.

PART II – NEUROLOGICAL DISORDERS

CHAPTER 8
NEUROLOGICAL ILLNESS IN HIV DISEASE

CONTENTS

CHAPTER 8

NEUROLOGICAL ILLNESS IN HIV DISEASE

Neurological disorders are a frequent manifestation of HIV infection in Africa. At least a fifth of infected persons will present with a major neurological illness either as the first clinical manifestation of HIV or occurring during the course of symptomatic HIV disease. The proportion of patients with clinical evidence of neurological dysfunction and have abnormal neurological findings is however much higher at 40-70%. At post mortem examination, over 90% of AIDS cases have pathological changes in their nervous system. Neurological disorders affect all parts of the nervous system including the brain, spinal cord, peripheral nerves, muscle and eye. This chapter outlines the main neurological illnesses arising from HIV infection. After reading the chapter the student should aim to understand the main mechanisms, clinical presentations, diagnosis and management of these illnesses.

INTRODUCTION

Neurological disorders in HIV infection are caused by three main processes: **loss of cell-mediated immunity**, **direct HIV infection,** and **inflammation/autoimmunity**. Adverse effects of drugs used to treat HIV and its co infections are also a cause.

Disorders related to loss in immunity are caused by opportunistic processes (OP), mostly infections and occasionally neoplasms. These occur mostly but not exclusively when the CD4 count is <200 cells/cm³. The main opportunistic infections (OI) are cryptococcosis, toxoplasmosis and tuberculosis (Chapters 6 & 7) and main opportunistic neoplasm is cerebral lymphoma. The main neurological presentations occurring as a result of those processes are **meningitis, focal neurological disorder (FND)** and **altered level of consciousness** or **coma** depending on the cause and CNS site involved.

Neurological disorders also arise from direct HIV infection of the nervous system and muscle. These include **HIV-associated dementia (HAD), distal sensory neuropathy (DSN), vacuolar myelopathy, retinopathy** and **myopathy**. These also occur mostly during the later stages of HIV infection when CD4 count is <100 cells/cm³.

Other neurological disorders that may occur throughout the course of HIV infection include **herpes zoster, Bell's palsy, Guillain-Barre Syndrome (GBS)** and **polymyositis**. These by contrast occur mostly during the asymptomatic stage when immunity is still relatively intact with CD4 counts typically >200 cells/cm³. GBS and polymyositis are caused by inflammation and autoimmunity. The general characteristics of the main HIV related neurological illnesses are summarized below in Table 8.1.

Table 8.1 Characteristics of main neurological illnesses in HIV disease

Cause	Clinical presentation	CD4 cells/cm³ ( ) = range	Estimated frequency in HIV
Opportunistic processes		**(0-200)**	**20-30%**
Infections			
Cryptococcus neoformans	meningitis	<100	10-20%
Mycobacterium tuberculosis	meningitis, *FND, paraplegia	(0-500)	1-10%
Toxoplasma gondii	*FND	<100	5-15%
Cytomegalovirus	retinitis, radiculopathy, encephalitis	<50	1-1.5%
JC virus (progressive multifocal leucoencephalopathy)	quadriplegia, encephalopathy	<100	uncommon
Tumours			
Primary CNS lymphoma (PCNSL)	*FND	<100	<1%
Direct HIV infection		**(0-200)**	**40-70%**
	HIV associated dementia (HAD)	<50	20-30%
	vacuolar myelopathy	<100	5-20%
	distal sensory neuropathy (DSN)	<200	20-30%
	retinopathy	<200	5-10%
	frontal lobe release signs	<200	50-70%
Inflammatory/autoimmune		**(200-500)**	
	Bell's palsy		common
	GBS		rare
	polymyositis		rare
Others		**(0-500)**	
Varicella	zoster	(2-500)	5-10%
	seizures		5-10%
	stroke		<1%
	paraplegia		1-2%

FND: hemiparesis, seizures, ataxia, cranial nerve palsies, coma

The main clinical presentations are **meningitis, focal neurological deficits, seizures** and **altered level of consciousness;** these are mostly caused by opportunistic infections and frequently occur, when more than one HIV related illness is present. Disseminated TB occurs in >50% of patients with advanced HIV disease in Africa.

CLINICAL PRESENTATIONS

MENINGITIS

Meningitis is one of the common neurological presentations of HIV infection in Africa. The main causes are *C. neoformans* and *M. tuberculosis* (Chapter 6). Both cause chronic meningitis and occur predominantly in patients with CD4 counts <100/cm³ although TB meningitis (TBM) may also occur at higher CD4 levels. Acute forms of meningitis also occur but these are much less common; the main acute forms are *acute bacterial (ABM)* secondary to pneumococcus and viral meningitis. Cryptococcal meningitis (CM) is now the most common type of meningitis in many parts of Africa and after TB it is the leading cause of death in AIDS in parts of Africa, accounting for up to a quarter of all HIV related deaths there (Fig. 8.1). TBM is also common and has been shown at post-mortem in West Africa to be present in >10% of AIDS patients (Fig. 8.2).

Clinically, CM and TBM may be indistinguishable from each other, although the onset of headache coupled with fever, nausea and vomiting evolving during the preceding week or two is more suggestive of CM. Definite signs of meningism are typically absent in CM in up to 75% of patients. Raised intracranial pressure with papilloedema is more common in CM but occurs in both types of meningitis.

Laboratory investigations can help to distinguish the different types of meningitis. In both types of meningitis the CSF shows an elevation in cells (mainly mononuclear) and protein but CSF can also be normal in 10-20% of patients. Distinguishing features in the CSF in CM are the presence of encapsulated yeast cells on India ink (60-80 %) and cryptococcal antigen (95%) and in TBM, AFB (<5% routine ZN staining). The percentage of positive AFB in CSF in TBM can be significantly improved (60%) by increasing the volume of CSF to 20 mls, centrifuging the sample and by microscopy for 20 minutes. The presence of cryptococcal antigenaemia may be detected in the blood during the 2-3 weeks preceding the onset of CM in some patients allowing for the possibility of earlier treatment. CT of the brain is usually not helpful but may show more basal meningeal enhancement in TBM and occasionally the presence of a tuberculoma. Supporting evidence for TBM includes the presence of concurrent systemic TB, (chest radiograph 40%) or failure to improve after 1-2 weeks of treatment for CM. Treatment of either or both CM or TBM is started immediately for suspected or confirmed infection as outlined in Table 8.2.

Pathology   **Histopathology**   **Microscopy**

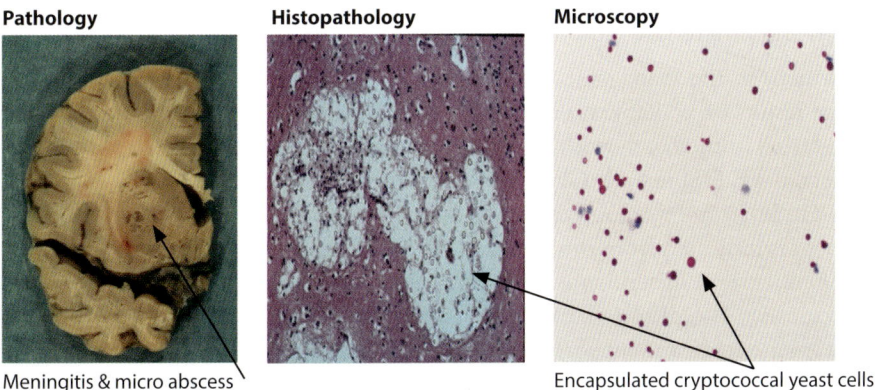

Meningitis & micro abscess   Encapsulated cryptococcal yeast cells

Figure 8.1 Brain & CSF in cryptococcal meningitis

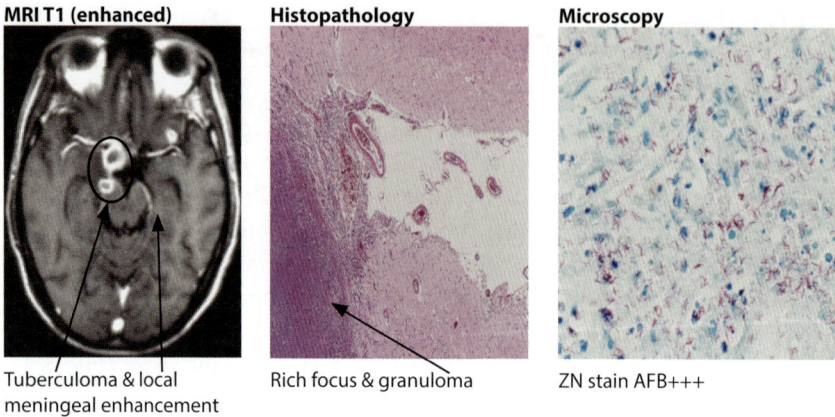

MRI T1 (enhanced)   **Histopathology**   **Microscopy**

Tuberculoma & local meningeal enhancement   Rich focus & granuloma   ZN stain AFB+++

Figure 8.2 Brain in CNS tuberculosis

FOCAL NEUROLOGICAL DISORDERS (FND)

Focal neurological disorders are among the most common neurological disorders in HIV disease. The main causes are *Toxoplasma* encephalitis (TE), tuberculoma and lymphoma. FNDs occur typically in patients with CD4 counts <100 cells/cm³ but can occur at higher CD4 counts. The main clinical presentations are hemiparesis, cranial nerve palsies and ataxia (50-60%), seizures, lethargy, confusion (40%) and coma. TE causing brain abscess is usually the most common cause of FND (Chapter 7), occurring in 5-15% of AIDS patients, although its frequency within Africa, will vary depending on the local prevalence of toxoplasmosis. Tuberculoma was reported to be the most common cause of focal brain lesions in HIV in one study area in South Africa. In TE there is usually a history of headache (60%) and fever (40-70%) over the preceding days or 1-2 weeks. Other indicators of TE include positive *Toxoplasma* serology and multiple ring-enhancing mass lesions on CT. A negative *Toxoplasma* serology makes the diagnosis of TE unlikely.

The main differential diagnosis in TE includes tuberculoma and lymphoma. However tuberculoma and primary cerebral lymphoma (PCL) are much less common and both have a slower clinical course than TE. On CT, while both tuberculoma and lymphoma can appear to be similar to TE, (Figs. 8.3-5) they may differ in their site and distribution in the brain (Chapter 7). Other less common causes of FND in HIV to be considered include stroke, occasionally syphilis and progressive multifocal encephalopathy (PML).

The choice of treatment in the management FNDs is based mostly on clinical suspicion and likely cause and the results of available investigations including a CT scan of the head (Table 8.2). Treatment is started immediately with high dose trimethoprim-sulfamethoxazole in those patients with suspected TE (Table 8.2). Clinical improvement is expected by day 3 in around 50% and by day 14 in 90% and if resources allow a follow up CT confirming improvement is helpful. TB treatment is indicated from the outset in all those suspected TB cases particularly if there is evidence of concurrent disseminated TB (e.g. AFB in sputum/typical chest radiograph findings for tuberculosis). The diagnosis of CNS TB should also be considered, if there is a failure or a poor response to treatment for TE after 7-14 days. If there is any indication from the start of either CM or ABM, then appropriate antimicrobials should be added from the start of treatment.

MRI T1 (enhanced)

Ring enhancing abscess

Histopathology

Inflammation (non granulomatous)

Microscopy

ZN stain AFB+++

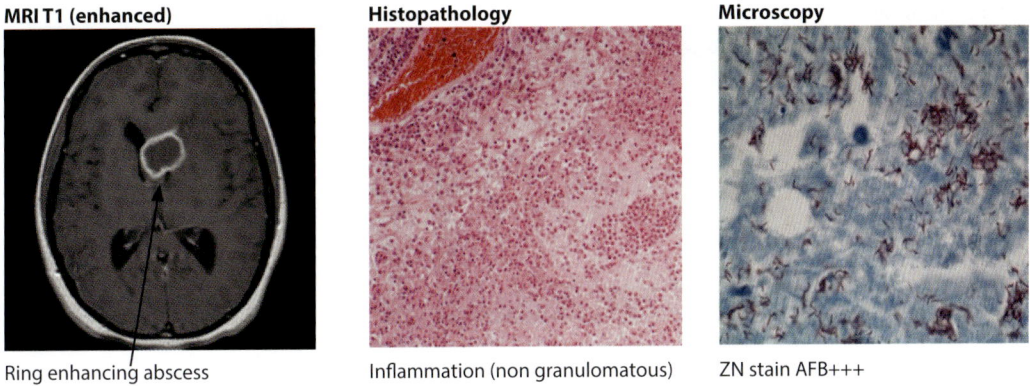

Figure 8.3 Brain in tuberculoma

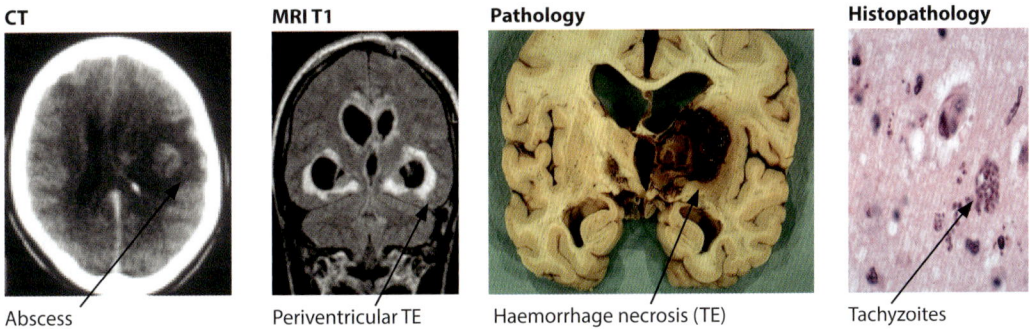

CT

Abscess

MRI T1

Periventricular TE

Pathology

Haemorrhage necrosis (TE)

Histopathology

Tachyzoites

Figure 8.4 Brain in toxoplasmosis

CONFUSION AND COMA

States of confusion, altered level of consciousness and coma are common clinical presentations particularly in the advanced stages of HIV disease in Africa. These states are mostly caused by the same opportunistic processes, usually infections that result in meningitis and FNDs but representing more advanced disease. Other causes of confusion and coma in HIV should also be considered, including metabolic disorders, organ failure particularly renal and cardiac, and side effects of ART medication, in particular efavirenz. If the cause is not known, then presumptive treatment should be started for the main OIs, **CM, TE** and **ABM** together until the precise diagnosis becomes clear (Chapters 6-7). If there is clinical evidence of **TB,** then TB treatment should also be added (Table 8.2).

STROKE

Stroke typically occurs during the otherwise asymptomatic phase of HIV infection when CD4 counts are 200-500 cells/cm^3. An association between stroke and the persistent generalized lymphadenopathy (PGL) stage of HIV has been shown in South Africa. The accumulated lifetime prevalence of stroke in HIV disease is <1%. Stroke can be difficult to diagnose clinically, mainly because the presentation is very similar to the non vascular causes of focal brain lesions in HIV infection. The clinical diagnosis of stroke is suggested by its acute onset, non progressive course and better clinical outcome. A CT scan of the brain may be necessary to

MRI T1 (enhanced)	Pathology	Histopathology

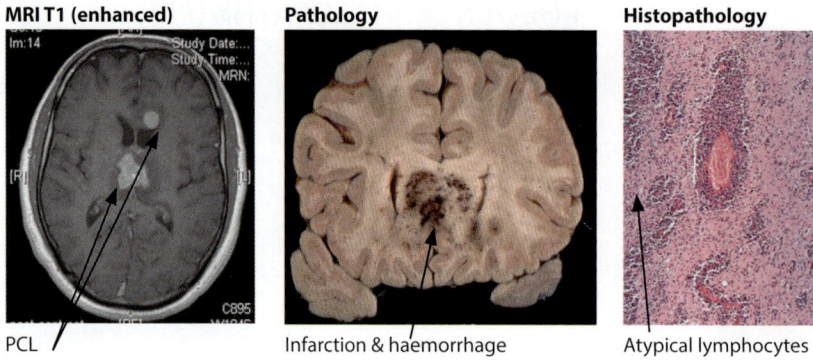

PCL	Infarction & haemorrhage	Atypical lymphocytes

Figure 8.5 Brain in lymphoma

confirm the correct diagnosis. The majority of strokes are ischaemic and occur in the anterior circulation. Mechanisms include vasculitis, coagulopathies, meningitis and emboli secondary to cardiac disease. Investigations and management are the same as for any stroke patient and should include a serology test for syphilis.

SEIZURES

New onset seizures occur in up to 5-9% of HIV infected persons at some stage throughout their long illness. Seizures occur most commonly during the later stages of HIV infection mostly as a complication of focal brain lesions secondary to opportunistic processes, in particular toxoplasmosis and tuberculoma. However, they may also occur at higher CD4 levels during the asymptomatic stage of HIV infection without any obvious underlying focal cause when their aetiology is related mostly to vasculitis. The seizures, although focal in origin are secondary generalized tonic-clonic in type. Management is directed at investigating and treating the suspected cause and suppressing the seizures (Table 8.2).

Table 8.2 Treatment based on presenting neurological disorder & likely cause

Neurological Disorder	Opportunistic infection	Treatment Regime	When to start
FND	toxoplasmosis (TE)	TMP-SMX#	immediate
Meningitis	cryptococcus (CM)	fluconazole/ amphotericin B	immediate
Coma	toxoplasmosis cryptococcus	TMP-SMX & fluconazole/ amphotericin B	immediate
Meningitis or FND or Coma	tuberculosis*	isoniazid pyrazinamide rifampicin ethambutol & steroids	immediate/or added@ 2/52**

 # trimethoprim/sulphamethoxazole
* TB treatment is started or added if chest radiograph or other findings indicate TB
** if there is treatment failure after 2/52 for either TE or CM

PROGRESSIVE MULTIFOCAL LEUCOENCEPHALOPATHY (PML)

PML is caused by the reactivation of a latent virus (JC virus) which is carried by most healthy people. It appears to be uncommon in AIDS in Africa (<1%). PML occurs in advancing states of immunosuppression when the CD4 count is <50/cm^3 but can occur in patients with higher CD4 counts <200 cm^3. The clinical presentation is one of a devastatingly severe progressive neurological disorder occurring over weeks and months. It is characterized by motor dysfunction (hemiparesis, quadriparesis), ataxia, seizures and cognitive changes (60-70%) and aphasia, visual problems and cranial nerve palsies (30-40%). CSF examination is usually normal. Neuroimaging may show hypodense disease in the white matter brain and cerebellum (15%). The diagnosis is confirmed by brain biopsy showing the typical JC inclusions in the oligodendrocytes (Fig 8.6). There is no effective treatment for PML but all suspected patients should start ART with some showing stabilization or improvement.

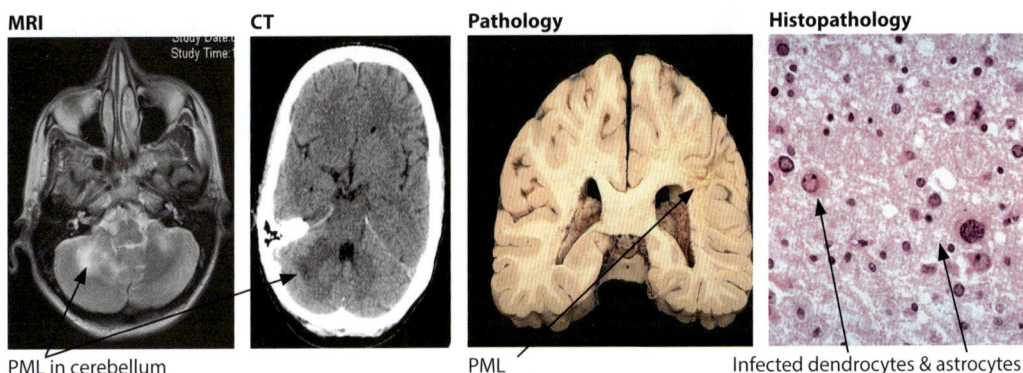

MRI **CT** **Pathology** **Histopathology**

PML in cerebellum   PML   Infected dendrocytes & astrocytes

Figure 8.6 Brain in PML

Key points

- major neurological disorders occur in >20% of HIV infected patients
- neurological infections are the leading cause of death in AIDS after systemic TB
- main presentations are meningitis, focal neurological disorder and coma
- main causes are cryptococcal meningitis, toxoplasmosis & tuberculosis
- management is frequently presumptive based on likely cause

VARICELLA-ZOSTER

The reactivation of latent varicella-zoster virus infection results in herpes zoster (HZ) or shingles. Primary infection causes chicken pox. The frequency of HZ is increased in HIV infection and characteristic residual scarring from previous zoster infection is present in 5-10% of AIDS patients in Africa. HZ occurs mostly during the otherwise asymptomatic stage of HIV infection (CD4 200-500 cells/cm^3). Acute HZ in HIV is recognizable clinically, by its local aggressiveness, involvement of multiple adjacent dermatomes and its tendency to occur at atypical sites including chest, face, back, neck, arms and leg (Fig. 8.7).

It also has a higher rate of complications including varicella dissemination (Fig. 8.7), myelitis, encephalitis and cranial nerve palsies. Post herpetic neuralgia is also more common.

Treatment for HZ involves both systemic and local measures. Aciclovir 800 mg/iv/po/tds for 5-7 days is recommended in the acute phase. The local application of a 1% gentian violet solution at the vesicular stage helps to prevent secondary infection and the application of a 1% phenol solution with calamine helps with local pain and itching. Analgesics may be required in addition to carbamazepine 200-400 mg/po/bid for post herpetic neuralgia. Survival in Africa in the pre ART era from onset was on average 3-4 years.

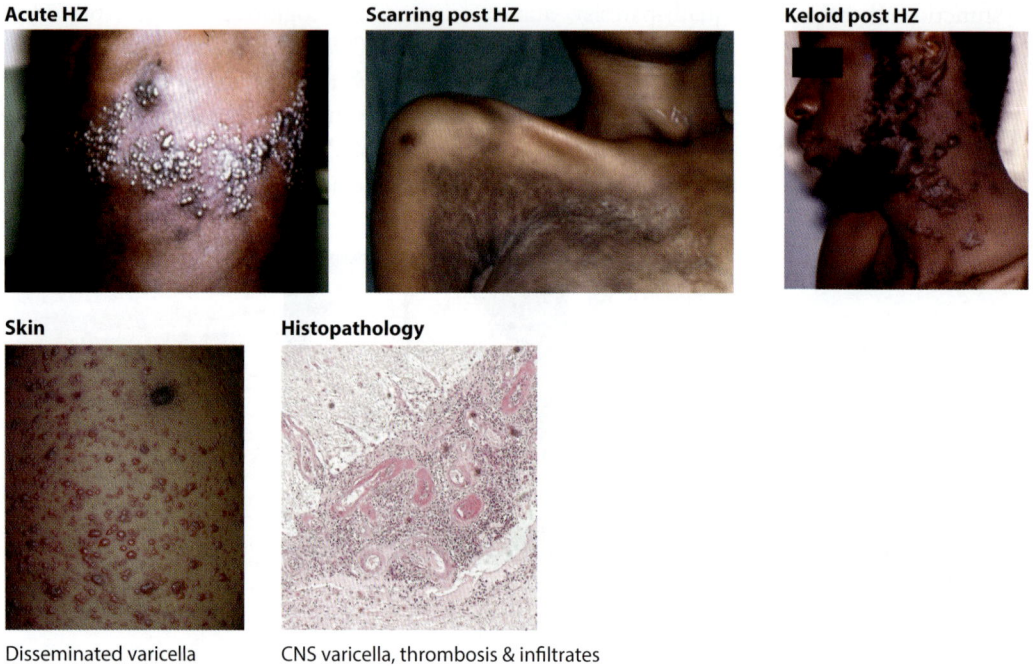

Acute HZ

Scarring post HZ

Keloid post HZ

Skin

Histopathology

Disseminated varicella   CNS varicella, thrombosis & infiltrates

Figure 8.7 Varicella-Zoster

CYTOMEGALOVIRUS (CMV)

CMV is a common virus affecting most persons in Africa. Primary infection is mostly acquired during early childhood, when it is either asymptomatic or associated with a mild febrile illness with a rash. Reactivation of CMV in HIV disease typically occurs during the later stages of infection when CD4 counts are <50 cells/cm^3. CMV retinitis affects around 1-1.5% of AIDS patients in Africa and although this figure may vary slightly with location, it is lower than that reported from high income countries. CMV retinopathy presents clinically with a characteristic painless haemorrhagic chorioretinitis, with loss of visual acuity first affecting one eye and later the other eye. Painless loss of vision is the main presenting complaint and blindness is inevitable unless treated. Fundoscopy appearance has been described as like that of a bush fire or pizza like and once seen is not subsequently easily missed (Fig.8.8). The main differential diagnosis is direct HIV retinopathy which is characterized by cotton wool spots and occasional haemorrhages which is seen in about 10% of patients with advanced disease (Fig. 8.9). However direct HIV retinopathy characteristically does not result in loss of vision. Other late but uncommon neurological presentations of CMV disease are encephalitis (Fig. 8.10) and infrequently a flaccid paraplegia secondary to lumbar radiculopathy.

The diagnosis of CMV in HIV is mainly clinical and treatment is with ganciclovir 5mg/kg/bd for 14 days and/or forscarnet. Thrombocytopenia is a side effect of treatment and blood counts should be checked regularly.

Haemorrhages & exudates

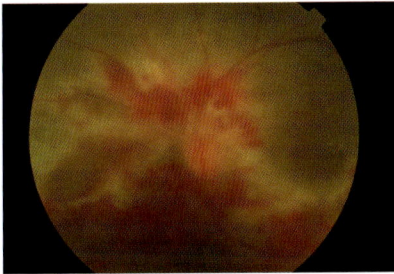

Cotton wool exudates

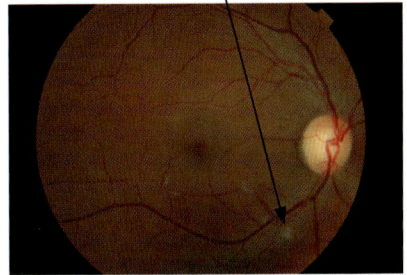

Figure 8.8 Retinopathy CMV

Figure 8.9 Retinopathy HIV

Pathology

Histopathology

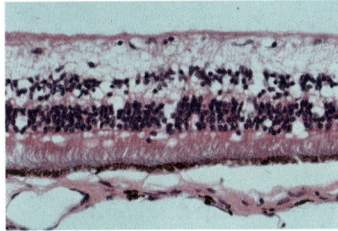

Microscopy

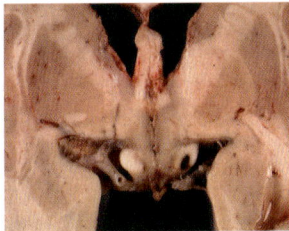

CMV ventriculitis

CMV retinitis

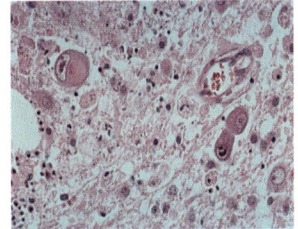

Owl eye inclusion bodies

Figure 8.10 Brain & retina in CMV

Key points

· HZ affects 5-10% of patients mostly during the asymptomatic stage of HIV infection
· HZ typically affects multiple adjacent dermatomes at atypical sites
· treatment is with local measures and aciclovir
· CMV infection results in characteristic retinopathy and blindness in about 1% of AIDS patients
· HIV retinopathy occurs in about10% of AIDS patients
· CMV may infrequently (<1%) cause a lumbar sacral radiculopathy resulting in paraplegia

IMMUNE RECONSTITUTION INFLAMMATORY SYNDROME (IRIS)

The immune reconstitution inflammatory syndrome is a complication of ART where the immune system directs an increased inflammatory response at an opportunistic infection. This results in paradoxical worsening in the patient's condition despite adequate treatment of the OI, hence the term paradoxical IRIS. It may also unmask other hidden OIs. IRIS may occur with several of the main neurological CNS OIs. These include CM, TB, TE, CMV and PML. It can occur in 20-30% of treated CNS OIs, usually occurring within the first weeks of starting TB treatment or sometimes months, in the case of CM treatment. Concurrent CNS TB IRIS may arise as a complication in treated pulmonary TB. Management of patients suspected of having IRIS frequently involves hospitalization and excluding other possible causes. Treatment with steroids for up to 2-3 months is frequently recommended, particularly in the case of TBM once other OIs have been excluded. The mortality rate in patients with IRIS is high, >30% in the case of treated CM and >10% in case of treated TB.

DIRECT HIV INFECTION

The HIV virus enters the CNS within days of primary infection and neurological disorders related to direct HIV infection have been observed occurring during all stages of the disease including early infection. Primary HIV infection of the nervous system is usually asymptomatic, but a viral meningoencephalitic illness can occur at this early stage. Also isolated self limiting aseptic meningitis can occur during the long period of asymptomatic HIV infection. The main clinically recognizable neurological disorders arising from direct HIV infection are HIV-associated neurocognitive dysfunction (HAND), HIV-associated dementia (HAD), peripheral neuropathies, vacuolar myelopathy and HIV retinopathy. These are found mostly during the later symptomatic stages of HIV disease when the CD4 counts are low.

HIV-ASSOCIATED DEMENTIA (HAD)

Chronic HIV infection of the brain leads to cognitive dysfunction in over 50% of patients (Fig 8.11). This is termed HIV associated neurocognitive dysfunction (HAND) and can range from mild impairment in functional performance to its severest form a frank dementia called HIV-associated dementia (HAD). HAD is reported to occur in up to a third of patients in high income countries but has virtually disappeared there because of the widespread use of ART. Varying frequencies of HAD have been reported from Africa with generally lower reported rates there (10-20%) being attributed to under diagnosis and poor survival outcomes. However, a recent study from South Africa, using appropriate investigations reported HAD in over one third of HIV patients. HAD occurs increasingly with advancing levels of immunosuppression and is most commonly seen in association with CD4 counts <100/cm^3. Factors associated with increased frequency of HAD include increasing age, treated CNS OIs and a history of substance abuse.

The defining early clinical characteristic of HAND/HAD is psychomotor retardation or a slowing down of both mental and motor activities. Established HAD presents typically with abnormalities in multiple domains including cognition, memory and motor function. The dementia ranges from early features such as mild apathy, disinterest and loss of attention with a general slowing of both mental and motor functions. In the later stages, there is a frank global loss of cognitive function with immobility and incontinence in end stage disease. Frequently associated neurological findings are frontal lobe release signs (FLRSs) (Fig. 8.12), signs of vacuolar myelopathy and distal sensory neuropathy (DSN). However, many patients in Africa die of opportunistic processes, mostly infections before reaching these later stages.

The clinical diagnosis of HAD may require a confirmatory CT of the brain to demonstrate the characteristic changes including cerebral atrophy and to exclude alternative causes, in particular opportunistic processes. In HIV encephalitis MRI of the brain shows increased signal in white matter (Fig. 8.11). Histopathology includes characteristic multi-nucleated giant cells and the presence of P-24 antigen on special staining. Management of HAD involves early diagnosis, treating any reversible cause and using ART treatment. The rate of HAD in Africa has been shown to significantly decrease after 6 months of ART treatment.

MRI T2

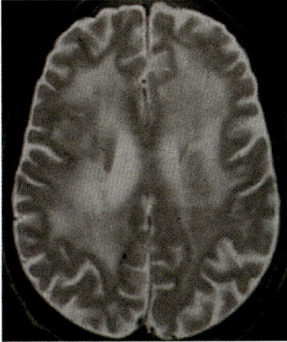

Increased signal in white matter

Histopathology brain

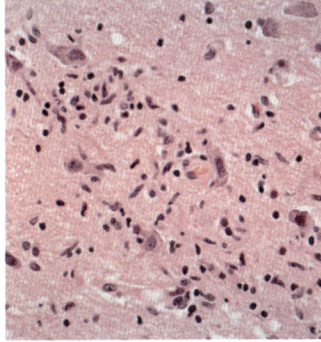

Multi-nucleated giant cells

Special stain for HIV

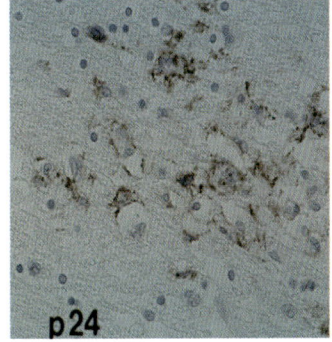

p24 antigen

Figure 8.11 Brain in direct HIV infection

Frontal lobe release signs (FLRSs)

The frequency of some primitive reflexes or FLRSs is increased in HIV disease and increases with advancing stages of HIV. The snout reflex (70%) and the palmomental reflex (50%) are found in the majority of patients with advanced HIV disease and in particular in association with HAD (90%) (Fig. 8.12). Their presence in a mainly younger age group helps to provide useful additional clinical evidence to help establish a diagnosis of HIV infection. It is however important to note that a snout or palmomental reflex may be present in association with other neurological disorders and are found occasionally in otherwise healthy persons. However, in healthy persons they are usually less pronounced and tire easily on repeated testing, this is in contrast to their presence in HIV disease when they are more pronounced and persist on repeated testing.

Control

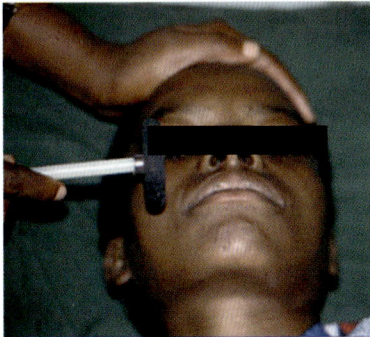

Snout reflex

A positive snout reflex

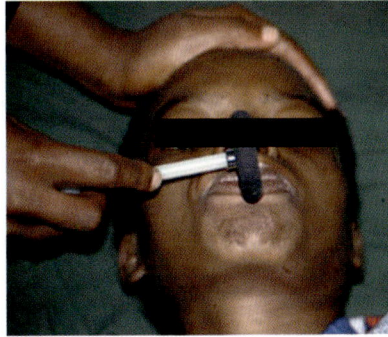

Figure 8.12 Frontal lobe release signs

The Snout reflex is elicited by pressing or tapping lightly on the patient's closed lips. In positive cases this causes a puckering or protrusion of the lips and occasionally the chin giving the appearance of a snout. (A slight or brief contraction of the lips may not be significant).

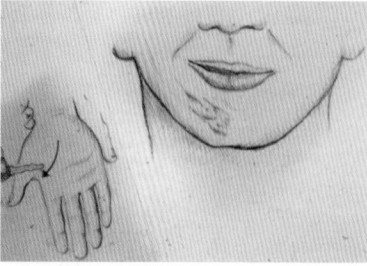

The palmomental reflex

Figure 8.12 Frontal lobe release signs

The Palmomental reflex is elicited by stroking in a distal direction the palm of the hand at the base of the thenar eminence. In positive cases it causes a brief contraction of the ipsilateral chin muscles and occasionally the corner of the mouth.

Key points

- HAND/HAD results from direct infection of the brain with HIV virus
- early HAND/HAD is characterised by slowing down of both mental & motor function
- late HAD is characterised by impairment/loss of cognitive function & memory
- affects >1/3 of patients in advanced HIV disease in Africa
- FLRSs are found in the majority of patients with AIDS & HAND/HAD
- HAD improves significantly 6 months after the start of ART

SPINAL CORD

The spinal cord is frequently involved in HIV disease. The causes vary with the stage of HIV infection and similar to the brain, are mostly related to either opportunistic processes (OPs) or to direct infection of cord with the HIV virus itself. Spinal cord disease presents clinically as paraparesis occurring typically in an otherwise asymptomatic person. The main opportunistic infections causing paraparesis are tuberculosis, herpes zoster, herpes simplex, CMV, syphilis and occasionally co-infection with HTLV-1 in endemic areas (Chapter 10). The main opportunistic neoplasm is lymphoma.

Direct infection of the spinal cord with HIV may result in **vacuolar myelopathy (VM)** of the cord which gives rise to clinical signs in about a fifth of HIV patients, particularly in those with advanced HIV disease. The main signs of VM are isolated brisk reflexes in the legs with extensor plantar responses, typically without any associated loss of power. Frequently, these upper motor neurone signs overlap with distal sensory neuropathy and then the ankle reflexes are absent. In <1% of patients, mainly in those with advanced HIV disease VM results in a spastic paraparesis with immobility and incontinence. Investigations of spinal cord disease are directed at diagnosing and treating the underlying cause.

Key points

- main spinal cord disorder in HIV is paraparesis
- paraparesis is caused mainly by opportunistic processes and infrequently by direct HIV infection
- main causes are TB, herpes zoster & simplex, syphilis, HTLV1 & lymphoma
- direct HIV infection of cord results in vacuolar myelopathy in >20% of patients
- signs of VM are isolated brisk knee reflexes, up going toes & rarely paraparesis

PERIPHERAL NEUROPATHIES

HIV frequently affects peripheral nerves. The main mechanisms are direct HIV infection, ART associated neuropathy and inflammation/autoimmunity (Chapter 11). The use of drug treatment in co-infections in HIV is also a cause of neuropathy e.g. isoniazid in TB treatment. The most common neuropathy in HIV disease is distal sensory neuropathy (DSN).

Distal sensory neuropathy (DSN)

DSN is the main HIV related neuropathy. It arises as a result of direct HIV infection of the dorsal root ganglion, thereby affecting peripheral nerves mostly on the sensory side. DSN affects about one quarter to one third of HIV patients, occurring mainly but not exclusively in those with advanced disease (Fig. 8.13). It can occur in association with CD4 >200/cm^3. The symptoms of DSN include painful, hot, burning, numbness or paraesthesia in feet and stocking distribution, developing slowly bilaterally over weeks or more commonly months. Power is usually maintained but may be decreased infrequently around the ankle joint. The ankle and very occasionally the knee reflexes are absent or decreased and areflexia may be the only finding to indicate the presence of DSN. Sensation involving light touch is mostly intact but is perceived as painful or dysaesthetic or hyperaesthetic particularly on the soles of the feet and palms. Vibration and pinprick are usually normal but may be impaired distally in the feet in advanced DSN. The upper limbs are mostly unaffected but the palms may be painful to touch.

Histopathology

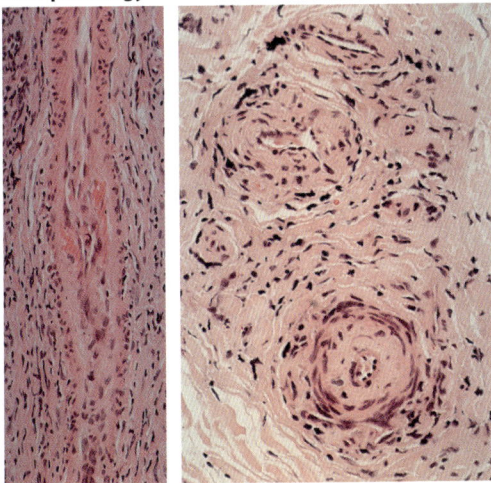

Perineural inflammation

Figure 8.13 Peripheral nerves in HIV

The mainstay of management is to start ART as early as possible. Symptomatic relief from pain may be obtained using simple analgesics and/or amitriptyline. The use of carbamazepine or gabapentin either alone or in combination with low dose tricyclics is helpful in some patients. However, opiates may be necessary in severe cases.

ART associated neuropathy

DSN may arise as an adverse effect of antiretroviral therapy. In particular this occurs with the use of the nucleoside reverse transcriptase inhibitors, stavudine (d4T). Other ART drugs associated with peripheral neuropathy include didanosine (ddI), lamivudine (3TC) and zalcitibine (ddC) and Efavirenz. The incidence of DSN in HIV has been shown to increase with the use of d4T and in particular the higher dosage (40 mg) and the duration of its use. ART neuropathy may affect up to 20% of patients who have been on dT4 for 6 months or more and increases the overall rate of DSN in HIV to >40%. The symptoms and signs are very similar to HIV related DSN, although sensory signs may be more marked in ART associated neuropathy. However, the two cannot easily be distinguished from each other clinically and hence they may both be termed DSN.

In Sub-Saharan Africa, DSN remains one of the main limiting side effects of first line ARTs. Management involves either reducing the standard dose of d4T from 40 to 30 mg (as recommended by WHO) or stopping and replacing d4T or the likely causal ART drug. Two thirds of patients may improve if switched to a non d4T regime. Many countries in Africa are now moving away from the use of stavudine based ART in order to reduce the problem of ART associated DSN. Other risk factors increasing the risk of DSN include a history of prior or active antituberculous therapy, older age, alcohol use and malnutrition. Care should be taken to ensure that pyridoxine 20 mg/po/daily has been prescribed in those patients taking isoniazid, and thiamine 100 mg/po/daily should be given in suspected cases of B-1 vitamin deficiency. Symptomatic management is otherwise the same as in HIV disease.

Key points

- HIV affects peripheral nerves by direct infection, ARTs and autoimmunity
- DSN secondary to direct HIV occurs in about 1/4 of patients & responds well to ART
- ART usage for >6 months with d4T, is associated with development of DSN
- majority of ART related neuropathies respond to stopping the offending drug
- analgesics may be necessary in both types of neuropathies

INFLAMMATION/AUTOIMMUNE

Bell's palsy, Guillain-Barre syndrome (GBS) and polymyositis occur mostly during previously asymptomatic HIV disease. With the exception of Bell's palsy these are uncommon illnesses but frequently prove to be the first indication of underlying HIV infection.

BELL'S PALSY

Bell's palsy is the most frequent presentation of mononeuritis in HIV in Africa. On screening for HIV in some high endemic areas in Africa, over 50% of patients presenting with idiopathic Bell's palsy early on in the epidemic tested positive for HIV. Therefore, an isolated Bell's palsy is now an indication for HIV screening. Bell's palsy typically occurs during otherwise asymptomatic HIV infection. A unilateral facial weakness develops over 24 hours and the clinical course is similar to that in non HIV associated Bell's palsy. However facial weakness may be bilateral in HIV infection (Fig. 8.14). The treatment and management is the same as for non HIV related Bells palsy (Chapter 12). Other cranial and mononeuropathies in HIV infection occur either individually or in combination (mononeuritis multiplex); but these are generally much less common than Bell's palsy.

Failure to smile   **Failure to close eyes fully**

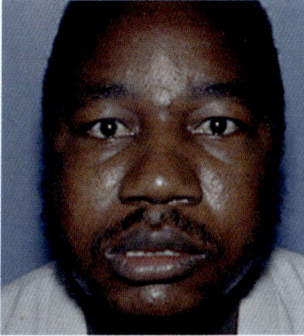

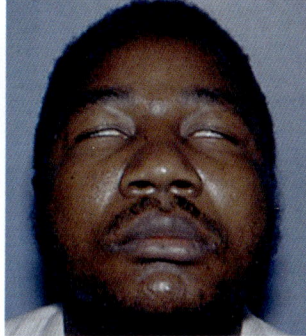

Figure 8.14 Bell's palsy in HIV (bilateral)

GUILLAIN-BARRE SYNDROME (GBS)

GBS or acute inflammatory demyelinating polyneuropathy (AIDP) is an uncommon form of autoimmune acute polyneuropathy and when it occurs in HIV, its onset is associated with a relatively intact immunity or an elevated CD4 count. Clinically, it is indistinguishable from classical or the non HIV associated GBS, apart from the increased number of lymphocytes found in the CSF in HIV infection. The clinical course and outcome are also similar (Chapter 11). Rarely, a more chronic form of polyneuritis occurs, this is called chronic inflammatory demyelinating polyneuropathy (CIDP).

MYOPATHY

There are two main types of muscle disease in HIV disease; myopathy and polymyositis (Fig 8.15). The most common type is myopathy which is characterised by painless, severe, generalised muscle wasting and weakness which occurs in association with systemic illness in advanced HIV infection. The severe wasting, myopathy (and diarrhoea) seen first in AIDS in East Africa gave rise to the name "Slim Disease". The second type of muscle disease, polymyositis is uncommon and occurs at an earlier stage, typically asymptomatic HIV infection. It is characterized by a painful marked proximal muscle weakness affecting the limbs and trunk. It is considered to be an autoimmune inflammatory disorder and responds well to steroids, although TB needs to be excluded before starting steroid treatment. Myopathies may also occur as a side effect of some ART medications.

Myopathy

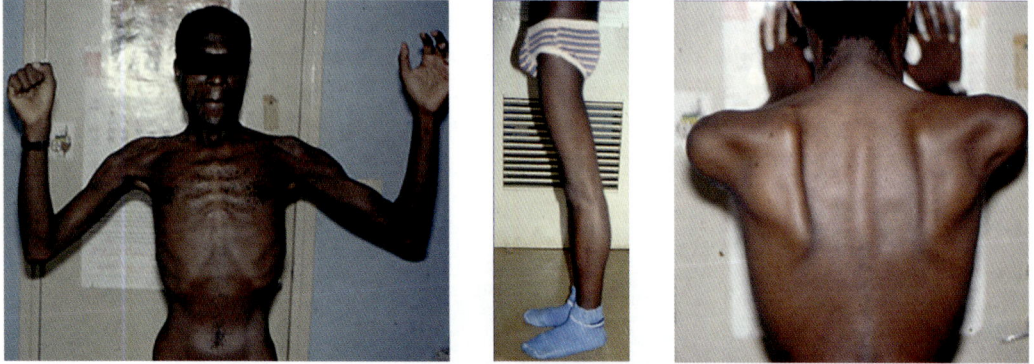

Proximal weakness & wasting

Figure 8.15 Polymyositis in HIV

Key points

- Bell's palsy, Guillain-Barre syndrome & polymyositis occur during asymptomatic HIV
- Bell's palsy is the most frequent mononeuropathy in HIV disease
- GBS is the same as in non HIV apart from increased lymphocytes in CSF
- myopathy is common in the later stages of HIV infection
- polymyositis is uncommon but responds well to steroids

References

Asselman V, Thienemann F, Pepper DJ, Boulle A, Wilkinson RJ, Meintjes G, et al. *Central nervous system disorders after starting antiretroviral therapy in South Africa.* AIDS. 2010 Nov 27;24(18):2871-6.

Balogou AA, Saka B, Kombaté D, Kombaté K, Mouhari-Toure A, Akakpo S, et al. *Causes of mortality associated with HIV/AIDS in health-care facilities in Togo: a six-month prospective study.* Trop Doct. 2011 Oct;41(4):215-7.

Beadles WI, Jahn A, Weigel R, Clutterbuck D. *Peripheral neuropathy in HIV-positive patients at an antiretroviral clinic in Lilongwe, Malawi.* Trop Doct. 2009 Apr;39(2):78-80.

Bhigjee AI. *Seizures in HIV/AIDS: a southern African perspective.* Acta Neurol Scand Suppl. 2005;181:4-7.

Bhigjee AI. *Neurological manifestations of HIV infection in Kwazulu-Natal South Africa.* J Neurovirol. 2005;11 Suppl 1:17-21.

Bhigjee AI, Madurai S, Bill PL, Patel V, Corr P, Naidoo MN, et al. *Spectrum of myelopathies in HIV seropositive South African patients.* Neurology. 2001 Jul 24;57(2):348-51.

Bicanic T, Meintjes G, Rebe K, Williams A, Loyse A, Wood R, et al. *Immune reconstitution inflammatory syndrome in HIV-associated cryptococcal meningitis: a prospective study.* J Acquir Immune Defic Syndr. 2009 Jun 1;51(2):130-4.

Brannagan TH, 3rd, Zhou Y. *HIV-associated Guillain-Barre syndrome.* J Neurol Sci. 2003 Apr 15;208(1-2):39-42.

Choi Y, Townend J, Vincent T, Zaidi I, Sarge-Njie R, Jaye A, et al. *Neurologic manifestations of human immunodeficiency virus-2: dementia, myelopathy, and neuropathy in West Africa.* J Neurovirol. 2011 Apr;17(2):166-75.

Dedicoat M, Livesley N. *Management of toxoplasmic encephalitis in HIV-infected adults--a review.* S Afr Med J. 2008 Jan;98(1):31-2.

Gannon P, Khan MZ, Kolson DL. *Current understanding of HIV-associated neurocognitive disorders pathogenesis.* Curr Opin Neurol. 2011 Jun;24(3):275-83.

Heckmann JM, Pillay K, Hearn AP, Kenyon C. *Polymyositis in African HIV-infected subjects.* Neuromuscul Disord. 2010 Nov;20(11):735-9.

Howlett WP, Luabeya MS, Kalula N, Kayembe NT. *Neurologic and psychiatric manifestations of HIV infection in Africa. AIDS in Africa,* edited Max Essex et al. Raven Press, Ltd., New York 1994 pp 393-422.

Howlett WP, Nkya WM, Kvale G, Nilssen S. *The snout and palmomental reflexes in HIV disease in Tanzania.* Acta Neurol Scand. 1995 Jun;91(6):470-6.

Howlett WP, Nkya WM, Mmuni KA, Missalek WR. *Neurological disorders in AIDS and HIV disease in the northern zone of Tanzania. AIDS.* 1989 May;3(5):289-96.

Jowi JO, Mativo PM, Musoke SS. *Clinical and laboratory characteristics of hospitalised patients with neurological manifestations of HIV/AIDS at the Nairobi hospital.* East Afr Med J. 2007 Feb;84(2):67-76.

Lucas SB, Hounnou A, Peacock C, Beaumel A, Djomand G, N'Gbichi JM, et al. *The mortality and pathology of HIV infection in a West African city. AIDS.* 1993 Dec;7(12):1569-79.

Modi G, Hari K, Modi M, Mochan A. *The frequency and profile of neurology in black South African HIV infected (clade C) patients - a hospital-based prospective audit.* J Neurol Sci. 2007 Mar 15;254(1-2):60-4.

Modi G, Modi M, Martinus I, Vangu M. *New onset seizures in HIV-infected patients without intracranial mass lesions or meningitis--a clinical, radiological and SPECT scan study.* J Neurol Sci. 2002 Oct 15;202(1-2):29-34.

Modi M, Mochan A, Modi G. *Management of HIV-associated focal brain lesions in developing countries.* QJM. 2004 Jul;97(7):413-21.

Mullin S, Temu A, Kalluvya S, Grant A & Manji H. *High prevalence of distal sensory polyneuropathy in antiretroviral-treated and untreated people with HIV in Tanzania.* Tropical Medicine and International Health. 2011Oct; 16(10):1291-6.

Oshinaike OO, Okubadejo NU, Ojini FI, Danesi MA. *The clinical spectrum of neurological manifestations in HIV/AIDS patients on HAART at the Lagos University Teaching Hospital, Lagos, Nigeria.* Nig Q J Hosp Med. 2009 Sep-Dec;19(4):181-5.

Patel VN, Mungwira RG, Tarumbiswa TF, Heikinheimo T, van Oosterhout JJ. *High prevalence of suspected HIV-associated dementia in adult Malawian HIV patients.* Int J STD AIDS. 2010 May;21(5):356-8.

Pepper DJ, Marais S, Maartens G, Rebe K, Morroni C, Rangaka MX, et al. *Neurologic manifestations of paradoxical tuberculosis-associated immune reconstitution inflammatory syndrome: a case series.* Clin Infect Dis. 2009 Jun 1;48(11):e96-107.

Rana FS, Hawken MP, Mwachari C, Bhatt SM, Abdullah F, Ng'ang'a LW, et al. *Autopsy study of HIV-1-positive and HIV-1-negative adult medical patients in Nairobi, Kenya.* J Acquir Immune Defic Syndr. 2000 May 1;24(1):23-9.

Robertson K, Kopnisky K, Hakim J, Merry C, Nakasujja N, Hall C, et al. *Second assessment of NeuroAIDS in Africa.* J Neurovirol. 2008 Apr;14(2):87-101.

Sacktor N, Nakasujja N, Skolasky R, Robertson K, Wong M, Musisi S, et al. *Antiretroviral therapy improves cognitive impairment in HIV+ individuals in sub-Saharan Africa.* Neurology. 2006 Jul 25;67(2):311-4.

Sotrel A, Dal Canto MC. *HIV-1 and its causal relationship to immunosuppression and nervous system disease in AIDS: a review.* Hum Pathol. 2000 Oct;31(10):1274-98.

Wong MH, Robertson K, Nakasujja N, Skolasky R, Musisi S, Katabira E, et al. *Frequency of and risk factors for HIV dementia in an HIV clinic in sub-Saharan Africa.* Neurology. 2007 Jan 30;68(5):350-5.

Zunt JR. *Central nervous system infection during immunosuppression.* Neurol Clin. 2002 Feb; 20(1):1-22.

PART II – NEUROLOGICAL DISORDERS

CHAPTER 9
COMA AND TRANSIENT LOSS OF CONSCIOUSNESS

CONTENTS

CHAPTER 9

COMA AND TRANSIENT LOSS OF CONSCIOUSNESS

Loss or alteration in consciousness is a very common clinical disorder. This can be transient lasting seconds or minutes as occurs in syncope and seizures or more prolonged as occurs in coma. *Coma is by definition a state of impaired consciousness during which the patient is unrousable by external stimuli.* In states of coma the patient remains in a sleep like state with no purposeful movements or response to any external stimuli. These can be measured by the Glasgow Coma Scale which defines coma as a GCS ≤ 8/15. Coma can be caused by disorders that affect either a part of the brain focally or the whole brain diffusely (Figs. 9.1-4). The causes of coma are generally classified as intracranial or extracranial and are outlined in Table 9.1. Episodes of transient loss of consciousness are by definition intermittent and usually sudden events from which the patient recovers fully. These arise either from the disorders of the cardiovascular system with an acute reduction of blood flow to the brain (syncope) or a disruption in brain electrical activity (seizure). The chapter outlines the main mechanisms, causes, investigations and management of coma and syncope. The student should aim to be familiar with these and be able to investigate and manage a patient presenting with loss of consciousness.

Pathophysiology

Consciousness is a person's awareness of themselves and their surroundings. Normal consciousness is maintained by an intact reticular activating system in the brain stem and its central connections to the thalamus and cerebral hemispheres. The reticular activating system keeps us awake and alert during the waking hours. Disorders that physically affect these areas can lead to disordered arousal, awareness and to altered states of consciousness. A focal brain lesion occurring below the tentorium (Figs.9.1 & 2) interfering with the reticular activating system can result in coma whereas a focal lesion occurring above the tentorium in one cerebral hemisphere results in coma only if the contralateral side of the brain is simultaneously involved or compressed (Fig.9.3) Diffuse lesions which affect the function of the brain as a whole including the reticular activating system can result in coma (Fig.9.4).

ASSESSMENT

Acute

Coma is an acute life threatening condition and evaluation needs to be quick, comprehensive and may involve starting emergency management even before the cause is established. Emergency management starts with an immediate assessment of airway, breathing and circulation (ABC) and involves the following steps. **Firstly** check that the airway is clear without secretions and that no cyanosis is present. This is achieved by rapid visual inspection and checking the vital signs. **Secondly** ensure that breathing rate is satisfactory (rate >10-12/min), that there are

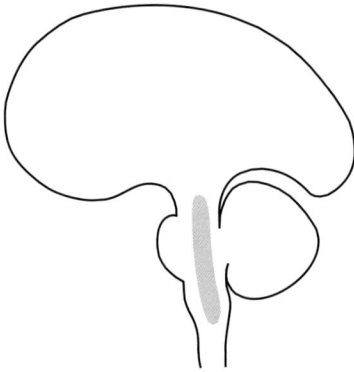

Figure 9.1 The reticular activating system

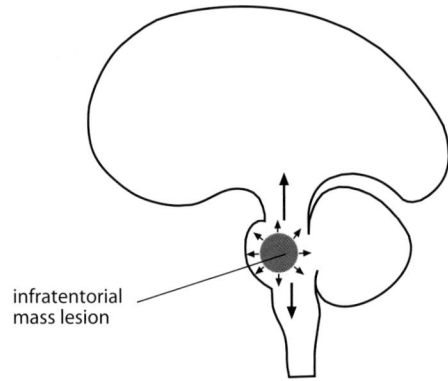

Figure 9.2 Sites that produce loss of consciousness

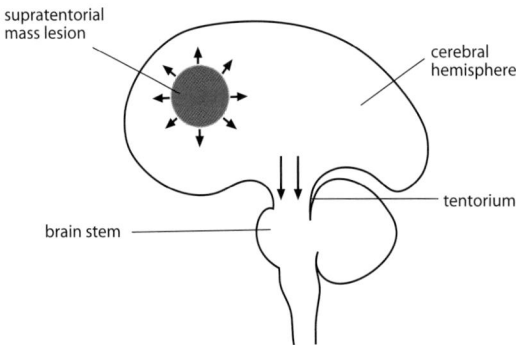

Figure 9.3 Sites that produce loss of consciousness

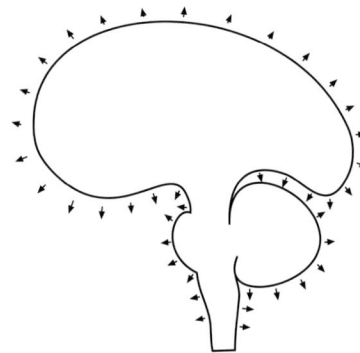

Figure 9.4 Encephalopathy diffuse

adequate breath sounds bilaterally on auscultation and that the oxygen saturation is >95%. If ventilation is inadequate or GCS is ≤8 then consider intubation and assisted ventilation. **Thirdly** check that the circulation is adequate by measuring pulse and BP. If the systolic blood pressure is <90 mm Hg then start immediate fluid resuscitation, and with inotropic support if BP remains persistently low despite adequate volume replacement. **Fourthly** insert an IV cannula and withdraw blood for laboratory studies. All comatose patients should have their blood glucose checked on arrival and treated immediately if hypoglycaemic (blood sugar <2.5 mmols/l) or hyperglycaemic. **Finally** treat any other immediately reversible cause without delay e.g. iv thiamine 100 mg in patients with history of alcoholism and naloxone 0.4-2 mg in patients with drug habituation (Table 9.4). If the patient is stable, then the clinical assessment can start.

Key points

- airway: make sure it is clear
- breathing: count RR & listen to the lungs, if respiration inadequate give O_2 & ventilate
- circulation: check pulse/BP and treat if systolic <90 mm Hg
- glucose: check urgently and treat any reversible cause immediately

Clinical assessment

This involves *history, general examination, level of consciousness* and *neurological examination.*

The history

The history is the most important part of the assessment as it frequently points to the underlying cause of coma. The diagnosis may already be obvious from the circumstances surrounding the coma e.g. head injury in a road traffic accident (RTA), stroke in hypertension or hyperglycaemia or hypoglycaemia in diabetes or a seizure in epilepsy. If the cause is not obvious then it is necessary to obtain a history from the patient's family members, friends or colleagues. The history should include information and details concerning the immediate circumstances and the possible cause of the coma. It should also include the patient's previous medical history, medications, allergies, possible toxins and details of social and family history including recent travel or anything relevant. In particular, ask if there was a recent preceding illness e.g. fever, headache, if the onset was sudden or gradual and check specifically for a history of trauma or fall, a history of epilepsy, alcohol or drugs. The main causes of coma are outlined below (Table 9.1).

Key points

- loss of consciousness is a medical emergency
- assessment needs to be brief and focused
- history is the most important part of the initial assessment
- cause may be obvious & reversible causes need to be considered
- main causes are head injuries, encephalopathies, infections & strokes

Table 9.1 Main disorders causing coma

Site/aetiology	Disorder
Intracranial	
Focal	
stroke	infarct, ICH, SAH
infections	brain abscess
trauma	haematoma (*ICH, EDH, SDH*)
tumours	primary or secondary
Diffuse	
infections	HIV, meningitis, malaria, encephalitis
seizures	post ictal/status epilepticus
trauma	traumatic brain injury
Extracranial	
hypoxia	cardiac, respiratory, renal, shock, anaemia
metabolic/toxic	hyper-hypoglycaemia, organ failure, hyponatraemia overdose, opiates, alcohol
hypertension	encephalopathy, eclampsia

Easy way to remember the causes of coma			
A	= anoxia/apoplexy	**I** = injury/infection	
		O = opiates	
E	= epilepsy	**U** = uraemia	

The general examination

This involves confirming the vital signs and checking for evidence of obvious injury or major underlying illness. Signs of head injury/basal skull fracture include lacerations or bruising to the head, around the eyes, behind the ear (Battle's sign) or CSF leak from the nose or ears (Chapter 19). Palpation of the head/neck may show signs of a fracture and swelling. Signs pointing to an underlying illness include paresis, hypertension, tongue biting, ketoacidosis, jaundice and evidence of infection including fever, meningitis, and pneumonia or discharging ear.

The level of consciousness (LOC)

This is the most important part of the assessment of the unconscious patient. Altered states of consciousness range from *confusion* and *delirium* to *stupor* and *coma* (**appendix 1**). *Confusion* is characterized by the patient being fully conscious but with impaired attention, concentration and orientation. Confusion can be tested at the bedside by checking if the patient is fully orientated in time, person and place with a score of 10/10 being fully orientated (Table 9.2).

Table 9.2 Testing for orientation 10/10*

Time	Person	Place
time	name	hospital
day	age	town/district
month	year of birth	country
year		

*score one for each correct answer

In a state of *delirium,* the patient although fully conscious is confused and restless with hallucinations. In a state of *stupor*, the patient is in coma but is rousable after intense stimulation; this is in contrast to coma where the patient is unrousable. In general the use of these terms has been replaced by the **Glasgow Coma Scale (GCS)** (Table 9.3).

Glasgow coma scale

The depth of coma can be measured by the **GCS**. This measures eye opening, best motor and verbal response, and is a reliable method for measuring and monitoring level of consciousness. It should be carried out and if necessary repeated on every comatose patient. When using the **GCS,** look carefully at the patient's face while assessing eye opening, and then check on the patient's ability to follow simple motor commands and listen to the patient's speech for content and orientation. If the patient is not responding to voice then test eye opening and limb movement response to deep pain by applying pressure to sternum or supra orbital ridge or nail beds. Record best eye opening, motor and verbal response as **E4, M6** and **V5.** Patients are considered comatose if the **GCS ≤ 8/15.**

Table 9.3 Glasgow Coma Scale

	Best response	**Score**
Eye opening (**E**)	spontaneously	4
	to speech	3
	to pain	2
	nil	1
Motor response (**M**)	obeys commands	6
	localizes stimulus	5
	flexes withdrawal	4
	flexes weak	3
	extension	2
	nil	1
Best verbal (**V**)	oriented fully	5
	confused	4
	inappropriate	3
	incomprehensible (sounds only)	2
	nil	1
Maximum score		15

The AVPU Method

A more simplified bedside assessment of the level of consciousness is the **AVPU method** (yes/no response). Its advantages are that it assesses the main levels of consciousness quickly and is easy and quick to use and communicate.

AVPU method

A: is the patient alert
V: is the patient responsive to voice

P: is the patient responsive to pain
U: is the patient unresponsive

Key points

- check the vital signs
- examine for signs of head injury or a systemic disorder
- assess the level of consciousness
- level of consciousness is the most important part of the assessment

THE NEUROLOGICAL ASSESSMENT

This frequently gives the clues towards establishing the aetiology of the coma. The neurological assessment in coma is necessarily shortened concentrating on the possible neurological causes of coma e.g. stroke, meningitis and the presence of any localizing signs. Note the level of consciousness and any obvious neurological abnormalities such as seizures, the pattern of breathing and the position of the eyes and posture of the trunk and limbs. In particular, record pupil size, equality, response to light and eye position or movements. Normal pupils are 3-4 mm in diameter and respond briskly to light. Abnormalities include fixed dilated pupil (s), >7 mm in size and non reactive to light. In states of coma the most common cause of a unilateral fixed pupil is herniation (Table 9.4.) and of bilateral fixed pupils is brain death. The presence or absence of the corneal reflexes should be noted and fundi checked for papilloedema. If there is no contra indication to moving the neck such as spinal or head injury neck stiffness should be tested although its absence is unreliable in coma.

In the comatose patient eye position and movements are observed and examined at rest and during head and neck movement. Eye movements may be checked by stimulating the vestibular system. The details concerning the methods of stimulation (Doll's eyes and caloric tests), are outlined in **appendix 1**. Note the presence of any cranial nerve palsies, the position of the limbs and any signs of limb paralysis. Motor response to pain can be checked by noting limb movement in response to a painful stimulus e.g. deep Achilles tendon pressure or knuckling the sternum. A flexor response in the arms and concurrent extension of the legs indicates a cortical site of origin **(decorticate)** whereas an extensor response at the elbow coupled with internal arm rotation and extension of the legs **(decerebrate)** indicates an upper brain stem injury. Unilateral or asymmetrical posturing indicates a contralateral focal brain lesion/injury. Tone and reflexes in the limbs are then examined in the routine manner. Main localizing neurological features in coma are summarized below in Table 9.4.

Table 9.4 Main localizing neurological features & causes in coma

Neurology finding	Localization	Main causes
Respiration pattern **Cheyne Stokes** (breathing progressively deeper and then shallower in cycles)	brain stem herniation/ encephalopathy	↑ICP, stroke
Eye position eyes looking to one side (conjugate deviation)	unilateral lesion	stroke, head injury & any focal lesion
Pupils		
fixed & dilated pupils	brain	anoxia, trauma, brain death
a fixed & dilated pupil	herniation of medial temporal lobe through tentorium compressing 3rd CN	unilateral mass lesion above tentorium due to any cause
pin point pupils	pontine lesion	stroke, organophosphorous poisoning, opiate overdose
Meningism	meningeal inflammation	infections & haemorrhage
Limb position		
hemiparetic/asymmetrical	unilateral lesion	stroke & any focal lesion
arms flexed, legs extended	decorticate posturing	cortical damage
all 4 limbs hyper extended & extensor posturing to pain	decerebrate posturing	brain, brain stem damage
Limb examination		
hypertonia & hyperreflexia & extensor plantars	brain/cord	any diffuse or focal lesion
bilateral extensor plantars	non localizing	coma any cause

Key points

- assessment of coma needs to be fast & focused
- history usually reveals the cause of coma
- general examination reveals the level of coma
- neurological examination may reveal the site
- don't forget fundoscopy

DIFFERENTIAL DIAGNOSIS

The differential diagnosis for persistent coma involves all causes of unresponsiveness including psychiatric and neurological disorders. These include unresponsiveness of psychogenic origin locked-in syndrome, persistent vegetative state and brain death **(appendix 1)**.

Psychogenic

This can be a manifestation of severe schizophrenia (catatonia), hysteria (conversion disorder) and malingering. These are all diagnoses of exclusion and should only be considered when other causes have been excluded and there is strong evidence in their favour. Neurological exam in these patients is invariably normal and most will exhibit resistance to eye opening and tensing or withdrawal to a painful stimulus. Investigations including caloric tests and EEGs if performed are normal. A return to full consciousness is usually the rule.

Locked-in syndrome

The term locked-in is a rare syndrome which describes patients who though fully conscious are quadriplegic and unable to speak. The main causes are stroke and trauma affecting the brain stem at the level of the pons/midbrain. The patients are usually able to see and hear but are unable to move or communicate apart from moving their eyes/eye lids. Only some of voluntary eye movements may be preserved e.g. looking upwards. This still allows for non verbal communication. The diagnosis can be confirmed by saying/indicating with your own eye movements to the patient to "open your eyes", "look up", "down" and "towards the tip of your nose". Using this method a way can then be established to communicate with the patient. If in doubt ask a senior colleague to examine and check the patient. EEG is normal. Survival for months and years is the rule.

Persistent vegetative state

Patient with this disorder are awake but not aware. Their eyes open and close normally and they have a sleep-wake cycle because of an intact brain stem but they show no purposeful response to any external stimuli. The cause is usually cerebral hypoxia or ischaemia or occasionally a structural lesion. Recovery is uncommon.

Brain death

Brain death is the irreversible loss of all brain stem function. This is loss of consciousness, respiration, response to pain and loss of all brain stem reflexes **(appendix 2)**. The patient should be unresponsive to any sensory input including pain and speech. The cause should be known, irreversible and sufficient to explain the death. Reversible causes of coma should be considered including CNS depressant drugs, metabolic disorders and hypothermia. If the patient is on assisted ventilation, the criteria for determining brain death are outlined in appendix 2.

INVESTIGATIONS

The main emergency investigations in patients presenting in coma are outlined below in Table 9.5. A blood glucose should be checked immediately and glucose given intravenously if <2.5 mmol/L. Screening for the presence of malaria parasites and checking of HIV status is routine practice in patients presenting in coma in Africa. When indicated bloods for other metabolic causes of coma should also be checked. A lumbar puncture is relatively contraindicated in states of coma. It is specifically contraindicated in states of undiagnosed deep coma **(GCS≤8)** until raised intracranial pressure and focal intracranial lesions have been excluded by fundoscopy and CT. Emergency X-rays are important in coma in particular in head injury. A skull X-ray may show a fracture and a CT a treatable cause of coma e.g. subdural haematoma.

Table 9.5 Emergency investigations

Bloods	blood sugar
	malaria parasite film
	FBC
	HIV
	biochemistry (renal & LFTs)
Urine	sugar & ketones
X-rays	
Skull/neck	may show fracture
Chest	may show pneumonia, PCP, TB
CT head	may show blood & fracture & structural lesion

MANAGEMENT

The emergency treatments of the main causes of coma are presented in Table 9.6. Medical and nursing care involves monitoring and regularly checking the vital signs, level of consciousness and pupils, usually every 15 minutes to four hourly depending on the clinical situation. It is important at this stage to avoid sedation and strong analgesics. General nursing care of eyes, mouth, bladder and bowels should be started early with special attention to avoiding pressure sores and prevention of deep vein thrombosis. The ongoing care of the comatose patient should ideally take place in an appropriate intensive care unit (ICU) setting, depending on the cause. The subsequent medical or surgical management will depend on the underlying cause. Consider intubation if GCS ≤ 8.

Table 9.6 Emergency treatment of coma

Disorder	Acute management
Stroke (ischaemic)	aspirin 300 mg/po/stat
Infections *cerebral malaria*	artemether* 2.4 mg/kg iv/im stat *or* quinine 600 mg/iv over 4 hours
acute bacterial meningitis	ceftriaxone 2 gm/iv infusion stat
cryptococcal meningitis	fluconazole 1200 mg/po/ng tube
toxoplasmosis	co-trimoxazole 80/400mg/4 tablets stat/po/ng tube
sepsis	ceftriaxone 2 gm/iv infusion stat gentamycin 80 mg/im/stat
Hypoglycaemia	25-50 ml of 50% dextrose/iv/stat *or* glucagon 1mg/im stat
Ketoacidosis	soluble insulin 5 iu/iv & 5 iu/im stat & start hydration
Raised intracranial pressure	mannitol 20%: 100-200 ml iv stat dexamethasone 16 mg/iv stat
Poisoning e.g. organophosphates	atropine 1.0 mg/iv/stat & repeat every 15-30 mins
Respiratory depression (secondary to suspected opiate overdose)	naloxone 0.4-2 mg iv every 2-3 mins to max of 10 mg
Wernicke's encephalopathy	thiamine 100 mg iv
Anaphylaxis	adrenaline 0.5-1 ml of 1:1000/im/stat *or* adrenaline 0.5-1 ml of 1:10,000/iv/stat

* artemisinin drugs are the first line drugs recommended for use in cerebral malaria although quinine is mostly available

Prognosis

The underlying cause of the coma is the most important factor in determining outcome. Acute reversible causes have the best prognosis; these include acute infections, seizure disorders, drug overdose and treatable head injury. Patients with reversible causes may remain unconscious for long periods. However significant recovery is very unlikely in those comatose patients without a reversible cause who remain unconscious for more than 24 hours after admission. The outcome is poorest in those patients with anoxic, ischaemic and structural lesions. In these patients the persistent absence of corneal and oculovestibular reflexes and absence of movement to pain are bad prognostic signs with the chances of meaningful recovery set at <3%.

Key points

- emergency treatment of the cause of coma should be started without delay
- patients with reversible causes can remain unconscious for long periods
- patients comatose for >24 hours without a reversible cause have a poor prognosis

TRANSIENT LOSS OF CONSCIOUSNESS

Transient loss of consciousness is a very common clinical disorder. The main causes are outlined below in Table 9.7. The most common type is vasovagal or simple faints which occur in all age groups. The main differential diagnosis for vasovagal syncope is an epileptic seizure (Table 9.8).

Table 9.7 Common causes of transient loss of consciousness

vasovagal syncope	pseudoseizure
cardiac syncope	hypoglycaemia
postural syncope	transient ischaemic attack (TIA)
epileptic seizure	

Vasovagal Syncope (Faint)

Syncope is a sudden episodic loss of consciousness and postural tone resulting from an acute reduction of blood flow to the brain. Syncope of vasovagal origin is the most common form of transient loss of consciousness and can affect all age groups especially teenagers, young adults and also older persons. It is of cardiovascular origin. There are many contributory causes and syncope is often triggered by prolonged standing in crowded warm, indoor surroundings e.g. schools, churches, hospitals. Psychogenic factors, emotion, tiredness, fear, pain and sometimes even seeing blood, needles or medical procedures may precipitate the syncope or fainting. Rarely, it is provoked by micturition or coughing.

During a typical faint, the person first describes feeling dizzy, hot and cold, sweaty; their vision becomes blurred and darkened and nearby voices become distant. This comes on relatively quickly over 10-15 seconds or at most a few minutes. The attack may be prevented at this stage, by lying flat or alternatively made worse by staying upright in either the standing or sitting position. If the attack is not prevented, there is a sudden loss of consciousness with a falling to the ground *(syncope).* The person then remains unconscious lying motionless, pale and sweaty for a short period, usually for less than 30 seconds but not more than a minute. There may be transient, brief ictal-like limb jerking and very rarely a seizure if there is prolonged anoxia. Bradycardia and dilated pupils are usually present. Persons then regain full consciousness remembering the events leading up to and immediately after the blackout. They may continue to feel sweaty and nauseated but are usually back to normal within 10-15 minutes or less. The attack of syncope may recur on attempting to stand up too soon. The differential diagnosis includes the other causes of transient loss of consciousness and in particular a seizure disorder. Management is one of reassurance and advice to avoid the precipitating factors.

Cardiac syncope

A cardiac cause is suspected when syncope occurs either in relation to exercise or alternatively occurs in the sitting or lying position or in a patient with known cardiac disease. *The syncope is characterized by its sudden onset usually without any warning* and then by an equally rapid recovery of consciousness on falling to the ground, the entire episode usually lasting a matter of seconds. The main causes are arrhythmias e.g. complete heart block and supra ventricular tachycardia and cardiac outflow obstruction e.g. aortic stenosis and hypertrophic cardiomyopathy. Investigations include ECG, monitoring for arrhythmias and cardiac Echo. Management is the treatment of the underlying cardiac disorder.

Cerebrovascular syncope

This is an uncommon cause of syncope. The main causes are basilar artery insufficiency, large vessel occlusive disease and carotid sinus compression or hypersensitivity. *Basilar artery insufficiency is characterized by sudden brief attacks of dizziness and vertigo, and sometimes transient symptoms of lower cranial nerve dysfunction.* These attacks last seconds to minutes and may be coupled with a loss of consciousness which can occasionally be more prolonged. Management is similar to that outlined in cerebrovascular disease (Chapter 5). Carotid syncope is caused by a tight collar or mass in the neck pressing on the carotid sinus or by an abnormally sensitive carotid sinus. It is more common in older males and in those taking antihypertensive medications, in particular beta blockers.

Postural syncope

The main causes are hypovolaemia, antihypertensive medications and polyneuropathies e.g. in DM. These result in either reduced blood volume or autonomic dysfunction. This may occur in any age group but is more common in the elderly on medications for hypertension. *Syncope secondary to posture should be suspected if the patient with a known risk factor complains of light-headedness or loss of consciousness when standing up rapidly which is relieved when either sitting or lying down.* The diagnosis is confirmed by a symptomatic drop in systolic blood pressure of >30 mm Hg on standing as compared to lying. Management includes changing or discontinuing any likely causal medications and giving clear instructions to the patient, concerning standing up gradually and the wearing of support stockings.

Hyperventilation syncope

Hyperventilation is a common cause of dizziness and faintness but rarely causes syncope. It occurs most commonly but not exclusively in teenage or young women, usually in response to stress and anxiety. *It is a benign disorder which is caused by over breathing in response to anxiety.* This results in a respiratory alkalosis and cerebral vasoconstriction which can cause light-headedness, dyspnoea, and a feeling of unreality, and may proceed to blackouts which mimic seizures. The diagnosis should be suspected if the patient is anxious and describes an episode of difficulty of getting their breath before and just as the attack develops. There is typically associated tingling on the lips, the tip of the nose and finger tips and rarely muscle twitches of the fingers, followed by a short episode of loss of consciousness usually lasting seconds. The symptoms can be reproduced by getting the patient to hyperventilate voluntarily and then stopped promptly by rebreathing from a paper bag.

Syncope and seizures

The main differential diagnosis of syncope is with epileptic seizures. Distinguishing these can be difficult but there are some differences. A clear description of the episode from both the patient and an observer is essential. Syncope of vasovagal origin is largely non recurring and tends to happen in stereotyped situations e.g. triggered by standing, heat, pain, blood, straining. Syncope arising from cardiac, posture and stress disorders is recurring but the underlying cause is usually apparent. Seizures are by their nature recurring and happen anywhere. The immediate preceding warning symptoms are different in both types of LOC. Patients with syncope have a characteristic set of vasovagal warning symptoms including light-headedness, nausea, blurred vision sweating and pallor lasting seconds or minutes. This is in contrast to the aura in seizures which if present is usually more stereotyped and of shorter duration lasting a second or less. The duration of LOC is also shorter in syncope lasting seconds to 1-2 minutes whereas in epilepsy it usually lasts 4-5 minutes or longer. During a syncopal attack the patient lies motionless with only occasional muscle twitching of the limbs and infrequently urinary incontinence and only very rarely if brain hypoxia occurs are there associated tonic clonic like limb movements and tongue biting. In contrast these are the characteristics of a seizure. In syncope recovery of full consciousness occurs within seconds of awakening whereas in seizures there is typically a period of postictal confusion which lasts for as long as 10-15 mins. These differences are summarized in Table 9.8.

Table 9. 8 Clinical differences between a fit and a faint

Clinical features	Vasovagal attack	Epileptic seizure
posture	upright	any posture
onset	gradual	sudden
incontinence/tongue biting	rare	common
period/unconsciousness	seconds	minutes
recovery	rapid within seconds	slow
precipitating factor	stereotyped	non stereotyped
recurring pattern	no	yes

Pseudoseizures

Some patients have unexplained seizure-like episodes of loss of consciousness. These episodes resemble seizures and are considered to be psychogenic or non epileptic in origin. The diagnosis should be suspected if there are *atypical episodes of loss of consciousness* occurring *mostly in teenagers* and *young adults, often females, usually lasting* longer than *5 minutes.* The attacks can mimic an epileptic seizure and may occur in association with known epilepsy. The main differences are already outlined in chapter 4.

HYPOGLYCAEMIA

The diagnosis should be suspected if there are *feelings of hunger, sweating, nervousness* and *palpitations* coupled with episodes of *confusion, abnormal speech* or *unusual* behaviour in a patient not at risk for seizures or syncope. A blood glucose <2.5 mmols/L is considered to be hypoglycaemia. These attacks occur most frequently in diabetics taking oral hypoglycaemic agents or insulin. Other less common causes include during or after a period of prolonged exercise, fasting, liver disease and malignancies including hepatoma and insulinoma. The loss of consciousness in hypoglycaemia can be prolonged (>30 mins) and seizures may occur. If untreated this may proceed to coma and brain damage. The diagnosis is confirmed by measuring blood glucose during the episode and by its response to treatment. While a blood sugar level should always be checked in the unconscious patient in whom hypoglycaemia is suspected, intravenous glucose should be given without waiting for the results of a confirmatory blood sugar.

TRANSIENT ISCHAEMIC ATTACK (TIA)

A TIA is a sudden ischaemic focal neurological deficit that *completely resolves in <24 hours* (Chapter 5). The neurological findings in TIA typically last for minutes and occasionally, hours and the presentations are the same as for stroke and include a loss of consciousness. They are mostly caused by thromboemboli arising from the internal carotid arteries or from the heart in atrial fibrillation or mitral valve disease. All TIAs should be treated with the same sense of urgency as stroke. The aim is to identify risk factors and prevent a stroke occurring as the risk over the following days and weeks is high (>10%). Antiplatelet drugs and anticoagulants are used as in stroke.

Key points

- transient loss of consciousness is a common outpatient problem
- main differential diagnosis is an epileptic seizure
- causes tend to be stereotyped
- history is the key to the correct diagnosis

APPENDIX 1 DESCRIPTIONS OF STATES OF ALTERED CONSCIOUSNESS

Confusion	disturbed consciousness and impairment of higher cerebral function
Delirium	confusion with motor restlessness, and transient hallucinations and delusions
Stupor	conscious but rousable only with intense stimulation
Coma	unrousable unresponsiveness (GCS ≤ 8/15)
Vegetative state	loss of consciousness with preservation of brain stem function
Death	loss of consciousness and capacity to breathe spontaneously: irreversible

APPENDIX 2 EXAMINING THE COMATOSE PATIENT FOR SIGNS OF BRAIN DEATH

Brain death is the irreversible loss of all brain stem function. This is loss of consciousness, respiration, response to pain and loss of all brain stem reflexes. In brain death the following brain stem reflexes must be absent:

- light reflex
- corneal reflex
- gag reflex
- cough to deep tracheal suction
- eye movements to testing (Doll's eyes)
- oculovestibular reflex (caloric test)

Doll's eyes or oculocephalic reflex

Check for the normal oculocephalic reflexes by rotating the head 180 degrees to the left or right (or up down) holding it there for 3-4 secs and observing the eyes. In the normal intact brain stem the eyes deviate to the side opposite to that of the head movement. In brain stem disease or deep coma the eyes remain fixed and move in the same direction as the head which is abnormal. The oculocephalic reflex is suppressed in the fully conscious patient so it can only be tested in the unconscious patient.

Caloric testing or oculovestibular reflex

First check that the external canal is clear and the tympanic membranes are intact. Then irrigate the tympanic membrane in each ear with 50-100 mls of iced cold water. The normal response is that the eyes deviate slowly towards the stimulated ear. In brain death and overdose there may be no response or if the brain stem is damaged the eyes may diverge.

Certifying brain death in a patient on a ventilator

In order to declare a patient brain dead whilst on a ventilator ideally two doctors must be certain that all brain stem reflexes are absent and that there is no reversible cause. The ventilation should have continued with the patient in this state for 24 hours. If a patient is on a ventilator there should be no spontaneous ventilation 10 minutes after disconnecting from the ventilator having preoxygenated the patient with 100% O_2 for at least 10 mins.

Selected references

Mapoure NY, Diouf FS, Ndiaye M, Ngahane HB, Doumbe J, Toure K, et al. *[A prospective longitudinal study of coma in the intensive care unit in an African setting: case of Dakar, Senegal].* Rev Med Brux. 2009 May-Jun; 30(3):163-9.

Adeleye AO, Olowookere KG, Olayemi OO. *Clinicoepidemiological profiles and outcomes during first hospital admission of head injury patients in Ikeja, Nigeria.* A prospective cohort study. Neuroepidemiology. 2009; 32(2):136-41.

Greenberg David, Aminoff Michael & Roger Simon, *Clinical Neurology,* McGraw Hill Fifth edition 2002.

Ginsberg Lionel, Neurology, *Lecture Notes,* Blackwell Publishing 8th edition 2005.

Gwer S, Thuo N, Idro R, Ndiritu M, Boga M, Newton C, et al. *Changing trends in incidence and aetiology of childhood acute non-traumatic coma over a period of changing malaria transmission in rural coastal Kenya: a retrospective analysis.* BMJ Open. 2012 Apr 1;2(2):e000475.

Manga NM, Ndour CT, Diop SA, Ka-Sall R, Dia NM, Seydi M, et al. *[Adult purulent meningitis caused by Streptococcus pneumoniae in Dakar, Senegal].* Med Trop (Mars). 2008 Dec; 68(6):625-8.

Mapoure NY, Diouf FS, Ndiaye M, Ngahane HB, Doumbe J, Toure K, et al. *[A prospective longitudinal study of coma in the intensive care unit in an African setting: case of Dakar, Senegal].* Rev Med Brux. 2009 May-Jun; 30(3):163-9.

Obiako OR, Ogunniyi A, Anyebe E. *Prognosis of non traumatic coma: the role of some socio-economic factors on its outcome in Ibadan, Nigeria.* Ann Afr Med. 2009 Apr-Jun; 8(2):115-21.

Obiako OR, Oparah S, Ogunniyi A. *Causes of medical coma in adult patients at the university college hospital, Ibadan Nigeria.* Niger Postgrad Med *J.* 2011 Mar; 18(1):1-7.

Plum F, Posner JB. *Diagnosis of stupor and coma.* 3rd edition. Davis, 1980.

Soumare M, Seydi M, Diop SA, Diop BM, Sow PS. *[Cerebral malaria in adults at the Infectious Diseases Clinic in the Fann Hospital in Dakar, Senegal].* Bull Soc Pathol Exot. 2008 Feb; 101(1):20-1.

Winkler AS, Tluway A, Schmutzhard E. *Aetiologies of altered states of consciousness: a prospective hospital-based study in a series of 464 patients of northern Tanzania.* J Neurol Sci. 2011 Jan 15; 300(1-2):47-51.

CHAPTER 10
PARAPLEGIA NON TRAUMATIC

CONTENTS

CHAPTER 10

PARAPLEGIA NON TRAUMATIC

Introduction

Paraplegia (PP) means paralysis of the legs. It is caused mainly by disorders of the spinal cord and the cauda equina. They are classified as traumatic and non traumatic. Traumatic paraplegia occurs mostly as a result of road traffic accidents (RTA) and falls (Chapter 19). Non traumatic paraplegia (NTP) has multiple causes (Table 10.1) and is the most common cause of adult neurological hospital admissions in Africa after stroke and infection. Paraplegia is among the most common community based neurological disorders in Africa. The aim of this chapter is to review the causes and management of NTP. The student should aim to be able to localise the site and classify the main causes of paraplegia and to investigate and manage a patient presenting with it.

AETIOLOGY

Paraplegia can arise from a lesion either within or outside the spinal cord or cauda equina. These are classified as **compressive** and **non compressive**. Compression is caused either by bone or other masses. The main compressive causes are Pott's disease (TB of spine) and tumours (usually metastases). The main non compressive causes are transverse myelitis secondary to viral infections, HIV, TB and very occasionally syphilis. Less common causes include Devic's disease, B-12 deficiency and helminthic infections. There also exists in Africa a large group of nutrition related non compressive paraplegias, termed the **tropical myeloneuropathies**. These include konzo, lathyrism and tropical ataxic neuropathy (TAN). The main causes of paraplegia are presented in Table 10.1.

Table 10.1 Main causes of nontraumatic paraplegia in Africa

Classification	Causes
Compressive	
Extradural	Pott's disease, metastatic ca/myeloma, cervical spondylosis, epidural abscess, echinococcus cyst
Subdural	
extramedullary	neurofibroma, meningioma
intramedullary	astrocytoma, ependymoma, tuberculoma, schistosome ova, syringomyelia
Non compressive	
transverse myelopathy	viral infections, HIV, TB, syphilis, HTLV-1, Devic's disease
nutritional	konzo, lathyrism, tropical ataxic neuropathy
vascular	sickle cell disease, dural AV fistula
hereditary	familial spastic paraplegia
deficiency	B-12

Common causes of paraplegia in Africa

- Pott's disease (TB)
- inflammation (transverse myelitis)
- malignancy (metastases)
- infection (HIV)
- nutritional (konzo)

Localization/anatomy

The spinal cord extends from C1 in the neck to the lower border of L1 (Fig. 10.1). The cauda equina extends from the end of the cord down to S5 within the sacral canal. Paraplegia arises from disorders affecting the thoracic spinal cord and the cauda equina, whereas quadriplegia or quadriparesis arises from disorders affecting the cervical cord. The most important information to elicit at the bedside is whether paraplegia is spastic or flaccid in type and whether there is a sensory level on the trunk above which sensation is normal (Chapter 2). This helps to localise the site of the lesion causing the paraplegia.

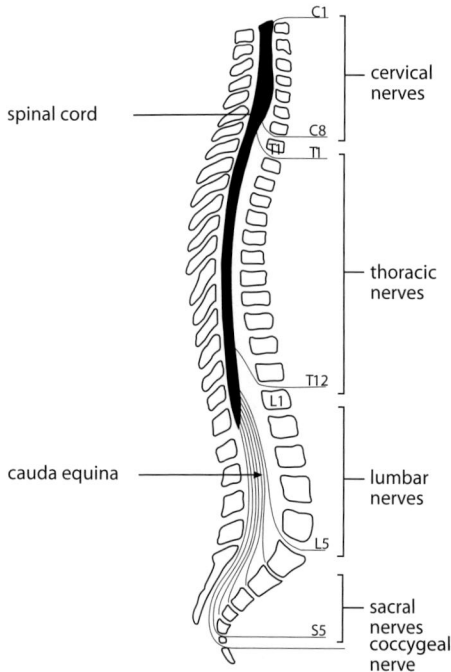

Figure 10.1 Spinal cord. Spinal nerves and vertebral column.

Key points

- paraplegia is a common neurological disorder
- clinically classified as compressive & non compressive
- main causes are Pott's disease, transverse myelitis & malignancy
- the most common community based cause is nutritional myelopathy
- disorders of the spinal cord result in a spastic PP
- disorders of the cauda equina result in a flaccid PP

COMPRESSIVE CAUSES

The causes of compressive paraplegia can be classified on neuroimaging (CT/MRI) as being either extradural or subdural in site. Subdural includes those arising from either within the spinal cord (intramedullary) or those arising outside the cord (extramedullary) (Table 10.1). The two main compressive causes in Africa are Pott's disease and metastatic malignancy, both of which are extradural. Acute cord compression is a medical emergency and needs rapid evaluation and intervention in order to prevent permanent disability. The history and neurological examination localise the level of weakness, and help to determine the likely cause of the paraplegia. However on their own without further laboratory and imaging investigations they may not reliably distinguish the cause.

Spinal TB

Spinal TB accounts for <10% of extrapulmonary TB. Extrapulmonary TB accounts for about 15% of all TB. Spinal TB can result in paraplegia in two main ways, either by infection of the spine (**Pott's disease**) accounting for the majority of cases of paraplegia or less commonly by direct infection of the spinal cord and cauda equina (**spinal cord tuberculosis**).

POTT'S DISEASE

Pott's disease is a leading cause of paraplegia in Africa and is the most common cause in childhood, adolescence and in young adults. It arises from haematogenous spread of the tubercle bacillus from pulmonary infection. The paraplegia occurs either at the time of the primary infection or more commonly 3-5 years later by reactivation. This results in infection of the spine affecting the intervertebral disc space and adjacent vertebrae which if not treated may result in characteristic extradural compression of the spinal cord causing paraplegia.

Clinical features

The main clinical features of Pott's disease are a history of localised back pain, over weeks or months, which is made worse by weight bearing and followed by a slowly progressive paraplegia. The paraplegia may be accompanied by low grade features of active systemic TB including fever, sweating and weight loss but this is not common. Neurological examination confirms paraplegia, the clinical signs depending on the level and the extent of the lesion. The lower thoracic and the lumbar spine are the most common sites affected. The spine should be carefully inspected for signs of local tenderness and the presence of any deformity, in particular a gibbus formation. A gibbus is a visible angular deformity of the thoracic or lumbar spine caused by collapse and anterior wedging of adjacent vertebrae. Local tenderness is best elicited by gently tapping the spines of the vertebrae with a finger tip or a patellar hammer.

Investigations

The ESR is typically elevated early on and throughout the course of Pott's disease and may be the only laboratory clue as to the likely underlying cause. Radiological evidence shows a characteristic loss of the disc space at the site of infection with destruction and wedging of adjacent vertebrae but the latter is a late finding. There may also be a paravertebral soft tissue swelling (Fig. 10.2) or uncommonly a psoas muscle abscess. A CT scan of the spine may also be helpful, particularly in early disease when plain X-rays may be normal. The diagnosis of Pott's disease is usually made by clinical suspicion, in combination with an elevated ESR and typical spinal X-rays. All suspected cases of Pott's disease should have a chest X-ray to exclude active pulmonary tuberculosis.

Treatment

Treatment is mostly carried out on clinical and X-ray grounds alone. Where possible a needle biopsy confirming the presence of acid fast bacilli should be performed and this is diagnostic. The standard anti tuberculous treatment for spinal TB is for a total of 18 months, however a shorter 12 month course has been recently recommended. Surgical treatment involving decompression of the cord and stabilization of the spine is helpful in a few mainly early cases of spinal cord compression.

Prognosis

The treated mortality rate is between 10-20% and full recovery rates of from 25 to 40%.

X-ray chest & spine

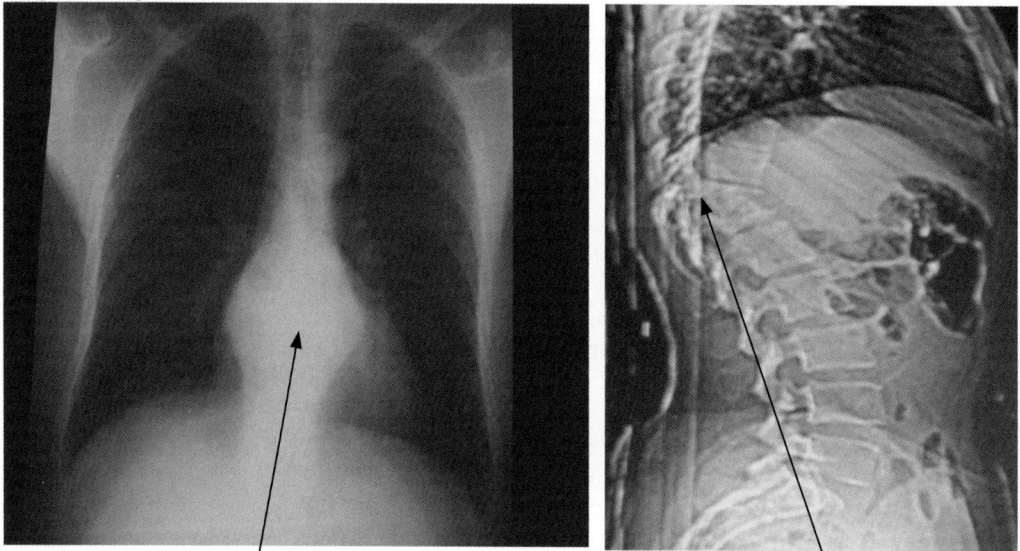

TB spine & paravertebral abscess

Vertebral collapse & wedging & gibbus

Figure 10.2 Pott's disease

SPINAL CORD TUBERCULOSIS

Direct infection of the spinal cord with TB presents clinically either as an acute myelitis developing over days or as a chronic radiculo-myelitis (Fig. 10.3) occurring over weeks to months. The resulting paraplegia is mostly lower motor neurone or flaccid in type with absent or depressed reflexes with urinary and faecal incontinence. Tuberculoma of the cord may also result in paraplegia but this is uncommon. TB meningitis may also arise from a source of infection within the spinal cord and the combination of TB meningitis and paraplegia is not uncommon in Africa. All patients presenting with paraplegia should be screened for HIV infection. The diagnosis and management of spinal cord tuberculosis is similar to that of TBM which is presented in chapter 6.

MRI T2 lumbar sacral spine

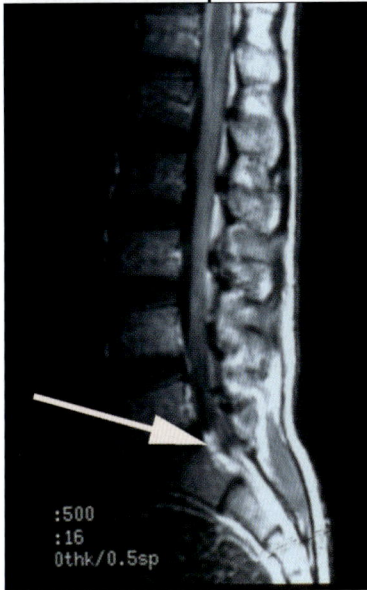

:500
:16
0thk/0.5sp

L5/S1 arachnoiditis

Figure 10.3 TB cauda equina

Key points

- Pott's disease is one of the most common causes of PP in Africa
- PP can also arise from direct TB infection of spinal cord or meninges
- clinical features of Pott's disease are back pain, spinal tenderness & progressive PP
- laboratory findings are a high ESR with typical spinal x-ray changes
- treatment is with anti TB Rx for at least 12 months
- CFR is 10-20% & morbidity rate is 25-40%

TUMOURS

Tumours affecting the spinal cord can be either primary arising from the cord, roots or meninges or secondary or metastatic arising from outside the cord. The most common overall cause of spinal cord tumours is secondary or metastatic. The main sources are prostate, breast, lung, kidney, lymphoma and multiple myeloma. They are mostly located extradurally and the most common sites affected are the thoracic followed by the lumbar spine. These are the main cause of paraplegia in older age groups (>50 years). Primary spinal cord tumours are very uncommon with an expected incidence of <1/100,000 per year and can occur in all age groups. These include meningioma arising from the meninges, neurofibroma arising from peripheral nerves and astrocytoma and ependymoma arising from the cord.

Clinical features

Patients presenting with paraplegia resulting from metastatic tumours typically have a history of localised back pain in combination with a mainly flaccid type paraplegia developing over a short period, usually days or weeks. Pain arising from the spinal site of metastasis is usually a distinctive feature. The paraplegia may be the first presenting complaint or a complication of known systemic malignancy. In contrast benign tumours tend to present with paraplegia evolving more slowly over months or years, and pain is less pronounced.

Investigation

Investigations help to confirm the suspicion of a malignancy with plain spinal x-rays showing lytic or blastic lesions or vertebral collapse depending on the primary (Fig. 10.4). CSF may sometimes show a high protein level and yellow discolouration particularly if there is a block to flow resulting in a concentration of CSF constituents. This is called the Froin syndrome. Neuroimaging (CT/MRI) of the spinal cord is necessary in all patients with suspected primary cord tumours and in some with suspected metastatic tumour.

Treatment

The treatment depends on the type of underlying tumour. Metastatic tumours causing cord compression initially require urgent steroids and analgesia if needed. More definitive treatments include local radiotherapy and occasionally surgical decompression. Chemotherapy may be helpful in patients with lymphoma and myeloma, whereas hormonal therapy can be very beneficial in those with metastatic breast and prostate cancer. Some benign tumours can be removed depending on their histology, size and local invasiveness. The prognosis for metastatic spinal cord tumour is generally poor.

X-rays spine & skull

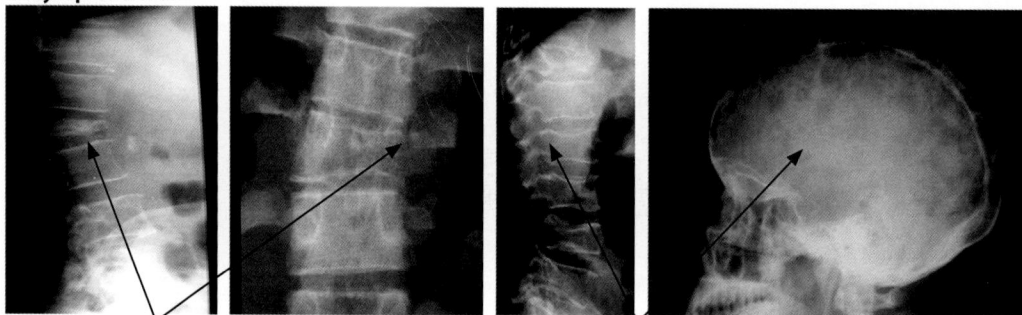

Metastatic carcinoma loss of height & pedicle   Multiple myeloma involving spine and skull

Figure 10.4 Malignancies

Key points

- metastatic malignancy is the most common cause of PP in the elderly
- prostate and breast are the most common primary sources
- paralysis is usually painful & flaccid with a sensory level on the trunk
- treatment includes steroids, analgesia, radiotherapy & chemotherapy

ACUTE EPIDURAL ABSCESS

Acute spinal epidural abscess is a relatively uncommon cause of paraplegia but is a medical emergency when it happens. It tends to occur in debilitated patients with diabetes, alcoholism or renal failure but may occur in an otherwise healthy person. *Staphylococcus aureus* is the most common organism accounting for 90% of cases, skin abscesses and boils are the most common sources of infection. It can affect all age groups.

Clinical features

The clinical features are those of a painful sub acute paraplegia developing over hours or days. The distinguishing features are very severe pain, sometimes radicular, and local tenderness at the site of the epidural abscess which is usually situated in the cervical or lumbar spine. These are frequently but not always coupled with fever and signs of infection with or without meningism.

Investigations

Investigations suggest a bacterial cause when the peripheral WBC (neutrophil count) and ESR are both elevated but these can be normal. CSF examination may reveal the presence of a few white blood cells and elevated protein level or be normal. Lumbar puncture should not be performed near the suspected abscess site as this may spread the infection to the CSF causing meningitis. A CT scan of the spinal cord with contrast may show epidural enhancement but can also be normal. MRI of the spinal cord with contrast is the investigation of choice.

Treatment

Emergency treatment is recommended on the grounds of clinical suspicion without waiting for the results of any investigations. Appropriate high dose intravenous antibiotics including cloxacillin are started and continued for a period of up to 6 weeks. High dose intravenous steroids may be of value if given early on during the first week or two of treatment. Urgent decompressive laminectomy may sometimes be indicated.

Key points

- epidural abscess is a medical emergency which requires urgent treatment
- sub acute painful PP occurring over hours or days
- occurs in DM, alcoholism, renal failure & skin infection & in healthy persons
- diagnosis is confirmed by contrast enhanced CT/MRI spinal cord
- treatment is iv antibiotics & steroids & sometimes surgery

CERVICAL SPONDYLOSIS

This is one of the most common causes of paraplegia in high income countries but appears to be a relatively uncommon cause in Africa.

Clinical features

Affected patients are usually older, >60 yrs and typically present with a slow insidious onset of weakness or stiffness in the legs, sometimes coupled with numbness and tingling in the upper limbs. There may be a history of previous neck injury or accident. Pain and bladder symptoms are uncommon. The main clinical findings are those of a spastic paraplegia coupled with wasting of the small hand muscles.

Investigations

Plain X-ray or CT of the cervical spine confirms the diagnosis, showing narrowing of one or two disc spaces with prominent osteophytes, narrowing of the cervical canal and evidence of cord compression (Fig. 10.5).

Management

Management is mostly conservative and includes analgesics, cervical collar and very rarely traction. Indications for consideration for decompressive surgery include progressive paraplegia, severe weakness and intractable pain. Surgery is aimed at the prevention of any further deterioration rather than making the patient better, although neurologic improvement is occasionally seen.

X- ray cervical spine	MRI T2 cord (lateral)	MRI T2 cord (axial)

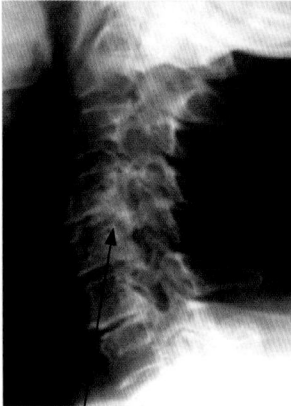

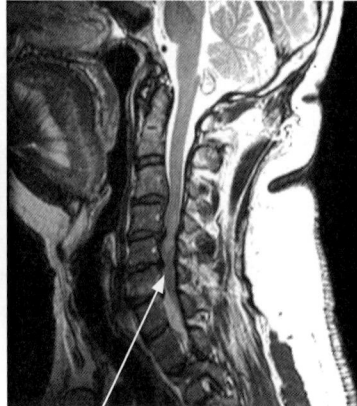

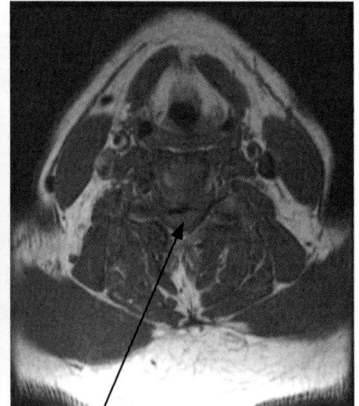

Narrowing & osteophytes   Compression   Compression

Figure 10.5 Cervical spondylosis

Key points

- cervical spondylosis is an uncommon cause of PP in Africa
- presents with slow onset spastic PP with numbness & wasting in hands
- occurs in older persons, often with a history of previous neck injury
- X-ray/CT neck: narrow disc spaces & canal with osteophytes & cord compression
- treatment usually conservative with analgesics & cervical collar

FLUOROSIS

Fluorosis is a disorder characterized by the deposition of excess fluoride in bones (osteofluorosis) and teeth (dental fluorosis). It results from chronic ingestion of fluoride rich waters over many years. Water contamination with fluoride occurs naturally in volcanic areas of the world. This is particularly the case in volcanic areas in the rift valley region of East Africa where there can be exposure to high levels of fluoride in drinking water. The degree of water contamination and exposure can vary enormously within adjacent areas in affected regions. Neurological disorders are uncommon and arise in fluorosis as consequence of the chronic deposition of fluoride in bone occurring over many years. This can result in narrowing of the diameter of the spinal canal and the intervertebral foramina which can cause compression. It mainly affects the cervical canal but may also affect the lumbar sacral canal. The resulting neurological disorders are mostly forms of spastic paralysis with or without associated radiculopathies. These lead to quadriplegia and paraplegia characterized by immobility, flexion deformities, severe spasms, and urinary incontinence. The diagnosis is usually suggested by the typical clinical and X-ray findings occurring in a person from a known volcanic area (Fig.10.6). Treatment is symptomatic. Primary prevention is the intervention of choice either by filtering all water at the point of access or drinking water at the point of usage.

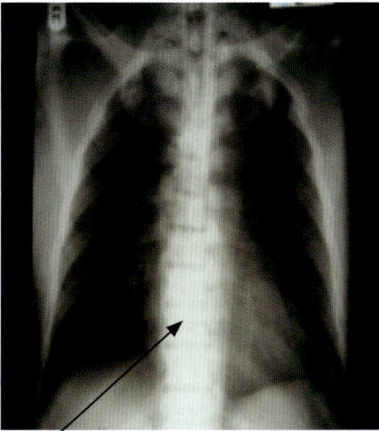

Whitening of bones

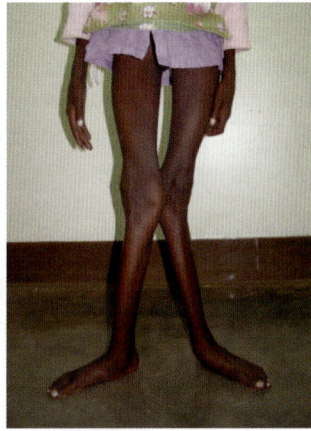

Severe skeletal fluorosis

Figure 10.6 Fluorosis

Key points

- skeletal fluorosis results from chronic high fluoride intake in drinking water
- cervical & lumbosacral spine are most commonly affected sites
- result in a quadri/paraparesis & radiculopathy
- PP is an uncommon complication of skeletal fluorosis
- skeletal X-rays confirm the diagnosis
- prevention is by filtering drinking water

SYRINGOMYELIA

This is an uncommon disorder in which a CSF filled cavity called a syrinx forms in the centre of the spinal cord. The time course of symptoms and signs is one of slow progression over many years. It typically starts slowly in the lower cervical cord and over many years, the cavity can involve the whole spinal cord down to T12 & L1. The cause is considered to be related to abnormalities in the dynamics of local CSF pressure and flow. Predisposing causes include a developmental abnormality of the skull base with flattening or platybasia coupled with variable protrusion of the lower brain stem and cerebellar tonsils through the foramen magnum. This is called the Arnold-Chiari malformation. Neck and cervical cord injury is another risk factor which is an important cause in Africa, particularly in women because of falls whilst carrying heavy loads on the head. There is usually a gap of 20-30 years from the time of the accident to the onset of first symptoms.

Clinical features

Syringomyelia results in a characteristic pattern of motor and sensory deficits with signs of a spastic paraplegia in the legs, and lower motor neurone signs in the upper limbs. Pain is a feature; this is often severe, burning or neuropathic in type and often in a radicular distribution in the limbs. The sensory findings are diagnostic, with involvement of the spinothalamic tracts producing loss of pain and temperature in a characteristic cape distribution over the shoulders. Sensory involvement occurs in the arms and legs depending on the site and extent of the syrinx. Because the cavity is situated in the centre of the cord there is sparing of the posterior columns with preservation of joint position, vibration and light touch. Characteristic clinical findings include neuropathic scars because of the loss of pain sensation, wasting of small hand muscles and claw hand deformities (Fig. 10.7). The clinical course in severe cases is a slowly progressive quadriplegia or paraplegia occurring over many years with the patient gradually becoming wheelchair and bedbound.

Treatment

Treatment is usually conservative. Neurosurgery, if indicated is aimed at stabilizing the condition with decompression of the foramen magnum and drainage of the syrinx.

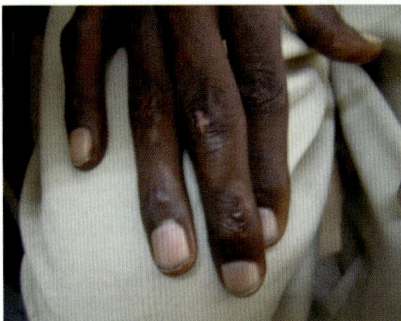

Neuropathic scars   Clawing

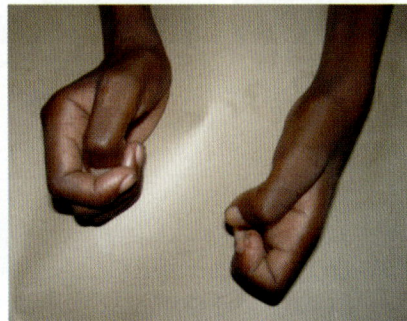

Figure 10.7 Hands in syringomyelia

Key points

- syringomyelia is uncommon cause of PP caused by a cavity within the spinal cord
- previous spinal injury & platybasia are the main risk factors
- history of injury is often >20 years earlier
- CFs are burning pains & wasting & neuropathic scars on the hands/arms
- & a slowly progressive SPP with loss of pain & temp but joint position/vibration are intact

NON COMPRESSIVE

The main non compressive causes of paraplegia in Africa are transverse myelitis, HIV, TB, schistosomiasis, syphilis, B-12 deficiency and HTLV-1.

TRANSVERSE MYELITIS (TM)

Transverse myelitis is a term used to describe an episode of inflammation affecting the spinal cord which results in an acute paraplegia. It is one of the major causes of paraplegia in young and middle aged persons in Africa. Mechanisms are considered to be infectious and autoimmune in origin, but in most cases the exact cause is not known. Viruses known to be involved are herpes zoster, herpes simplex, HIV and HTLV-1. Devic's disease (neuromyelitis optica) and systemic lupus erythematosis (vasculitis) are uncommon causes.

Clinical features

Transverse myelitis typically results in an acute devastating flaccid paraplegia, developing over hours or days with a sensory level on the trunk and loss of control of bladder and bowel. Pain though frequently present at onset is mild and usually clears. Spasticity usually develops later, but may not in very severely affected cases who remain flaccid because of involvement of the anterior horns in the spinal cord. At onset the CSF may show elevation in leucocytes and protein and MRI imaging may show high signal in the cord (Fig.10.9). CT examination of the spine is useful to exclude other causes.

Treatment

Treatment initially is with high dose intravenous steroids in combination with a course of antiviral medication e.g. acyclovir 10 mg/kg (800 mg) iv/po/3-4 times daily for 10 days if clinically appropriate. High dose steroids include methylprednisolone 1000 mg iv daily for 5 days followed by oral prednisolone 60 mg daily, tapering over 2-3 weeks. High dose dexamethasone, 24-32 mg daily can also be used if methylprednisolone is unavailable.

Prognosis

Recovery is variable, it may be rapid but in some cases can be slow and incomplete, occurring over months or years. However, most patients are permanently disabled and confined to a wheelchair.

Key points

- transverse myelitis is one of the common forms of PP in Africa
- affects mainly young & middle aged persons
- viruses are a known cause but in most cases the cause is not identified
- paraplegia occurs over hours or days with initial flaccidity, sensory level & incontinence
- treatment: antiviral medication & iv steroids but most persons are left permanently disabled

HIV

Paraplegia is a major neurological disorder in HIV disease (Chapter 8). It can occur during the asymptomatic stage of HIV infection when CD4 counts are >200/cm^3 and more commonly during the symptomatic stage when CD4 counts are very low <100/cm^3. The main causes are opportunistic processes and direct HIV infection of the spinal cord. Opportunistic infections (OIs) include tuberculosis, herpes zoster, herpes simplex, CMV, syphilis and co-infection with HTLV-1 in endemic areas. The main opportunistic tumour is lymphoma.

Direct infection of the spinal cord causes a **vacuolar myelopathy (VM)** in advanced HIV infection. (Chapter 8). This results in a progressive spastic paraplegia associated with urinary incontinence and sensory ataxia in <1% of patients. More common findings in vacuolar myelopathy are isolated hyperreflexia in the legs, usually the knees and extensor plantar reflexes. These isolated neurological signs are present in >20% of patients with advanced disease. Infection with cytomegalovirus can uncommonly cause a paraplegia during the later stages of HIV infection. This is due to lumbosacral radiculopathy and results in a flaccid paraplegia. Management of paraplegia in HIV is directed at finding and treating the underlying cause and starting ART depending on the degree of immunosuppression.

Key points

- PP is a major but a relatively uncommon neurological complication in HIV disease
- main mechanisms are OIs & direct HIV infection of the cord
- main OIs are TB, viral infections & syphilis
- vacuolar myelopathy arises from HIV infection of cord & causes PP in <1% of pts
- management is by treating the underlying cause & by starting ART

SCHISTOSOMIASIS

Involvement of the spinal cord is considered to be uncommon, although 1-5% of all cases of non traumatic paraplegia in schistosome endemic parts of Africa are reported to be caused by schistosomiasis (Chapter 7). Reports from schistosome affected areas of Malawi suggest that it may be even more common there. Paraplegia occurs mostly with *S. mansoni* (SM) and occasionally with *S. haematobium*. It happens particularly in early infection in the non immune host and when there is a heavy worm and egg load.

Pathogenesis

The paraplegia arises because of marked acute inflammatory response of the host to schistosome eggs being deposited in and around the spinal cord (Fig. 10.8). The likely source of the eggs are ectopic adult worms either living in veins around the cord or by retrograde flow of eggs through valveless spinal veins in connection with the iliac veins. The time between exposure and onset of the paraplegia is usually weeks to months and rarely years. The conus medullaris and the cauda equina are the most common sites affected (Chapter 7).

Clinical features

The clinical features include lumbar pain followed by difficulty passing urine, which may precede the other symptoms by days or weeks. The main presentation is that of a progressive flaccid paraplegia, occurring over days or weeks, usually with sensory and bladder involvement. Other neurological presentations include myeloradiculopathy and spastic paraplegia.

Diagnosis

The diagnosis should be considered in any patient with an acute onset paraplegia who is living in or has come from an endemic area. The diagnosis is difficult because the paraplegia mainly occurs during the early invasive phase of the adult worms, when there is little clinical or laboratory evidence of underlying schistosome infection. Stool examination for eggs may be negative and rectal snips are positive in only about 50% of cases. A positive serological test is useful in non endemic patients as an indicator of previous exposure. CSF examination may show lymphocytes and occasionally eosinophils as well as an elevation in protein. CT of the spinal cord is usually not helpful but MRI imaging with contrast may show hyper intense areas in the cord or irregular enhancement and dilation of the conus.

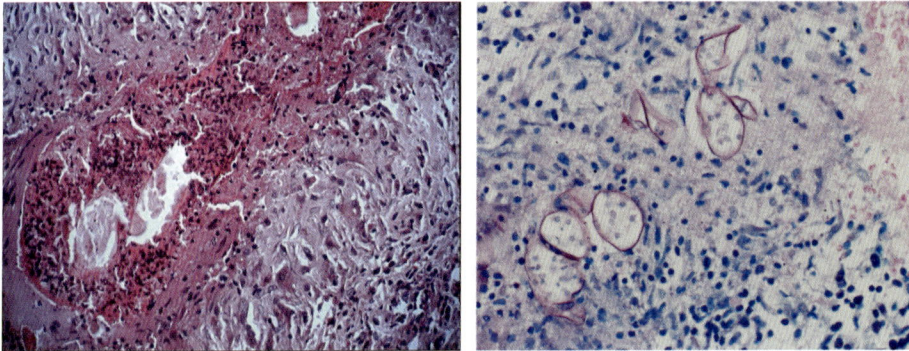

Granuloma around SM eggs   SM egg shells

Figure 10.8 Schistosome mansoni eggs in the spinal cord, histopathology

Treatment

Treatment is with praziquantel 40 mg/kg/day orally for up to 14 days in combination with oral prednisolone 60-90 mg daily for 3 weeks. Surgery has been tried for acute cases of failed medical treatment. The prognosis is guarded, with about 10% mortality, 30% remaining permanently paraplegic and 60% showing moderate to good recovery.

Key points

- schistosomiasis is a known cause of acute PP in endemic areas
- lower end of spinal cord & the cauda equina are the main sites affected
- flaccid PP is the main clinical presentation
- diagnosis is difficult because there is little laboratory evidence of infection
- treatment is with praziquantel & steroids for 2-3 weeks
- CFR is 10% & 30% left paralysed

Other causes of non compressive paraplegia include **syphilis, human T cell lymphotropic virus type 1 (HTLV-1), Devic's disease, vitamin B-12 deficiency**, ischaemia, sickle cell disease, vasculitis, arteriovenous malformation (AVM) and hereditary spastic paraplegia.

SYPHILIS

Syphilis is a sexually transmitted disease caused by the spirochete *Treponema pallidum* (Chapter 6). It is estimated that neurological involvement will occur in about 7% of patients 10-25 years after primary infection, if primary syphilis is untreated. However despite the frequency of primary syphilis in Africa, neurosyphilis remains uncommon in many countries there. The reason for this has been ascribed to the continued widespread use of antibiotics inadvertently treating early infection or altering the natural history of clinical disease. The incidence of neurosyphilis is increased when syphilis is associated with HIV infection.

Clinical features

Spinal syphilis typically presents either as a progressive spastic paraplegia or as tabes dorsalis with posterior column loss, lightning pains and Charcot's joints. However tabes dorsalis remains a distinctly uncommon clinical presentation in Africa.

Diagnosis

The diagnosis of neurosyphilis depends on the serological detection of antibodies in both blood and CSF. The Venereal Disease Research Laboratory (VDRL) is the screening test most commonly used in Africa although it may be negative in HIV infection. Limitations to VDRL include false positives in serum but not in the CSF which can however be negative in 20-30% cases. More sensitive and specific diagnostic antibody tests include the fluorescent treponemal antibody absorption (FTA) and the treponemal antibody immobilization test (TPI). The CSF may also show elevated leucocytes and protein.

Treatment

Treatment is with penicillin 2-4 million units i.v. 4 hourly for 14-21 days.

HUMAN T CELL LYMPHOTROPIC VIRUS TYPE 1 (HTLV-1)

HTLV-1 is a retrovirus which is endemic in some areas of western, southern and central Africa with just a few clusters reported in eastern Africa. It is endemic in areas of Japan, the Caribbean and South America. The serological prevalence rates are 3-6% in some of the worst affected communities. It is transmitted perinatally, sexually and by blood transfusion. Chronic infection for up to 20-30 years can result in a slow progressive form of tropical spastic paraplegia known as HTLV-1 associated myelopathy (HAM). However this occurs in only 1-5% of persons infected with the virus with the majority being asymptomatic carriers. The distinctive clinical feature of HTLV-1 is that of a progressive spastic paraplegia characterized by slow onset over years of stiffness and weakness affecting the legs with paraesthesiae, back pain and urinary symptoms. The diagnosis is confirmed by finding HTLV-1 antibodies in the blood and CSF. There is no effective treatment although steroids have been tried.

DEVIC'S DISEASE (NEUROMYELITIS OPTICA)

This is an uncommon but severe disease in Africa characterized by recurring attacks of acute severe demyelinating transverse myelitis and optic neuritis. This results in paraplegia and blindness. Occasionally, the disease is monophasic but this appears to be unusual in Africa. It occurs predominantly in females in their late teens or early 20s in Africa but may affect older women in their 30s and 40s in high income countries. The optic neuritis typically precedes the transverse myelitis but can also occur concurrently with it. The relapses are severe, occurring usually within 6 months of the first and subsequent episodes.

Diagnosis

The diagnosis in Africa is mainly clinical. Examination of CSF may show increased protein and the presence of lymphocytes. A highly specific immunoglobulin antibody to aquaporin (NMO –IgG) can now be detected in blood and CSF of infected persons but the test is only available in some specialised neurological centres in Africa. MRI imaging if available shows increased signal in the spinal cord often spanning several vertebral levels and almost complete withering of the cord in cases of long standing disease (Fig. 10.9).

MRI T2 cervical & upper thoracic cord

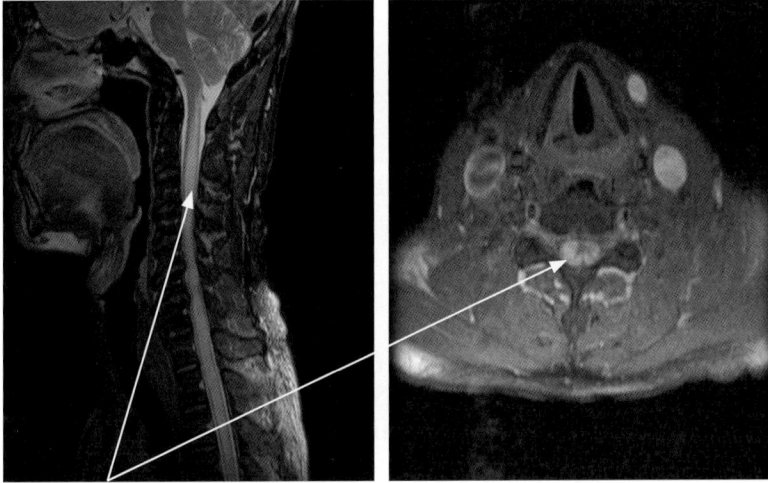

Inflammation within the cord

Figure 10.9 Transverse myelitis in Devic's disease

Treatment

Treatment for the acute attacks is with high dose steroids for periods of 4-6 weeks and if available, repeated plasma exchange or intravenous immunoglobulin for the non responders. Long term prophylaxis with a combination of steroids and azathioprine or other forms of immunosuppression has been tried but the response is variable. Residual disability after an attack is usual with many patients becoming wheelchair or bed bound within 1 to 2 years of onset.

VITAMIN B-12 DEFICIENCY

Vitamin B-12 deficiency causes a peripheral neuropathy, sub acute combined degeneration of the cord (SACD), optic atrophy, dementia and pernicious anaemia. The main spinal findings are those of a myelopathy with brisk knee reflexes and up going plantars. These typically occur in combination with signs of neuropathy, including absent ankle jerks and loss of peripheral sensation including joint position sense. All or some of the above may be present in any one patient. The main causes of SACD are nutritional deficiency, seen most commonly in vegetarians, and malabsorption. Malabsorption may be caused either by a lack of intrinsic factor which seems to be quite uncommon in Africa and also by diseases of the terminal ileum.

Diagnosis

Diagnosis is by finding the typical neurological findings in combination with evidence of megaloblastic anaemia i.e. elevated mean corpuscular volume (MCV) and low serum B-12.

Treatment

Treatment is with intramuscular injections of B-12. The dose is 1 mg on alternate days for a total of five injections followed by 1 mg injections every 3 months for life. If intramuscular injections are not available then B-12 can sometimes be given orally, in a dose of 1 mg po daily.

This may provide adequate replacement particularly in cases secondary to nutritional or dietary deficiency.

Key points

- neurosyphilis is uncommon in many countries in Africa
- HTLV-1 is endemic in selected areas of South, West & Central Africa
- Devic's disease is uncommon but severe demyelinating disorder of CNS
- B-12 deficiency is a treatable but uncommon cause of neuropathy & paraplegia

TROPICAL MYELONEUROPATHIES

These are a group of paraplegias and peripheral neuropathies that are considered to be nutritional in origin. They include the tropical spastic paraplegia (TSP) group, **konzo** and **lathyrism**, and the peripheral neuropathy group, **tropical ataxic neuropathies (TAN)**. These disorders represent a distinct group of community based myeloneuropathies which result in paraplegia. They occur largely as epidemics and are the commonest cause of neurological disability in the rural communities in which they occur in Africa. These are non curable when they happen and their management lies mainly in prevention.

KONZO

Konzo is a distinct form of tropical myeloneuropathy characterized by abrupt onset of a non progressive but permanent spastic paraplegia related to cassava consumption. It occurs mainly as epidemics in exclusively cassava growing areas of the east, central and western Africa. Epidemics have been known to occur in cassava growing of the former Belgian Congo as far back as 1928 and possibly earlier. In epidemics as many as 1-30/1000 persons are affected, mainly growing children and fertile women. It also occurs in an endemic form but at much lower rates.

Aetiology

The cause of konzo has been attributed to the combined effect of months of high cyanide and low protein (methionine and cysteine, sulphur based amino acids) intake from exclusive consumption of insufficiently processed bitter cassava (Fig. 10.11). The bitter cassava grow well in poor soils but contain increasing amounts of cyanogenic glycosides mainly linamarin. Processing disrupts the root tissue and releases volatile hydrogen cyanide and this makes the food safe for human consumption. The main processing methods used in Africa involve hydrolysis or soaking in water, crushing and fermentation or sun drying. Safe processing takes days in the case of hydrolysis and fermentation, to weeks for sun drying. Shortening of these methods is a risk factor for the disease.

Clinical features

The clinical features are characterized by an abrupt (usually <24 hours) onset of a permanent but non progressive spastic paraplegia (Figs. 10.10). The upper limbs and optic nerves may also be involved in some cases. The bladder, bowel and sensation are all spared. The range of disability varies from very mild upper motor neurone findings in the legs to spastic paralysis of all four limbs in very severe cases. The majority of persons with konzo can walk with the aid of crutches.

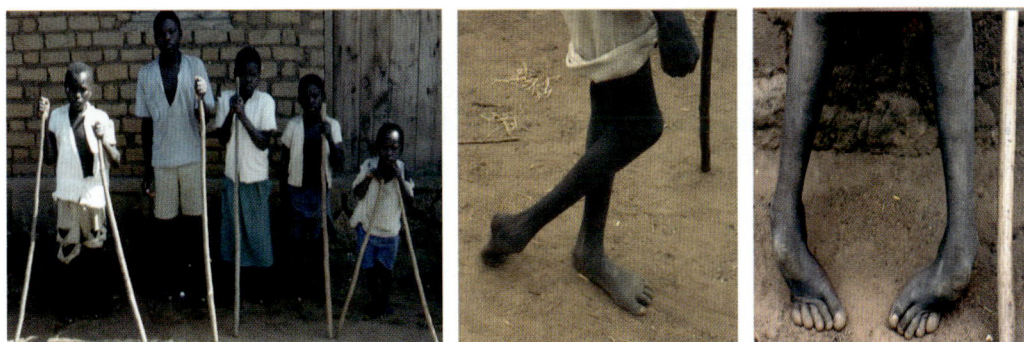

Konzo patients (all from same family)   Typical spastic gait in konzo   Spastic feet in konzo

Figure 10.10 Konzo patients

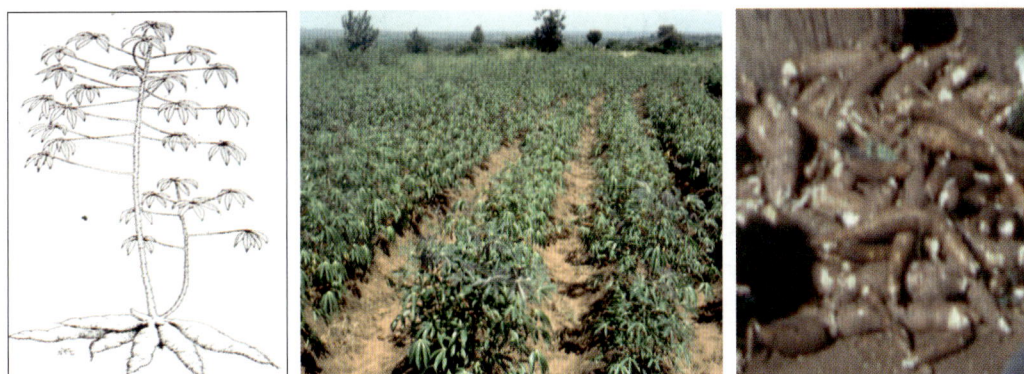

Cassava shrubs & harvested tubers

Figure 10.11 Cassava

Diagnosis

The clinical criteria for diagnosis are an abrupt (<1/52) onset of spastic paraparesis in the absence of any other cause in a patient coming from a cassava growing area. Supportive investigations include elevated blood or urine thiocyanate levels and low levels of the essential amino acids methionine and cysteine. These investigations are only available in specialist or research laboratories.

Clinical criteria for diagnosing konzo

- spastic paraplegia
- abrupt onset in <one week
- occurring in a cassava growing area
- no other cause is found

Treatment and prevention

There is no medical treatment for the condition. Prevention is mainly directed at growing cassava with lower cyanide content and public education concerning safer methods of cassava processing. A newer and safer "wetting method" of cassava processing has recently been promoted in some affected communities in East Africa. Additional measures include establishing early warning systems of potentially high cyanide levels in cassava tubers and of pending epidemics and the provision of supplementary protein before or early on during epidemics. Surgical treatment involving Achilles tendon lengthening operations have proved successful in increasing mobility in some patients.

LATHYRISM

Lathyrism is an epidemic form of spastic paraplegia found almost exclusively in parts of India, Bangladesh and South East Asia where large quantities of the grass pea (*Lathyrus sativus*) a drought resistant crop are grown and consumed. In Africa it is found only in parts of North Western Ethiopia where the grass pea is widely grown and consumed. The association of paraplegia with grass pea consumption was already recognized in ancient Greece.

Aetiology

The disease is caused by a neurotoxic amino acid found in the grass pea called beta-N-oxalylamino-L-alanine (BOAA). Lathyrism occurs after weeks or months of almost exclusive consumption of the grass pea.

Clinical features

It occurs mostly as epidemics and occurring with about the same frequency and age distribution as Konzo. It is clinically almost identical to konzo, apart from the mild sphincter involvement occasionally found in lathyrism (Fig. 10.12). However, they are distinguishable from each other because they both occur in geographically distinct areas which do not overlap.

Treatment and prevention

The management and prevention are along the same principles as that for konzo.

Illustration & photos

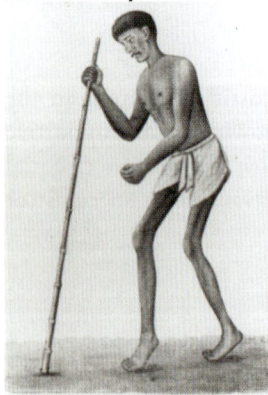 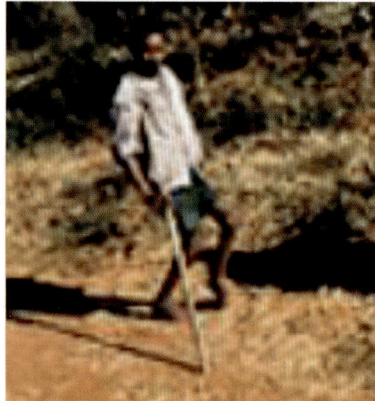 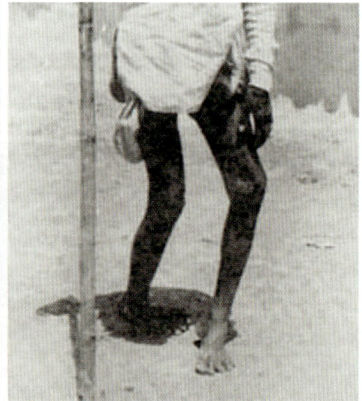

India (1922) Ethiopia India

Figure 10.12 Lathyrism

Key points

- konzo and lathyrism are distinct forms of tropical spastic paraplegia
- occur mainly as epidemics in different areas in Africa
- konzo occurs only in cassava growing & lathyrism occurs only in grass pea growing areas
- each is caused by weeks/months of almost exclusive consumption of a staple food
- both result in permanent spastic paraparesis & are prevented by similar measures

TROPICAL ATAXIC NEUROPATHY (TAN)

This is another distinct form of tropical myeloneuropathy. It has originally been described in cassava eating populations in Nigeria and Tanzania in the 1960s and more recently again in Nigeria and in southern India. The disease is characterized by a combination of gradual onset in older adults of peripheral neuropathy, sensory ataxia, optic neuritis, deafness and sometimes spastic paraplegia. The presence of any two or more of these findings is sufficient to make the diagnosis. The cause is not known but is linked to chronic cyanide exposure from chronic cassava consumption in combination with possible vitamin B nutritional deficiency. Management includes vitamin B supplementation.

MANAGEMENT OF PARAPLEGIA

There are four major principles governing the management of patients presenting with paraplegia.

Do not delay

The early establishment of correct diagnosis, treatment and the prevention of complications are critical to the outcome for the patient. It is important to preserve whatever neurological function is still remaining.

Establish the cause

The cause is established by history, physical examination, laboratory and radiological investigations. The main investigations are outlined below in Table 10.2.

Table 10.2 Main investigations in paraplegia

Type of investigation	Investigation	Disease
Bloods *Haematology*	FBC, ESR, B-12, sickle cell test	TB, malignancy, SACD, sickle cell disease, abscess
Biochemistry	glucose, creatinine, electrolytes, calcium, total protein and electrophoresis	myeloma, malignancy
Serology	HIV, VDRL, schistosome, cysticercosis and echinococcosis serology	HIV disease, syphilis, helminthic infections

continues

Imaging		
X-rays: plain	spine, chest skeletal survey myelography	TB/abscess malignancy
CT/MRI	spinal cord	cord compression: TB, malignancy transverse myelitis
Procedures		
Lumbar puncture	opening pressure, colour, cells, protein, glucose, culture, VDRL	malignancy, TB, transverse myelitis, other infections

Treat the cause

The treatments for the main causes of paraplegia are outlined below in Table 10.3. There is a low threshold for starting TB treatment in Africa, particularly in younger patients presenting with paraplegia.

Table 10.3 Summary: Treatment for some reversible causes of PP

Disease	Treatment
Potts disease	TB Rx
TB spinal cord	TB Rx & steroids
metastatic malignancy	steroids & analgesia
transverse myelitis	steroids & acyclovir
HIV	treat the cause & ART
cervical spondylosis/disc	surgical decompression if indicated
schistosomiasis	praziquantel & steroids for 2 weeks
syphilis	penicillin for 21 days
Devic's disease	steroids
SACD	B-12
acute epidural abscess	iv antibiotics

Prevent complications

The patient needs assistance to care for skin, limbs, bladder and bowels. This is best achieved by the early involvement of the patient's family in cooperation with the nurses and physiotherapists.

Skin

The prevention of pressure sores is critical to the patient's survival. In immobile patients pressure sores develop quickly over bony prominences particularly the sacrum, hips and heels. This is more likely to occur during the first days of the illness. Specially designed air mattresses that minimize this risk are unavailable in most hospitals in Africa. Prevention of bed sores can best be achieved by a rigorous approach which involves 2 hourly turning of the patient day and night and starting immediately on admission. This task should be entrusted to a family carer or carried out by the nursing staff.

The skin should be inspected frequently and always be kept dry and clean. Attention early to adequate nutrition and measures to prevent infection are also very important. These measures include the use of mosquito bed nets to prevent malaria and a bed cage to keep weight of blankets off the paralysed legs. If bed sores do become established they require vigorous cleaning, surgical debridement and possible skin grafting.

Bladder and bowels

Urinary catheterization is necessary when there is a non functioning bladder. This typically occurs during the first days of an acute paraplegia and persists particularly in patients with flaccid paraplegia. The bladder is innervated by both the autonomic and the somatic or voluntary nervous system. Loss of control of bladder function or neurogenic bladder arises because of lesions situated in either the spinal cord or cauda equina. Patients with spinal cord lesions and usually a spastic paraplegia may eventually after months develop satisfactory reflex bladder emptying or require intermittent self catheterization and treatment with antispasmodic or anticholinergic drugs. Patients with a cauda equina lesion and flaccid paraplegia usually require permanent catheters. It may be necessary to use antibiotics for urinary tract infections.

Constipation is a feature of both flaccid and spastic paraplegia with the bowels opening every week or less often. Measures to prevent it include satisfactory fluid intake, adequate fibre/bulk in the diet, and the early use of laxatives usually the combination of a lubricant and an irritant. Manual evacuation may be necessary when there is faecal impaction.

Limbs

Care of paralysed limbs involves frequent passive movements. This helps to prevent thrombosis, joint stiffness, spasticity and contractures, and to exercise the non affected muscles. The management of spasticity and avoidance of contractures is best done by a physiotherapist and trained family members, and also through the use of antispasmodics.

The main antispasmodics available are baclofen and diazepam. The starting dose of baclofen is 5 mg twice daily increasing slowly over weeks to 20-40 mg twice daily as required. The limiting adverse effects are drowsiness, fatigue, and the fact that it can sometimes take away the spasticity that the patient needs and uses to be able to stand and mobilise. The starting dose of diazepam is 2-5 mg three times daily, increasing to a maximum of 20 mg three times daily. The limiting adverse effects are drowsiness and fatigue, and anxiety may occur on sudden withdrawal. Other drugs used for spasticity include dantrolene and tizanidine. Further measures include the use of support stockings and low dose heparin which help to prevent deep vein thrombosis.

Key points

- treat the cause without delay & aim to prevent complications
- main complications are bedsores, urinary retention, infection & spasticity
- 2 hourly turning should start immediately on admission
- entrust care to a relative or carer

LONG TERM MANAGEMENT

Paraplegia is a devastating illness which results in disappointment, depression, shame, resentment, anger and an altered role in family. Patients with chronic paraplegia have to come to terms with the loss of function of the lower half of their bodies. They need support in the activities of daily living (ADL), mobility, work and family life. They benefit particularly from specialized knowledge, support and encouragement. In a medical setting, this is usually provided by medical staff including nurses, doctors, physiotherapists, occupational therapists and carers. In order to cope at home, the person and their family need the wider support of carers, friends and the community. Longer term measures should include plans for social and recreational activities and employment in order for the patient to be more able to participate as fully as possible in everyday life. Some specific measures are outlined below.

Motor

The provision of a wheelchair is often both necessary and essential for mobility. The patient needs to be educated about the use of a wheelchair and learn the skills needed for independent transfers. This will involve the patient learning some knowledge about the level of cord involvement and injury and the extent and severity of any resulting paralysis and disability. The patient needs to train to strengthen the non paralysed muscles and family members need to be instructed and trained to regularly passively move paralysed limbs in order to prevent contractures and bed sores. House adaptation is usually necessary for use of a wheelchair.

Skin

Great care needs to be taken to prevent the development of pressure sores. A routine of avoiding prolonged periods of weight bearing will need to be established and maintained. This is helped by the person regularly taking the weight of the body off the seat of chair or wheelchair a couple of times every hour and by using protective cushions to guard against pressure points. Regular inspection of skin is essential and may of necessity have to be carried out by the carer.

Bladder and bowels

The patient needs training in reflex bladder emptying, condom drainage, intermittent self catheterization, indwelling catheter management, anticholinergic drugs and early recognition and treatment of urinary tract infections. The patient needs a healthy wholesome and regular diet with laxatives and suppositories to avoid constipation.

Sex and fertility

This needs to be discussed and explained with the patient and partner. Erectile potency may be retained in upper motor neurone spinal cord disorders and respond to oral medications phosphodiesterase inhibitors e.g. sildenafil. In contrast erectile potency is lost in cauda equina or lower motor neurone disorders. In female patients local spasticity in the thigh adductors may be helped by local antispasmodic injections or medications.

Weight and calories

Paraplegic patients need on average 40-50% less calories. This needs to be explained clearly to the patient in order to avoid excessive weight gain.

Key points

- assist & support the person to recover functional independence
- involves prevention of bed sores, urinary tract infection & weight gain
- includes provision, use and maintenance of a wheelchair
- long term aim is to participate as fully as possible in everyday life
- needs support of carers, family, friends & community

Selected references

Bhigjee AI, Moodley K, Ramkissoon K. *Multiple sclerosis in KwaZulu Natal, South Africa: an epidemiological and clinical study.* Mult Scler. 2007 Nov;13(9):1095-9.

Bradbury JH, Cliff J, Denton IC. *Uptake of wetting method in Africa to reduce cyanide poisoning and konzo from cassava.* Food Chem Toxicol. 2011 Mar;49(3):539-42.

Brinar VV, Habek M, Zadro I, Barun B, Ozretic D, Vranjes D. *Current concepts in the diagnosis of transverse myelopathies.* Clin Neurol Neurosurg. 2008 Nov;110(9):919-27.

Carod-Artal FJ. *Neurological complications of Schistosoma infection.* Trans R Soc Trop Med Hyg. 2008 Feb;102(2):107-16.

Carod-Artal FJ, Mesquita HM, Ribeiro Lda S. *Neurological symptoms and disability in HTLV-1 associated myelopathy.* Neurologia. 2008 Mar;23(2):78-84.

Cliff J, Muquingue H, Nhassico D, Nzwalo H, Bradbury JH. *Konzo and continuing cyanide intoxication from cassava in Mozambique.* Food Chem Toxicol. 2011 Mar;49(3):631-5.

Cooper S, van der Loeff MS, McConkey S, Cooper M, Sarge-Njie R, Kaye S, et al. *Neurological morbidity among human T-lymphotropic-virus-type-1-infected individuals in a rural West African population.* J Neurol Neurosurg Psychiatry. 2009 Jan;80(1):66-8.

Dean G, Bhigjee AI, Bill PL, Fritz V, Chikanza IC, Thomas JE, et al. *Multiple sclerosis in black South Africans and Zimbabweans.* J Neurol Neurosurg Psychiatry. 1994 Sep;57(9):1064-9.

de-The G, Giordano C, Gessain A, Howlett W, Sonan T, Akani F, et al. *Human retroviruses HTLV-I, HIV-1, and HIV-2 and neurological diseases in some equatorial areas of Africa.* J Acquir Immune Defic Syndr. 1989;2(6):550-6.

Ghezzi A, Bergamaschi R, Martinelli V, Trojano M, Tola MR, Merelli E, et al. *Clinical characteristics, course and prognosis of relapsing Devic's Neuromyelitis Optica.* J Neurol. 2004 Jan;251(1):47-52.

Godlwana L, Gounden P, Ngubo P, Nsibande T, Nyawo K, Puckree T. *Incidence and profile of spinal tuberculosis in patients at the only public hospital admitting such patients in KwaZulu-Natal.* Spinal Cord. 2008 May;46(5):372-4.

Haimanot RT, Fekadu A, Bushra B. *Endemic fluorosis in the Ethiopian Rift Valley.* Trop Geogr Med. 1987 Jul;39(3):209-17.

Haimanot RT, Kidane Y, Wuhib E, Kalissa A, Alemu T, Zein ZA, et al. *Lathyrism in rural northwestern Ethiopia: a highly prevalent neurotoxic disorder.* Int J Epidemiol. 1990 Sep;19(3):664-72.

Howlett WP, Brubaker GR, Mlingi N, Rosling H. *Konzo, an epidemic upper motor neuron disease studied in Tanzania.* Brain. 1990 Feb;113 (Pt 1):223-35.

Kayembe K, Goubau P, Desmyter J, Vlietinck R, Carton H. *A cluster of HTLV-1 associated tropical spastic paraparesis in Equateur (Zaire): ethnic and familial distribution.* J Neurol Neurosurg Psychiatry. 1990 Jan;53(1):4-10.

Lambertucci JR, Silva LC, do Amaral RS. *Guidelines for the diagnosis and treatment of schistosomal myeloradiculopathy.* Rev Soc Bras Med Trop. 2007 Sep-Oct;40(5):574-81.

Lekoubou Looti AZ, Kengne AP, Djientcheu Vde P, Kuate CT, Njamnshi AK. *Patterns of non-traumatic myelopathies in Yaounde (Cameroon): a hospital based study.* J Neurol Neurosurg Psychiatry. 2010 Jul;81(7):768-70.

Modi G, Mochan A, Modi M, Saffer D. *Demyelinating disorder of the central nervous system occurring in black South Africans.* J Neurol Neurosurg Psychiatry. 2001 Apr;70(4):500-5.

Modi G, Ranchhod J, Hari K, Mochan A, Modi M. *Non-traumatic myelopathy at the Chris Hani Baragwanath Hospital, South Africa--the influence of HIV.* QJM. 2011 Aug;104(8):697-703.

Ndondo AP, Fieggen G, Wilmshurst JM. *Hydatid disease of the spine in South African children.* J Child Neurol. 2003 May;18(5):343-6.

Oluwole OS, Onabolu AO, Link H, Rosling H. *Persistence of tropical ataxic neuropathy in a Nigerian community.* J Neurol Neurosurg Psychiatry. 2000 Jul;69(1):96-101.

Owolabi LF, Ibrahim A, Samaila AA. *Profile and outcome of non-traumatic paraplegia in Kano, northwestern Nigeria.* Ann Afr Med. 2011 Apr-Jun;10(2):86-90.

Parry O, Bhebhe E, Levy LF. *Non-traumatic paraplegia in a Zimbabwean population--a retrospective survey.* Cent Afr J Med. 1999 May;45(5):114-9.

Pittock SJ, Lucchinetti CF. *Inflammatory transverse myelitis: evolving concepts.* Curr Opin Neurol. 2006 Aug;19(4):362-8.

Solomon T, Willison H. *Infectious causes of acute flaccid paralysis.* Curr Opin Infect Dis. 2003 Oct;16(5):375-81.

Tshala-Katumbay D, Eeg-Olofsson KE, Tylleskar T, Kazadi-Kayembe T. *Impairments, disabilities and handicap pattern in konzo--a non-progressive spastic para/tetraparesis of acute onset.* Disabil Rehabil. 2001 Nov 10;23(16):731-6.

Tylleskar T, Howlett WP, Rwiza HT, Aquilonius SM, Stalberg E, Linden B, et al. *Konzo: a distinct disease entity with selective upper motor neuron damage.* J Neurol Neurosurg Psychiatry. 1993 Jun;56(6):638-43.

Zellner H, Maier D, Gasser A, Doppler M, Winkler A, Dharsee J, et al. *Prevalence and pattern of spinal pathologies in a consecutive series of CTs/MRIs in an urban and rural Tanzanian hospital–a retrospective neuroradiological comparative analysis.* Wien Klin Wochenschr. 2010 Oct;122 Suppl 3:47-51.

Zenebe G. *Myelopathies in Ethiopia.* East Afr Med J. 1995 Jan;72(1):42-5.

CHAPTER 11
DISORDERS OF PERIPHERAL NERVES

CONTENTS

CHAPTER 11

DISORDERS OF PERIPHERAL NERVES

Peripheral neuropathies are a major cause of neurological disability in Africa. They occur as a result of disease or injury and can affect nerve roots, individual nerves and peripheral branches of nerves (Fig.11.1). The main causes are HIV, leprosy, diabetes mellitus, drugs, nutrition and alcohol (Table 11.1 & 2). This chapter reviews the main clinical presentations, investigations and management of peripheral nerve disorders. The student should aim to be able to recognize the different types of neuropathies and know their main causes and management.

Pathophysiology

Peripheral nerves are made up of multiple axons surrounded by myelin, Schwann cells and their covering sheaths. Individual axons are either myelinated or nonmyelinated. In neuropathies the nerves may be damaged at three main sites: the axon, the myelin and the cell body. If the axon is damaged, it is called an axonal neuropathy. This is the most common form of peripheral neuropathy and usually affects sensation greater than power and has a mainly distal distribution. If the myelin is damaged this is called a demyelinating neuropathy. This affects power more than sensation and the weakness is usually proximal as well as distal. If the cell body is damaged then either sensory or motor nerve fibres or both may be damaged permanently depending on which cell body is involved. Recovery occurs if the basement membrane survives but is faster in demyelinating than in axonal neuropathies.

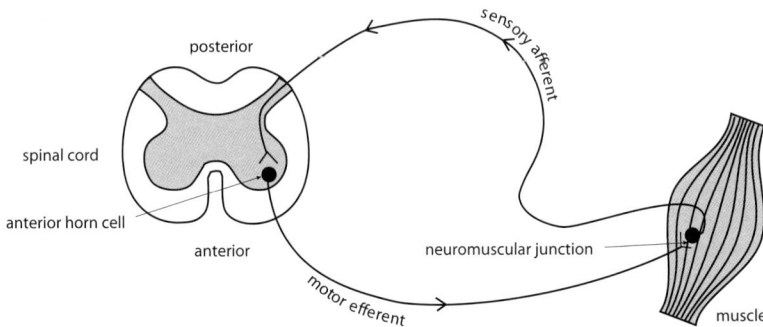

Figure 11.1 The peripheral reflex pathway

TYPES OF PERIPHERAL NERVE DISORDER (PND)

Peripheral neuropathies are divided into two main groups: mononeuropathies which involve single nerves and polyneuropathies which involve many nerves.

MONONEUROPATHY

This describes a group of focal peripheral nerve disorders (FPNDs) where individual nerves or their branches are affected. The main mechanisms are compression, entrapment, vasculitis, infiltration and infection. In the upper limbs, this happens mostly at the wrist, elbow and occasionally the upper arm. In the lower limbs, the most common sites are at the level of the inguinal ligament, the knee and the buttocks. A misplaced injection in the buttocks in young children is the main cause of sciatic nerve injury in Africa. If more than one nerve is involved, this is called multiple mononeuropathy or mononeuritis multiplex. Leprosy is a common cause of both mononeuropathy and mononeuritis multiplex in Africa. Other causes include HIV, diabetes and vasculitis. The main clinical features of the most common focal nerve lesions are outlined in Table 11.1 and illustrated in Figs 11.2-5.

Table 11.1 Common focal peripheral nerve disorders

Nerve	Main site	Mechanism	Main Cause	Clinical Features
Median	wrist	entrapment	carpal tunnel syndrome, leprosy	pain, tingling hand/wrist, arm, numbness radial 3 & 1/2 fingers, wasting thenar muscles, weakness of thumb abduction
Ulnar	elbow	compression	trauma/injury, leprosy	pain, tingling hand wrist, numbness ulnar 1 & 1/2 fingers, wasting hypothenar muscles, weakness little finger flexion, claw hand deformity
Radial	arm	compression	sleep	wrist drop, weakness wrist, dorsiflexion
Sciatic	buttock	infiltration	injection	pain buttock, leg, foot, numbness leg and foot, weakness knee flexion & muscles below knee, absent ankle jerk
Femoral	thigh	vascular	diabetes	pain thigh (severe), numbness anteromedial thigh & medial leg, weakness hip flexion & knee extension, absent knee jerk
Lateral cutaneous nerve thigh	inguinal ligament	compression	occupational, carrying baby on hip	numbness, tingling and pain over anterolateral thigh (meralgia paraesthetica)
Common peroneal	knee	compression infiltration	illness, leprosy, leg crossing	numbness dorsum foot, foot drop, weakness foot eversion

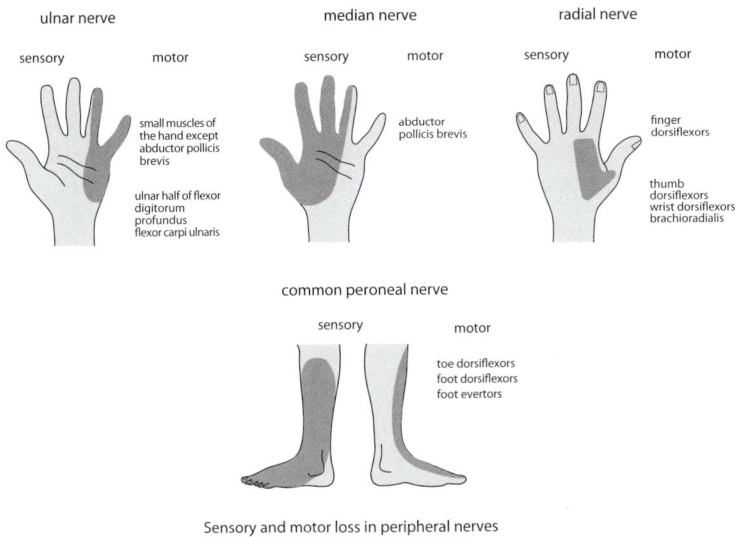

Figure 11.2 Sensory and motor loss in main mononeuropathies

Median nerve compression occurs mostly at the wrist as the median nerve passes through the carpal tunnel resulting in carpal tunnel syndrome (CTS). CTS is characterized by tingling pain in the hand or arm particularly at night. The pain and paraesthesiae are in the distribution of the median nerve and involve the thumb, index, middle and half the ring finger but may extend up the forearm and arm. It often wakes the patient from sleep at night and is relieved by hanging the arm down and shaking the hand. CTS is frequently provoked by manual tasks. Sensory loss in CTS usually affects the lateral (radial) three and a half fingers and spares the palm. Sensation to the lateral fingers and palm are lost in median nerve lesions located in the forearm (Fig. 11.2). In long standing cases there is wasting of the thenar eminence and weakness of thumb abduction and opposition (opponens pollicis) (Figs 11.2 & 3). **Tinel's sign** may be positive i.e. tapping the carpal tunnel at the distal crease of the wrist reproduces pain and tingling. Alternatively there may be tingling on extreme wrist flexion for one minute (**Phalen's sign**). However, in clinical practice these signs, although useful when present are unreliable when absent. Treatment is by local injection of steroids, wearing a night time wrist splint or by surgical decompression if necessary

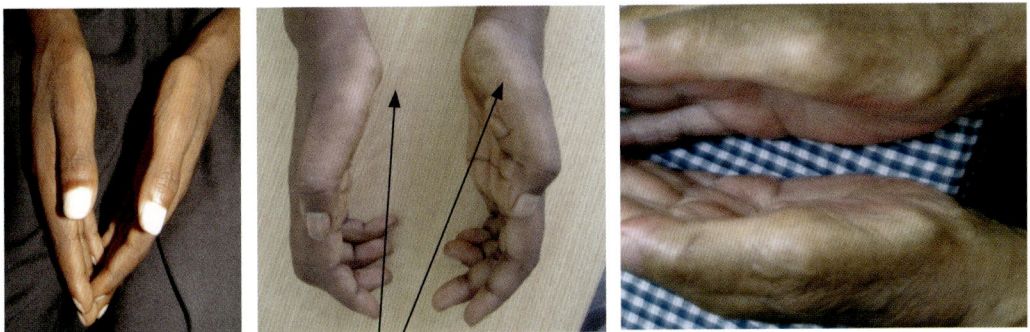

Typical wasting of thenar muscles

Figure 11.3 Median neuropathy (bilateral)

Ulnar nerve is prone to compression along its path. The main site of pressure or stretching is at the elbow within the cubital tunnel or the ulnar groove. This results in dyasthesia/paraesthesia and sensory impairment/loss in the distribution of the little finger and adjacent half of the ring finger and ulnar aspect of the hand front and back. There is wasting and weakness of the intrinsic muscles of the hand and the deep flexors of the 4th and 5th finger with sparing of the thenar muscles (Figs. 11.2 & 4). This gives rise to the characteristic claw hand deformity seen in chronic ulnar lesions.

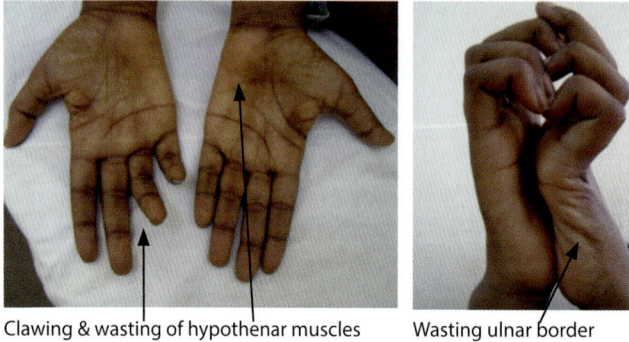

Clawing & wasting of hypothenar muscles   Wasting ulnar border

Figure 11.4 Ulnar neuropathy

Radial nerve compression arises mostly from prolonged abnormal posture with resulting compression of the radial nerve in the radial groove above the elbow e.g. drunkard's palsy. It can also arise from compression in the axilla, e.g. using crutches, and from fracture of the shaft of the humerus. Compression results in wrist drop with weakness of the finger and wrist extension and sometimes a small patch of sensory loss on the dorsum of the hand and web of the thumb (Fig. 11.2).

Lateral cutaneous nerve of thigh travels under the lateral part of the inguinal ligament. Compression results in a patch of sensory loss over the anterolateral aspect of the thigh of variable size ranging from a palm sized patch to an area extending from the hip to the knee but never crossing the midline of the axis of the thigh (**meralgia paraesthetica**). This is one of the most common mononeuropathies and its onset is associated with weight gain e.g. pregnancy and also occupational e.g. chronic abnormal posture, bending (e.g. plumber). It is usually self-limiting.

Sciatic nerve injury most commonly occurs as a result of a misplaced injection in the buttocks in early childhood. The sciatic nerve (tibial & common peroneal nerves, L4,5,S1,2) is responsible for sensation below the knee involving the entire anterolateral aspect of leg and the sole and dorsum of the foot. It is responsible for the following movements, hip extension, knee flexion and ankle plantar and dorsiflexion. Injury results in loss of sensation and power in these distributions along with a decreased or absent ankle jerk.

Common peroneal nerve compression at the fibular head results in foot drop and sensory loss on the dorsum of foot and lateral leg (Figs 11.2 & 5). The main causes are trauma and pressure. It occurs more commonly in immobile patients who are prone to compression.

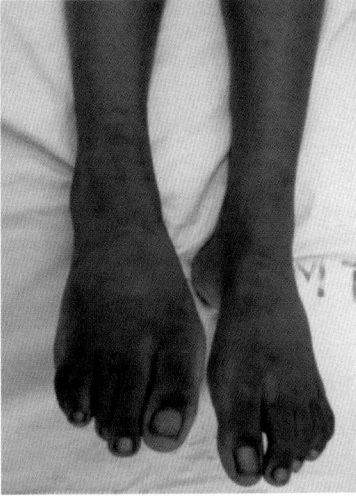

Figure 11.5 Common peroneal nerve neuropathy. Bilateral foot drop (left > right)

Femoral neuropathy most commonly occurs in association with diabetes mellitus. The main symptoms are thigh pain, weakness of hip flexion and decreased or absent knee jerk. Treatment is pain relief and treating the underlying cause.

Key points

- mononeuropathies are recognised by their clinical setting & pattern of sensory & motor loss
- include CTS: ulnar injury, peroneal palsy, meralgia paraesthetica, sciatic injury & femoral ischaemia
- main mechanisms: trauma, entrapment, compression, infection & inflammation
- leprosy is a major cause of mononeuropathies
- a misplaced injection is main cause of sciatic nerve injury

POLYNEUROPATHIES

Polyneuropathies are diffuse, symmetrical disorders usually affecting the limbs distally to a greater extent than proximally. Clinically, they are classified as acute or chronic, motor or sensory or mixed and also autonomic. Patients presenting with polyneuropathics typically present with impairment or loss of sensation in a distal or peripheral glove and stocking distribution. Distal weakness may occur later in the feet and legs followed by the hands and arms. Neurological examination usually reveals wasting, fasciculation, distal weakness with absent reflexes and loss of light touch. Vibration and joint position sense may also be involved. The sphincters involving bowel and bladder are typically spared. The main causes of polyneuropathy are outlined in Table 11.2.

Table 11.2 Main causes of polyneuropathies in Africa

Classification	Cause	Crude frequency
Infection	HIV, leprosy	very common
Metabolic	diabetes, (renal failure)	common
Drugs	ARTs (stavudine, didanosine), isoniazid, dapsone, vincristine	common
Toxic	alcohol, (chronic cassava consumption)	common
Deficiency	vitamin B-1 (alcoholics), B-6 (isoniazid), B-12 (pernicious anaemia)	uncommon
Inflammatory	Guillain-Barre Syndrome (GBS), chronic inflammatory demyelinating polyradiculoneuropathy (CIDP)	very uncommon
Vasculitis	rheumatoid arthritis, systemic lupus erythematosus (SLE), polyarteritis nodosa (PAN)	uncommon
Hereditary	Charcot-Marie-Tooth disease, others	uncommon
Neoplastic paraproteinaemia paraneoplastic	monoclonal gammopathy, carcinoma lung, breast, ovary	very uncommon
Idiopathic (>50% of all peripheral neuropathies)	unknown	most common

Main causes of polyneuropathy in Africa

- HIV
- diabetes
- leprosy
- drugs
- alcohol
- nutrition

Clinical features

The history may provide the first clue as to the aetiology of a neuropathy. There may be a history of a known risk factor for neuropathy, e.g. HIV, use of antiretroviral drugs (ART) in particular stavudine, diabetes, alcohol abuse, renal failure or very rarely a family history. The history provides essential information concerning the mode of onset, time course, distribution, character and pattern of symptoms.

The clinical distribution will indicate whether it is confined to just one nerve or is more generalised affecting all peripheral nerves. An acute onset over days with both proximal and distal weakness suggests a demyelinating disorder like GBS, whereas a more chronic onset over months suggests a distal sensory motor axonal neuropathy as occurs in DM or HIV. Burning or pain in the feet is very characteristic of the neuropathy in HIV, diabetes, vitamin deficiencies and alcoholism. Additional clinical findings may also indicate the cause; the peripheral nerves may be thickened in leprosy, or clawing of the feet or pes cavus is seen in hereditary neuropathies or the low blood pressure on standing characteristic of autonomic neuropathies. The predominance of either sensory or motor findings is also helpful.

Motor

Muscle weakness suggests motor neuropathy. Motor symptoms include mild to severe weakness in the limbs, problems with walking or running, and difficulties manipulating or using fingers and hands. The main causes of motor neuropathy are GBS, polio and very rarely lead poisoning. Main findings on neurological examination include wasting, weakness and loss of reflexes in the limbs (Fig.11.6).

Sensory

Numbness, tingling or pain in a glove and stocking distribution suggest a mainly sensory neuropathy. Terms used to describe the superficial sensory symptoms include: paraesthesia, meaning abnormal tingling sensation; hyperaesthesia, meaning increased sensitivity to a stimulus and dysaesthesia, meaning unpleasant tingling. The term allodynia means painful sensation from light non painful stimulus e.g. stroking. Sensory symptoms tend to occur before motor symptoms and typically involve the feet earlier than hands. Findings on neurological examination include loss of light touch, pain and joint position sense distally in the limbs mostly the feet. A sensory polyneuropathy may also cause poor balance and unsteady gait due to a loss of position sense in the feet. This is called sensory ataxic neuropathy. When the neuropathy involves loss of pain then trophic changes and digital loss can occur (Fig. 11.7)

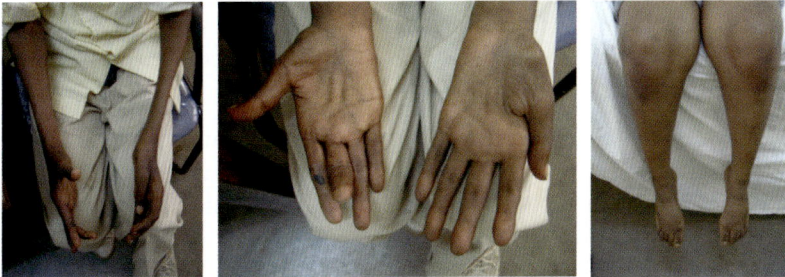

Wasting forearms & small hand muscles · Distal wasting & foot drop

Figure 11.6 Motor and sensory neuropathy

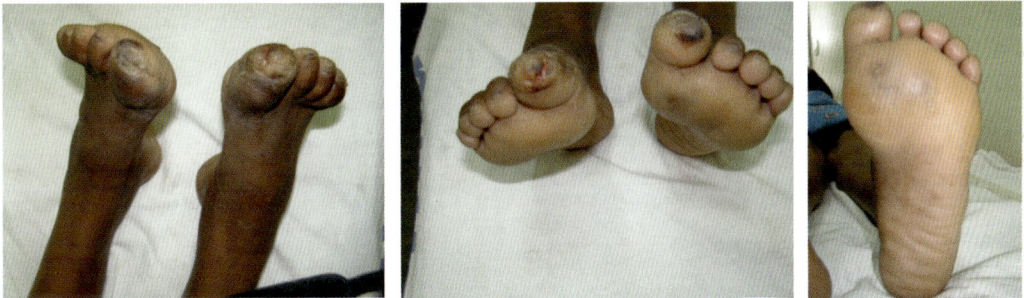

Loss of terminal digits, ulcers & trophic changes

Figure 11.7 Sensory neuropathy

Differential Diagnosis

The differential diagnosis of neuropathies includes diseases affecting muscle, neuromuscular junction and occasionally myelopathy and rarely motor neurone disease. Polymyositis and myopathy may sometimes mimic a neuropathy but skin involvement and the mainly proximal pattern of weakness should suggest underlying muscle disease. Fatigability after exercise, a mainly truncal-axial pattern of weakness, ptosis and intact reflexes all point to myasthenia gravis. While myelopathy symptoms may sometimes mimic neuropathy, the predominantly upper motor neurone signs, the sphincteric involvement and pattern of sensory loss or alteration should all suggest spinal cord involvement. Exclusive motor involvement with weakness and fasciculation are pointers towards progressive muscular atrophy (PMA), a form of motor neurone disease, although this is uncommon.

Diagnosis

The diagnosis of peripheral neuropathy relies mainly on the clinical findings and in as many as half the cases no underlying cause is found. Investigations should include laboratory screening tests for the common causes as outlined in Table 11.3. Simple blood tests exclude causes such as HIV, diabetes and B-12 deficiency. CSF examination may show an elevated protein in GBS and CIDP. Nerve conduction studies and electromyography are very helpful if available.

Nerve conduction studies (NCS) and Electromyography (EMG)

These are used mainly to determine whether there is a disease of the peripheral nerves, neuromuscular junction or muscle and to distinguish between them. NCS can also determine whether the neuropathy is purely sensory or also affects the motor fibres and whether the primary disease is axonal (causing death of axons) or demyelinating (affecting Schwann cells and myelin sheaths) or a mixture of both.

NCS involve stimulating a nerve with an electrical impulse and measuring the speed of conduction at two points along the nerve. This is called the conduction velocity. NCS also involves recording and measuring the amplitude of muscle action potential (MAP). NCS can distinguish demyelinating from axonal neuropathies. In general, a reduction in conduction velocity and normal MAP favours demyelination whereas normal conduction velocity and reduced MAP favours axonal neuropathies. Most neuropathies are axonal in type and largely untreatable. The most common type is termed distal symmetrical polyneuropathy (DM and HIV). In contrast demyelinating neuropathies (GBS) are uncommon but are largely treatable.

EMG involves insertion of a needle electrode into muscle and measures electrical activity in muscles. The patterns of electrical recordings at rest and during activity can determine the likely origin of the disorder.

Table 11.3 Laboratory investigations in peripheral neuropathy

Type	Investigation	Disorder
Haematology	FBC, B-12, folate, HIV, VDRL, ESR	vit deficiency, HIV, syphilis infection, vasculitis
Biochemistry	glucose, renal, liver, thyroid function tests, protein electrophoresis	diabetes, renal failure, myxoedema, paraproteinaemia
Urine	cells, protein casts	
Immunology	auto antibodies: ANCA, rheumatoid factor, antinuclear antibody	RA, SLE, PAN
X-ray	chest, bones	malignancy, myeloma
Lumbar puncture	protein	GBS, CIDP
Electrical	NCS	axonal versus demyelinating
Skin slit smears/biopsy	acid fast bacilli	leprosy

Management of neuropathy

The first principle of management is to diagnose and treat the underlying cause of neuropathy. High dose corticosteroids are used in neuropathies complicating vasculitis and chronic inflammation. Other forms of immunosuppression include intravenous immunoglobulin (IVIG) and plasma exchange (PE). These are used in GBS but these are unavailable to all but the largest medical centres in Africa. Pain is controlled by local and general measures. Local measures include application of heat, and topical anaesthetics. General measures include analgesics, anti inflammatories, tricyclics, the antiepileptic drugs carbamazepine, pregabalin and gabapentin and also opiates (Chapter 20). Weak or paralysed limbs may be assisted with orthoses. General advice is given to prevent ulcers by wearing protective foot wear and avoiding injury. The most common or important individual neuropathies are presented below.

Key points

- main causes of neuropathy are HIV, diabetes, leprosy & ART
- history and examination provide clues to diagnosis & aetiology
- neuropathies are either sensory or motor or a mixture of both
- investigations involves bloods, csf examination and X-rays
- main aim is treat the underlying cause & to control symptoms

INDIVIDUAL NEUROPATHIES

HIV

HIV frequently affects peripheral nerves. The main mechanisms are direct HIV infection and autoimmunity (Chapter 8). The most common neuropathy in HIV is a distal sensory neuropathy (DSN) secondary to HIV infection itself and to ART. Less common neuropathies include Bell's palsy and inflammatory neuropathies including Guillain-Barre syndrome.

Distal sensory neuropathy (DSN)

DSN is the main HIV related neuropathy and occurs as a result of direct HIV infection triggered immune activation affecting peripheral nerves (Fig.11.8). It affects about one quarter of AIDS patients, occurring mostly but not exclusively in more advanced HIV disease with CD4 counts <200/cm³.

The main symptoms of DSN are a painful, hot, burning, numbness or paraesthesia like sensation occurring symmetrically in a foot and stocking distribution, developing slowly over weeks and months. Power is usually maintained but may very occasionally be decreased around the ankle joint. The ankle and infrequently the knee reflexes are absent or decreased and this may be the only sign to indicate the presence of DSN. Sensation involving touch is mostly intact but touch is characteristically perceived by the patient as painful or dysaesthetic, particularly when touched crudely on the soles of the feet and the palms of the hands. Vibration and pinprick may be impaired distally in the feet in advanced disease. The upper limbs are typically unaffected apart from the dyaesthesia in the palms.

The mainstay of management is to start ART as soon as possible. Symptomatic relief of pain may be obtained using simple analgescics and/or amitriptyline; gabapentin or lamotrogine are more expensive alternatives. However opiates may be necessary in severe cases.

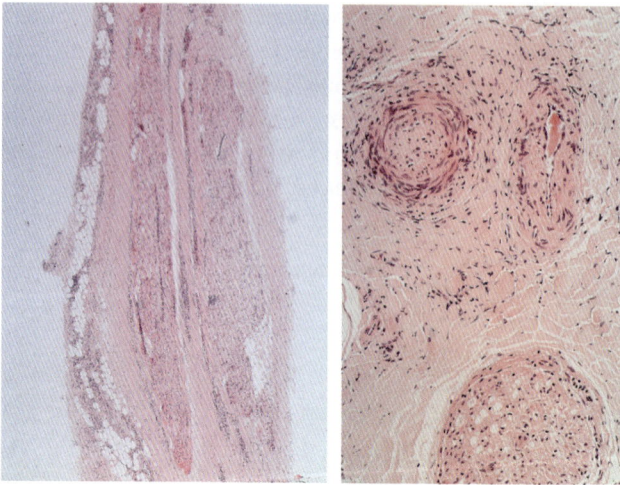

Figure 11.8 DSN in HIV, histopathology. Perineural inflammation.

ART associated neuropathy

Peripheral neuropathy may also occur as an adverse effect of antiretroviral therapy. The symptoms and signs are very similar to HIV related neuropathy, although the sensory signs may be more marked in ART neuropathy. Both HIV and ART related neuropathy are termed DSN. In Sub-Saharan Africa, DSN is one of the main limiting side effects of first line ART. In particular this occurs with the use of the nucleoside reverse transcriptase inhibitor, stavudine (d4T). The incidence of DSN in HIV has been shown to increase with the use of d4T, in particular with 40 mg dosage and its duration of use. DSN may affect up to 20% of patients who have been on dT4 for 6 months or more and this increases the overall rate of DSN in HIV to >40%.

Management involves either reducing the standard dose of d4T from 40 to 30 mg (as recommended by WHO) or stopping and replacing d4T or the likely causal ART drug. Two thirds of patients may improve if switched to a non d4T regime. Other ART drugs associated with peripheral neuropathy include didanosine (ddI), lamivudine (3TC) and zalcitibine (ddC). Known risk factors for DSN include a history of previous or active antituberculous therapy, older age, alcohol use and malnutrition. Care should be taken to ensure that pyridoxine 20 mg/po/daily has been prescribed in all patients taking isoniazid, and that thiamine 100 mg/po/daily should be given in suspected cases of B-1 vitamin deficiency. Otherwise symptomatic management is the same as in HIV disease.

Bell's palsy

Bell's palsy or facial nerve palsy is the most frequent presentation of mononeuritis in HIV infection (Chapter 8). On screening during the acute phase of the HIV epidemic in some areas in Africa as many as 50% of patients presenting with Bell's palsy tested positive for HIV. Bell's palsy occurs typically during the asymptomatic phase of HIV infection when the patient feels otherwise well and is still relatively immunocompetent. The facial weakness develops over 24 hours and the clinical course is similar to that in non HIV associated Bell's palsy, however it may occasionally be bilateral. Facial nerve palsy onsets during the later stages of

HIV infection occur mostly in association with opportunistic infections involving the CNS, mainly meningitis.

Inflammatory neuropathies

Guillain Barre Syndrome (GBS) and chronic inflammatory demyelinating polyneuropathy may also occur in association with HIV infection. These occur during the otherwise asymptomatic phase of HIV infection when immunity is relatively intact. They are both relatively uncommon forms of neuropathy but may be the first clinical indication of underlying HIV infection. Their mechanism is considered to be autoimmune based. Clinically GBS in HIV is indistinguishable from non HIV associated GBS apart from the presence of a number of lymphocytes in the CSF possibly due to the concurrent HIV infection. The management and the prognosis is the same as in non HIV associated demyelinating neuropathies.

Key Points

- neuropathy in very common in HIV disease
- most common is DSN in 40% of patients
- mechanisms are direct HIV infection, ART toxicity & autoimmunity
- management includes starting ART & reducing/stopping offending drug
- frequency of GBS & Bell's palsy are increased in HIV infection

LEPROSY

Leprosy is a chronic progressive potentially disabling granulomatous disease of the skin, and or peripheral nerves caused by *Mycobacterium leprae*. It causes damage to nerves which results in characteristic deformity and disability. It used to be the commonest cause of neuropathy worldwide but since the introduction of multi drug therapy (MDT) in the late 1980s over 15 million cases of leprosy worldwide have been treated successfully. Despite a reported decline in the incidence of leprosy, there are still a quarter to half a million new cases reported worldwide each year with most occurring in India. Africa accounts for over 40,000 newly reported cases annually. The countries with the highest incidence in Africa are the DRC and Mozambique.

Transmission

Leprosy is transmitted by inhalation of aerosolized nasal secretions from an infected person. Effective transmission requires regular prolonged close household or community contact with an infected person. The incubation period from infection to clinical disease varies from months to up to 30 years. The average incubation of contracting the disease from contact household cases is estimated to be about 5 years. Touching does not spread the disease.

Clinical features

The clinical features are determined by the host immune response. The main clinical presentations are anaesthetic skin lesions and peripheral neuropathy.

Host response

The majority of persons infected with *M. leprae* never develop clinical disease and this represents an effective host response. When disease does develop the clinical spectrum corresponds with the degree of T cell mediated immunity of the patient. Leprosy has a wide range of clinical presentations ranging from polar tuberculoid (TT) through borderline to polar lepromatous

(LL) (Figs. 11.9-10). While TT leprosy represents a good but still ineffective cell mediated immunity, LL represents little or no cell mediated immunity.

In TT at histology there are high levels of cell mediated immunity with granuloma formation and very few if any bacilli seen on histology, which limits the disease to a single or few well defined anaesthetic skin patches or palpable nerve trunks. This is in contrast to LL where there are no granuloma and many bacilli which result in multiple, bilateral, symmetrical skin and nerve lesions which are consequently more extensive and slowly progressive (Fig. 11.10).

In between, there are borderline states ranging from paucibacillary disease in borderline tuberculoid (BT) with 3-5 skin lesions with local palpable enlarged nerves to multibacillary disease in borderline lepromatous (BL) with multiple skin lesions with variable sensory loss and symmetrical nerve enlargement.

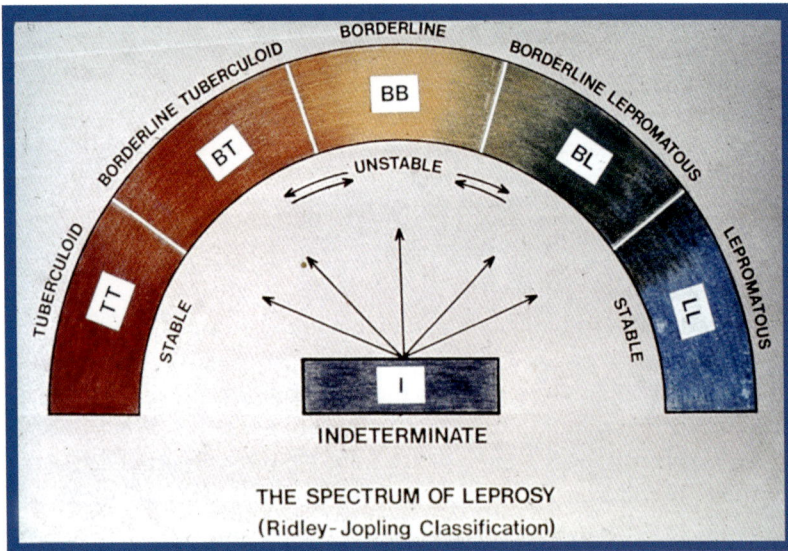

Figure 11.9 Immunological spectrum of leprosy

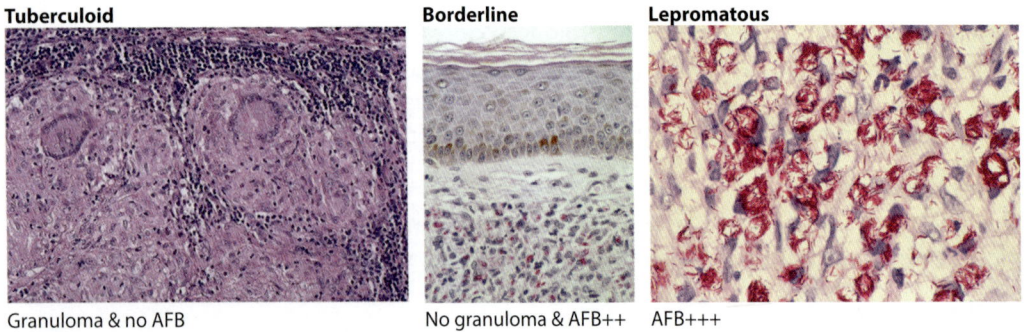

Figure 11.10 Histopathology leprosy

Skin

The skin lesions in leprosy vary with type, stage and immunity. The most common are plaques and macules but papules and nodules also occur. In tuberculoid leprosy there are single or few well circumscribed hypopigmented lesions with sharp borders. These are macular or plaque-like hypoanaesthetic patches often with loss of sweating and occurring usually on the trunk (Fig. 11.11). In lepromatous leprosy there are multiple, widespread, symmetrical, hypopigmented lesions with mostly intact sensation and/or infiltrated patches, papules and nodules. Widespread skin infiltration of the face results in the classical "leonine facies" of lepromatous leprosy (Fig. 11.11). All suspected skin lesions should be tested carefully for light touch, pain, temperature and for sweating.

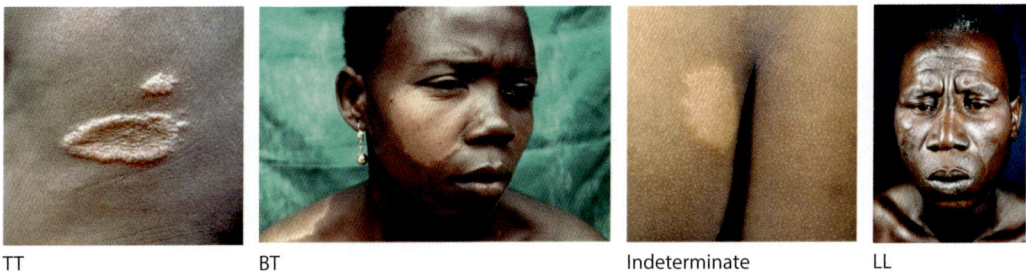

TT   BT   Indeterminate   LL

Figure 11.11 Skin in leprosy

Nerves

The main sequela of untreated leprosy is chronic disability secondary to nerve damage. Patients with leprosy present with skin lesions, muscle wasting, weakness or numbness in a peripheral nerve distribution or a burn or an ulcer in an anaesthetic hand or foot (Fig. 11.19). Nerve damage in leprosy occurs at two main levels; at the level of peripheral nerves and their main branches in TT and at the level of the small nerve twigs in skin and subcutaneous tissues in LL.

In TT, there is localized and asymmetrical involvement of the peripheral nerves. This occurs near the surface of the skin, where they present with palpable, thickened sometimes tender nerves and loss of neurological function in the distribution of the nerve. The common sites are the greater auricular in the neck, the ulnar at the elbow, median at the wrist, radial cutaneous at the wrist, common peroneal at the knee and posterior tibial behind the medial malleolus (Figs. 11.12-13).

In LL the dermal nerves are destroyed and there is a symmetrical peripheral neuropathy with a peripheral glove and stocking sensory loss.

Borderline leprosy produces most nerve damage as multiple nerves are involved earlier and more rapidly than in LL. Patients typically present with new skin lesions, nerve pain and sudden nerve palsies.

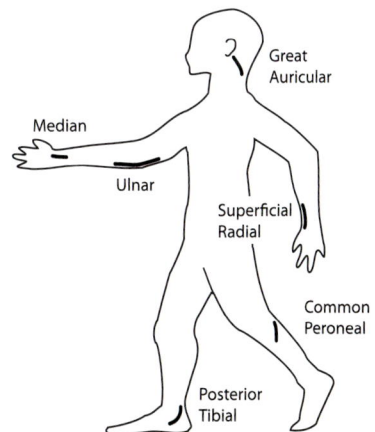

Figure 11.12 Sites to examine for enlarged nerves in leprosy

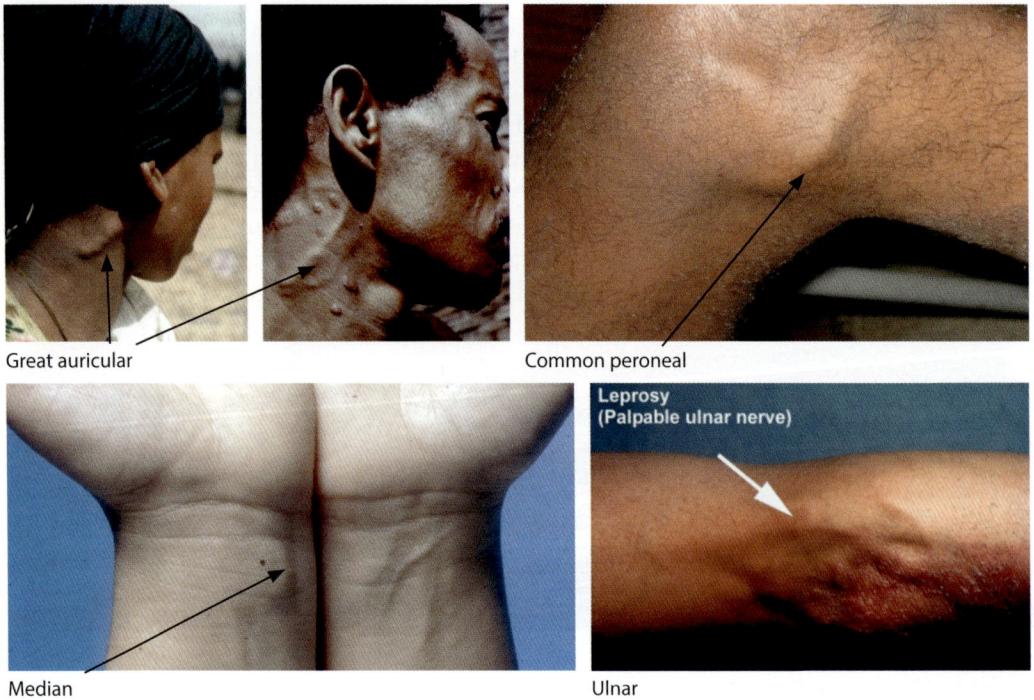

Great auricular

Common peroneal

Median

Leprosy
(Palpable ulnar nerve)

Ulnar

Figure 11.13 Nerve enlargement in leprosy

Neurological findings

There is a wide spectrum of sensory and motor neurological findings in leprosy. The sensory findings range from a subtle loss or decrease of temperature, pain, touch and sweating in a single skin patch in TT to a widespread peripheral neuropathy with evidence of sensory loss in the cooler extremities in LL. The sensory loss in LL may involve the extensor surface of the legs, feet, forearms and hands, nose, cheeks, breasts, abdomen and buttocks with sparing of the palms soles and scalp. An abrupt transition to normal sensation on the scalp is called the "hairline sign". Marked single or multiple peripheral nerve damage can occur in TT leprosy resulting in wrist drop, claw hand, dropped foot or failure to close an eye (lagophthalmos) (Figs.11.14-15). Motor findings in LL present as distal weakness of the intrinsic muscles of hands and feet. Loss of peripheral reflexes, joint position and vibration sense are typically late findings in leprosy being preserved early on in the disease.

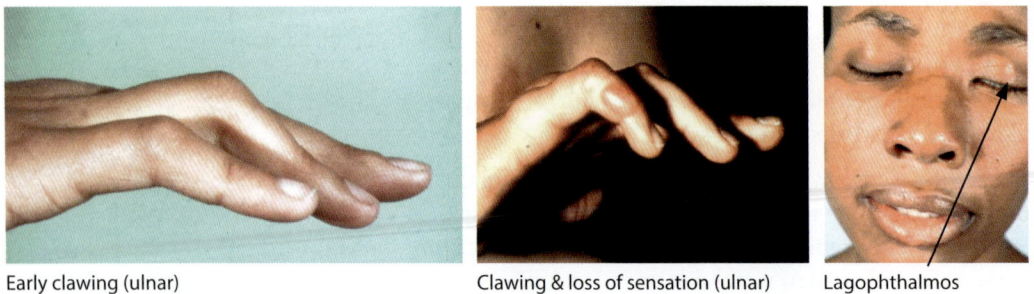

Early clawing (ulnar)

Clawing & loss of sensation (ulnar)

Lagophthalmos

Figure 11.14 Nerve damage in leprosy

Eyes

Damage to the eye results from involvement of both trigeminal and facial nerves. This results in a loss of sensation on the cornea and inability to close and protect the eye (Fig. 11.14). A minor injury may result in corneal scarring and blindness. Direct massive invasion of the cornea can occur mainly in LL causing conjunctivitis, iritis and eventually blindness (Fig. 11.15).

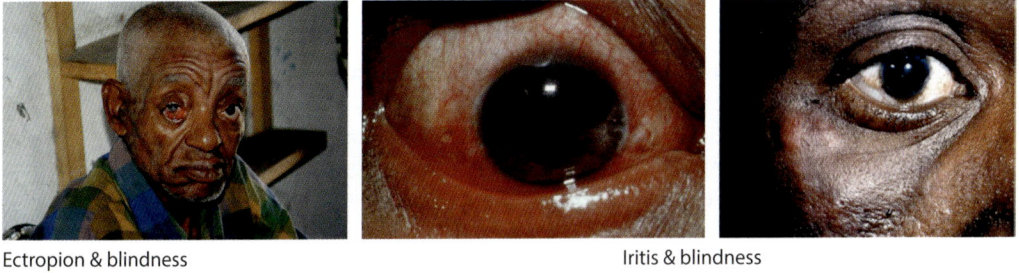

Ectropion & blindness   Iritis & blindness

Figure 11.15 Eye damage in leprosy

Diagnosis

The diagnosis of leprosy is above all a clinical one and early diagnosis is crucial to management. The diagnostic features are hypopigmented patches with definite loss of sensation (Fig. 11.11) (however skin lesions in BL/LL may not have sensory loss), palpably thickened peripheral nerves (Figs. 11.12-13) and the presence of acid fast bacilli in slit skin smears or biopsy. Samples are taken from the ear lobes (Fig. 11.16), eye brows and the edges of active lesions. The density of bacilli on slit skin smears is called the bacterial index (BI). WHO classifies leprosy as paucibacillary (PC) when no bacilli are seen and multibacillary (MB) when bacilli are seen. If more than five skin lesions are seen, this is also classified as MB disease regardless of the absence of bacilli on skin smear. This method is used when slit skin smears are not available.

Diagnostic features of leprosy

- skin lesions with sensory loss
- thickened peripheral nerves
- acid-fast bacilli on slit skin smears or biopsy

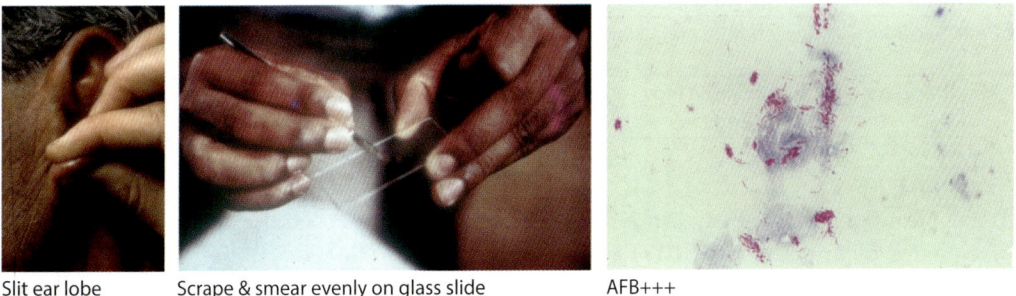

Slit ear lobe   Scrape & smear evenly on glass slide   AFB+++

Figure 11.16 Slit skin smear

Differential diagnosis

The differential diagnosis for neuropathy in leprosy includes mononeuropathies, sensorimotor polyneuropathies, hereditary neuropathies and syringomyelia. Amyloid and neurofibromatosis also can cause nerve thickening mimicking leprosy. While the typical pattern of skin and neurological involvement help to establish the diagnosis in leprosy particularly in endemic areas, a keen index of suspicion is always necessary especially in non endemic areas.

Key points

- leprosy is chronic infection of skin and nerves caused by M. leprae
- a major cause of disabling peripheral neuropathy in Africa
- findings explained by variation in degree of cell mediated immunity
- neurological features: numbness or weakness in individual nerves & polyneuropathy
- diagnosis: anaesthetic skin lesions, thickened peripheral nerves & AFBs in skin snips

Treatment

Education of the patient about their disease has been identified as the most important strategy in successful management of leprosy. The key areas are an understanding of its low infectivity, importance of drug compliance, an awareness of reversal reactions, the critical need for care of anaesthetic feet and hands and social issues.

The main aim of treatment is to cure the patient without residual permanent disability. The treatment of leprosy depends on whether it is lepromatous or tuberculoid in type. All patients should receive multiple drug treatment (MDT); for 6 months in TL or paucibacillary disease and for 12-24 months in LL or multibacillary disease. The treatments include dapsone, clofazamine and rifampicin and are outlined in Table 11.4. Patients are no longer infectious after 72 hours of treatment. Relapse rates range from 0 to 2.5% in paucibacillary disease to 0-8% in multibacillary disease. The main side effects of MDT include red urine discolouration with rifampicin, red-brown discolouration of the skin with clofazamine and haemolysis with dapsone, particularly in patients with G6PD deficiency. Nerve damage in leprosy can occur before, during and after MDT. The main mechanism of nerve damage after starting MDT is by reactions (Table 11.5).

Table 11.4 MDT regimes (WHO)

Type of Leprosy	Drug Treatment				
	Daily (self administered)		Monthly (supervised)	Length, months	Side effects
Paucibacillary	dapsone 100 mg	and	rifampicin 600 mg	6	haemolysis (G6PD), allergy, hepatitis, red urine
Multibacillary	clofazimine 50 mg dapsone 100 mg	and	rifampicin 600 mg clofazimine 300 mg	12-24	red skin, ichthyosis

Reactions

The clinical course of leprosy can be made acutely worse by reversal reactions. These can be precipitated by drug therapy (MDT), pregnancy and other illnesses. These are two main types of reactions, type 1 reversal reactions and type 2 erythema nodosum leprosum (ENL) reactions (Table 11.5). Type 1 reactions tend to occur in immunologically unstable borderline patients, (BT, BB and BL) upgrading towards tuberculoid leprosy during the first or second year of

MDT or after treatment. It occurs in about 30% of BL patients. The peak time is within the first 2 months of treatment. They present with acute inflammation, erythema, oedema and tender nerves, sometimes with dramatic loss of nerve function (Fig.11.17). Short course steroids are used for 3-4 months in BT and 6 months in BL patients. Erythema nodosum leprosum (ENL) type 2 reaction occurs in about 20% of LL and in 10% of BL patients (Fig.11.18). Patients with a high bacterial load are more at risk. It presents with fever and crops of small pink nodules mainly over the extensor surfaces. Systemic and nerve involvement are also common. To suppress the inflammation repeated short courses of steroids may be necessary and clofazamine is also used. Thalidomide has been successfully used in young men. However, it is relatively contraindicated in young females because of the high risk of teratogenesis mainly phocomelia and has not therefore been licensed in the majority of centres.

Table 11.5 Reversal reactions on treatment

Classification	Leprosy risk group	Frequency	Clinical features	Occurrence	Management
Type 1 (reversal)	borderline leprosy	30%	**skin:** erythema, oedema hands and face mainly	1) within the first 2 months of treatment	prednisolone 40-60 mgs daily decreasing by 5 mg every 2-4 weeks for 3-6 months
			nerves: tender & loss of function in nerve distribution	2) within 12/12 or after Rx	
				3) puerperium	
Type 2 (ENL)	lepromatous	20%	**skin**: crops of painful pink nodules	1) within the first or second year of treatment	prednisolone 1mg/kg/day/2-3/52 weeks only
	borderline lepromatous	10%	**others:** fever uveitis/iritis, arthritis neuritis orchitis	2) may occur years after treatment	clofazimine 300 mg daily for 2/12, followed by 200 mg daily for 2/12
				3) pregnancy, lactation	thalidomide 400 mg daily (use in men) for months

Complications

The complications of leprosy arise as a result of nerve damage leading to deformity and disability. This occurs through loss of pain sensation leading to trauma, burns, tissue damage, injury and secondary infection. The main complications are ulceration, osteomyelitis, foot and wrist drop, contractures, loss of digits and blindness (Fig. 11.19). Prevention is by patient education about the early recognition of the disease, reactions, complications and the initiation of appropriate treatment. Teaching patients about their disease is most important. The patient needs to be particularly aware of risk and guard an anaesthetic limb by protective measures including special footwear and routine daily inspection for signs of trauma. Ulcers should be treated with rest, surgical debridement and antibiotics if infected. Reconstructive surgery is helpful in contractures and in eye complications.

Swelling & acroderma of face and feet

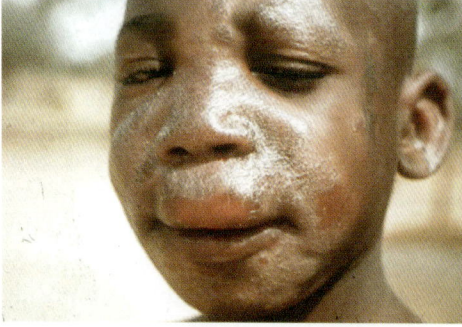
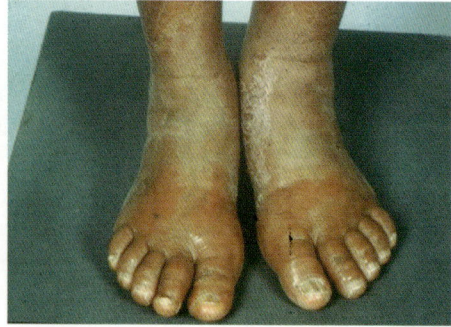

Histology

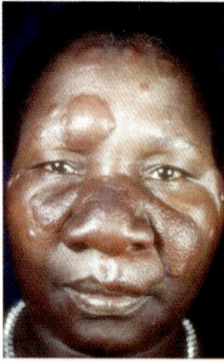
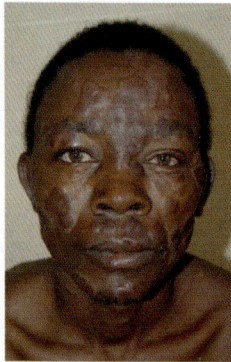
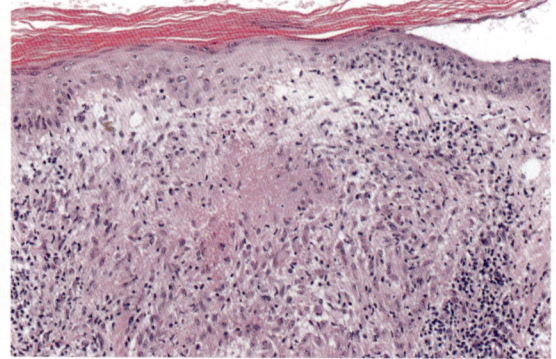

Lepra reactions

Granuloma like & no AFB

Figure 11.17 Type 1 reversal reactions

Histology

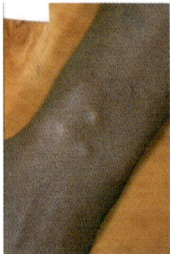
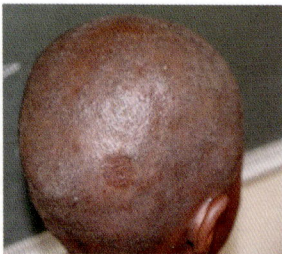
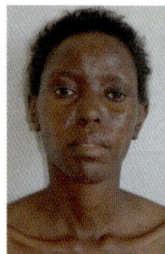
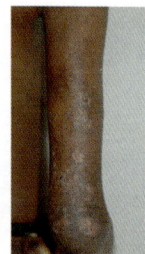
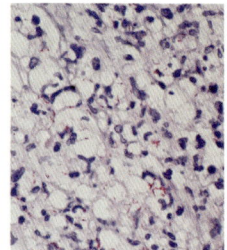

Nodules

Ulcers

No granuloma & AFB ++

Figure 11.18 Type 2 reversal reactions, ENL

Prevention

The mainstay of the prevention of leprosy in endemic areas is by passive case finding and then directly observed treatment (DOTS) rendering the patient non-infectious to others. Chemoprophylaxis of close contacts may also be an effective strategy in the future and studies are underway to assess its role. BCG gives variable (>50%) protection against clinical leprosy.

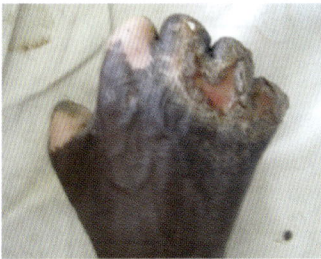

Ulceration & loss of digits

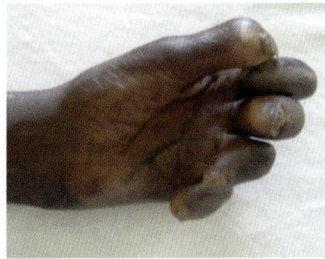

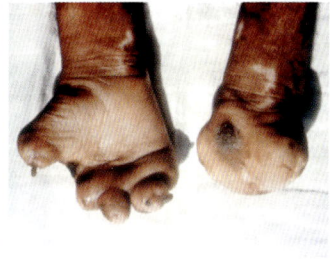

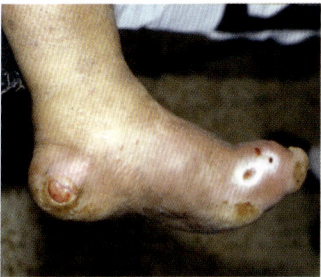

Ulceration & osteomyelitis

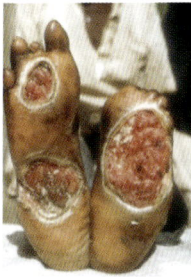

Figure 11.19 Complications of leprosy

Key points

- educating the patient about their disease is best way to manage leprosy
- Rx includes MDT & compliance, awareness of reactions & prevention of disability
- complications occur as a result of nerve damage causing anaesthesia and weakness
- they include ulcers, osteomyelitis, foot/wrist drop, contractures, loss of digits & blindness
- prevention of leprosy is by passive case finding, DOTS & BCG vaccination

DIABETES

Diabetic neuropathy is the most common type of neuropathy worldwide. It is present in about one in ten diabetic patients at diagnosis and in the majority of patients 25 years later on. The main finding is a slowly progressive distal sensory neuropathy (DSN) starting in toes and gradually spreading up to knees and later to fingers and hands. It is characterized by numbness, tingling, pain, decreased sensation in the feet and legs and areflexia. Autonomic neuropathy may occur and its main clinical features include orthostatic hypotension, gastroparesis and impotence. Infrequently diabetes may cause isolated mono and multiple neuropathies. The most common ones are 6th and 3rd cranial neuropathies, femoral neuropathy and radiculopathies affecting the lumbar and sacral nerve roots. Management is by strict control of blood glucose levels, treatment of neuropathic pain and the prevention of foot and leg ulcers much in the same way as in leprosy.

Key points

- neuropathies are very common in diabetes
- DSN is the most common neuropathy
- isolated mononeuropathies may also occur
- treatment involves control of glucose, pain and prevention of complications
- blood sugar should be checked in all patients with unexplained neuropathies

VITAMIN DEFICIENCY

The main causes of neuropathy due to vitamin deficiency are B-1 (thiamine), B-6 (pyridoxine) and B-12 (cobalamin).

Vitamin B-1 deficiency

Thiamine (B-1) deficiency causes beriberi and Wernicke-Korsakoff-Syndrome (WKS). Beriberi can be dry or wet. Dry beriberi results in a sensory motor polyneuropathy while wet beriberi results in cardiac failure and generalised oedema. Beriberi in Africa is mainly caused by malnutrition arising from food shortages and also occasionally from alcoholism. WKS is an encephalopathy which can be acute or chronic. The usual cause is thiamine deficiency in alcoholism. Acute WKS is characterized by confusion, amnesia, ataxia and nystagmus and ocular paralysis. When WKS becomes chronic, it is characterized by an irreversible confabulatory type dementia with a devastating loss of short term memory. Treatment for both conditions is by thiamine replacement either intravenously or orally. The response is variable in acute or mostly none at all in chronic WKS. The dose of thiamine is 100 mg/daily. It is essential to first replace the missing thiamine before giving intravenous dextrose or treating infections or replacing other vitamins, as failure to do this can precipitate an irreversible WKS.

Vitamin B-6 deficiency

Pyridoxine (Vit B-6) deficiency causes a mainly sensory neuropathy. The main cause in Africa is isoniazid in TB treatment. It can be prevented by giving pyridoxine 20-50 mg orally daily, whenever isoniazid is used. Overdoses of vitamin B-6 may actually cause neuropathy so it is important to avoid doses greater than 100 mg daily.

Vitamin B-12 deficiency

Cobalamin (Vit B-12) deficiency causes a polyneuropathy, sub acute combined degeneration of the cord (SACD), optic atrophy, dementia and pernicious anaemia. Vitamin B-12 deficiency may be less common in Africa than in high income countries. The main clinical findings of the neuropathy are absent ankle jerks, loss of peripheral sensation (especially joint position and vibration) in combination with brisk knee reflexes and up going plantar responses. The main causes are nutritional deficiency and malabsorption of B-12. Malabsorption may be due to lack of intrinsic factor and diseases of the terminal ileum. Treatment is with hydroxycobalamin (Vit B-12) 1 mg (1000 micrograms) intramuscular injections on alternate days for a total of five injections or 5 mg. This is followed by 1 mg injections every 3 months for life. In the absence of severe malabsorption, replacement can be given orally at a dose of 1 mg daily.

ALCOHOL

Alcohol misuse is an increasingly common cause of neuropathy worldwide. Apart from malnutrition related thiamine deficiency, alcohol causes a direct effect on nerves by the toxic effect of its metabolites. It presents with a history of a slowly progressing burning dysasthesia mainly in the feet and legs over months or years in a person misusing alcohol. On examination, there are signs of a distal sensory motor neuropathy usually without significant loss of power. Treatment is to stop the alcohol and replace thiamine (Vit B-1) although painful symptoms frequently persist. Tricyclics and/or the antiepileptics may be helpful for treatment.

Key points

- Vitamin B deficiencies occur mainly because of food shortages & disease
- B-1 (thiamine) deficiency causes beriberi and WKS
- B-6 (pyridoxine) deficiency occurs with isoniazid in TB treatment
- B-12 (cobalamin) deficiency causes neuropathy treatable with B-12 injections
- chronic excessive alcohol may result in a painful persistent sensory neuropathy

GUILLAIN-BARRE SYNDROME (GBS)

GBS is an immune mediated demyelinating polyneuropathy. It is an uncommon disease affecting about 2/100,000 each year. It presents as an acute progressive usually ascending flaccid paralysis that reaches its peak usually around 10-14 days but always by definition in less than 4 weeks. This is followed by a plateau phase and eventual recovery for most patients after 3-6 months. Two thirds of cases are associated with a history of preceding febrile illness, diarrhoea, immunization or surgery during the previous 2-3 weeks. Preceding causes of fever associated with GBS include campylobacter jejuni, cytomegalovirus, and other respiratory and gastrointestinal infections. HIV infection is associated with an increased risk of GBS and patients with suspected GBS should be screened for HIV.

Clinical features

The presenting complaint is that of a rapidly developing motor weakness occurring over days and sometimes hours. Sensory symptoms, mainly paraesthesiae, often painful may accompany the weakness but these are usually mild. Motor weakness is usually marked early on both proximally and distally. Reflexes are diminished or absent. Sensation is mostly intact but may be impaired. There is no sensory loss on the trunk. Sphincters are spared. Lower motor neurone type facial weakness occurs in about half the patients but may be mild and is frequently bilateral. Other cranial nerves may be involved. Respiratory failure and autonomic symptoms occur in over a fifth of patients. The main complications and cause of death in GBS are respiratory failure, pneumonia, cardiac arrhythmias and pulmonary embolism. The differential diagnosis includes other causes of acute flaccid paralysis. These include transverse myelitis, organophosphorous poisoning, diphtheria, polio, botulinum and lead poisoning. Chronic inflammatory demyelinating polyneuropathy is a more chronic form of GBS with a slower onset, over 2-3 months and responds well to steroids.

Investigations

These include a full blood count, HIV test, blood glucose, creatinine and electrolytes. A lumbar puncture should be carried out to check for the characteristic elevation in CSF protein in the absence of white blood cells (WBC <5/mm³). The CSF protein may be normal during the first week of the illness and this may need repeating during the second or third week. If available, nerve conduction studies will show marked slowing of motor conduction velocities characteristic of a demyelinating polyneuropathy.

Key points

- GBS typically presents with acute rapidly progressing limb weakness over 1-2 weeks
- lower back and proximal limb pain may be an initial presenting complaint
- facial nerve palsies may be present
- approximately two thirds have a recent (2/52) history of either diarrhoea or a febrile illness
- diagnosis is supported by elevated csf protein without WBCs

General management

The outcome of GBS depends on the quality of nursing care. The patient should be initially placed in an intensive care unit. Nursing care is directed at checking for signs of increasing weakness, respiratory failure and the prevention of bedsores and contractures. The vital signs and in particular the vital capacity should be measured 4 hourly for the first few days of the illness. If the vital capacity falls to the range of 1.5-1 litre, then assisted ventilation must be considered. The heart should be monitored for arrhythmias and any surges in blood pressure treated with beta blockers. Compression stockings and low dose heparin are used to prevent deep vein thrombosis and pulmonary emboli. A nasogastric tube may need to be passed if swallowing is a concern. The patient may need analgesia for pain and psychological support. Physiotherapy should be started on admission.

Specific treatments

Steroids have no role in the treatment of GBS. Specific treatments include intravenous immunoglobulin (IVIG) or plasma exchange (PE). IVIG is the treatment of choice but both are equally beneficial. Disease progression, respiratory failure and significant disability are all indications for their use and they should be administered within the first 2 weeks of onset of the illness, as they are not of value after that time. Their main role is to halve the average period of hospital stay from about 12 to 6 weeks. However, these treatments are mostly unavailable because of their high cost and limited resources.

Prognosis

The mortality in GBS in Africa is around 10%. Recovery in the remaining 90% is good but some (10-20%) remain partially disabled at 12 months.

Key points

- acute care involves regular monitoring for respiratory failure i.e. FVC <1.5 litres
- main complications are respiratory failure, pneumonia, arrhythmia & pulmonary emboli
- specific treatments include IVIG & PE
- CFR in Africa is about 10%, with most patients recovering fully after 3-6/12

CHRONIC INFLAMMATORY DEMYELINATING POLYNEUROPATHY (CIDP)

CIDP is similar to GBS but follows a chronic progressive course over months rather than weeks. It is very uncommon but represents a treatable neuropathy. The cause is not known. The clinical features are characterized by a mixed motor sensory peripheral neuropathy usually with proximal as well as distal weakness. Cranial nerves and autonomic system are not usually involved. The results of investigations are similar to GBS with elevated protein in CSF and evidence of demyelination on NCS.

Treatment is with high dose steroids prednisolone initially 60 mg/od for 4-6 weeks, reducing slowly over months until on a minimum maintenance dose of 5-20 mg on alternate days. IVIG or plasma exchange can also be used as in GBS. Azathioprine or methotrexate can be added as steroid sparing agents. Response to immunosuppression is good but may have to be continued in the longer term.

Selected references

Agrawal A, Pandit L, Dalal M, Shetty JP. *Neurological manifestations of Hansen's disease and their management.* Clin Neurol Neurosurg. 2005 Oct;107(6):445-54.

Bademosi O, Osuntokun BO. *Diseases of peripheral nerves as seen in the Nigerian African.* Afr J Med Med Sci. 1981 Mar-Jun;10(1-2):33-8.

Britton WJ, Lockwood DN. *Leprosy.* Lancet. 2004 Apr 10;363(9416):1209-19.

de Freitas MR. *Infectious neuropathy.* Curr Opin Neurol. 2007 Oct;20(5):548-52.

Evans D, Takuva S, Rassool M, Firnhaber C, Maskew M. *Prevalence of peripheral neuropathy in antiretroviral therapy naïve HIV-positive patients and the impact on treatment outcomes-a retrospective study from a large urban cohort in Johannesburg, South Africa.* J Neurovirol. 2012 Jun;18(3):162-71

Haimanot RT, Abdulkadir J. *Neuropathy in Ethiopian diabetics: a correlation of clinical and nerve conduction studies.* Trop Geogr Med. 1985 Mar;37(1):62-8.

Haimanot RT, Melaku Z. *Leprosy.* Curr Opin Neurol. 2000 Jun;13(3):317-22.

Howlett WP, Vedeler CA, Nyland H, Aarli JA. *Guillain-Barre syndrome in northern Tanzania: a comparison of epidemiological and clinical findings with western Norway.* Acta Neurol Scand. 1996 Jan;93(1):44-9.

Koike H, Sobue G. *Alcoholic neuropathy.* Curr Opin Neurol. 2006 Oct;19(5):481-6.

Lockwood DN. *Leprosy—a changing picture but a continuing challenge.* Trop Doct. 2005 Apr;35(2):65-7.

Lockwood DN, Suneetha S. *Leprosy: too complex a disease for a simple elimination paradigm.* Bull World Health Organ. 2005 Mar;83(3):230-5.

Maritz J, Benatar M, Dave JA, Harrison TB, Badri M, Levitt NS, Heckmann JM. *HIV neuropathy in South Africans: frequency, characteristics, and risk factors.* Muscle Nerve. 2010 May;41(5):599-606.

McGrath CJ, Njoroge J, John-Stewart GC, Kohler PK, Benki-Nugent SF, Thiga JW, et al. *Increased incidence of symptomatic peripheral neuropathy among adults receiving stavudine- versus zidovudine-based antiretroviral regimens in Kenya.* J Neurovirol. 2012 Jun;18(3):200-4.

Melaku Z, Zenebe G, Bekele A. *Guillain-Barre syndrome in Ethiopian patients.* Ethiop Med J. 2005 Jan;43(1):21-6.

Ooi WW, Srinivasan J. *Leprosy and the peripheral nervous system: basic and clinical aspects.* Muscle Nerve. 2004 Oct;30(4):393-409.

Radhakrishnan K, Thacker AK, Maloo JC. *A clinical, epidemiological and genetic study of hereditary motor neuropathies in Benghazi, Libya.* J Neurol. 1988 Sep;235(7):422-4.

Sitati FC, Naddumba E, Beyeza T. *Injection-induced sciatic nerve injury in Ugandan children.* Trop Doct. 2010 Oct;40(4):223-4.

Van Veen NH, Lockwood DN, Van Brakel WH, Ramirez J, Jr., Richardus JH. *Interventions for erythema nodosum leprosum.* A Cochrane review. Lepr Rev. 2009 Dec;80(4):355-72.

Wadley AL, Cherry CL, Price P, Kamerman PR. *HIV neuropathy risk factors and symptom characterization in stavudine-exposed South Africans.* J Pain Symptom Manage. 2011 Apr;41(4):700-6.

Walker SL, Lockwood DN. *Leprosy.* Clin Dermatol. 2007 Mar-Apr;25(2):165-72.

Walker SL, Lockwood DN. *Leprosy type 1 (reversal) reactions and their management.* Lepr Rev. 2008 Dec;79(4):372-86.

PART II – NEUROLOGICAL DISORDERS

CHAPTER 12
CRANIAL NERVE DISORDERS

CONTENTS

CHAPTER 12

CRANIAL NERVE DISORDERS

Cranial nerve disorders are common neurological disorders. The clinical skills needed to examine the individual cranial nerves are presented in chapter 1. The overall aim of this chapter is to present the main cranial nerve disorders and to integrate examination and localization in their diagnosis. After reading the chapter the student should be able to localize and diagnose main disorders affecting pupils, vision, eye movements, facial sensation and movements, hearing, speech and swallowing.

OLFACTORY NERVE

Smell

Neurological disorders involving the olfactory nerve are uncommon and the olfactory nerve is rarely tested in day to day clinical practice. During a routine neurological examination it is sufficient to ask the patient if there is a loss or decrease in the sense of smell (anosmia). Frequently patients are unaware of a loss of smell or may only complain of losing their sense of taste. This is because both smell and taste are used together to appreciate the flavors of food and drink. If there is a loss or deterioration in smell, then each nostril should be tested separately as outlined in chapter 1. The most common cause of transient loss of smell is mucosal swelling in the nose or sinuses as a result of local infection e.g. head cold, allergy or smoking. Anosmia may occur after a head injury when there is a shearing injury to the olfactory bulb and its central connections through the cribriform plate. A rare cause of unilateral anosmia is a meningioma in the olfactory groove. Olfactory hallucinations are a feature of temporal lobe epilepsy.

Optic nerve

Disorders affecting the optic nerve are common and clinical assessment involves a history and examination. The history involves asking about a loss or decrease in vision, double vision, pain and headache and their mode of onset, progression and time course. The examination of the optic nerve includes testing the *pupillary responses, visual acuity, visual fields* and *fundoscopy*. Details concerning the technique of examination have already been set out in chapter 1.

PUPILLARY RESPONSES

Pupillary size and reactions

Both pupils should be normal in size (2-6 mm), equal, central and circular (ECC). The iris controls the size of the pupil. It does this by means of two groups of muscle fibres supplied by the autonomic nervous system. The sphincter pupillae is a circular constrictor smooth muscle supplied by the parasympathetic and the dilator pupillae is a radial smooth muscle supplied by the sympathetic nervous system. The balance between these accounts for normal pupil size.

The important aspects in their examination are summarized below.

Key points

- look at the pupils and note their size & whether they are equal or not
- shine a bright light into one eye and look at pupil reaction in that eye (direct light reflex)
- repeat and look at the pupillary reaction in the other eye (consensual reflex)
- do the same for the other eye

THE LIGHT REFLEX

Pathway for pupillary constriction (parasympathetic)

A light (torch) is shone in each eye separately whilst asking the patient to fix on an object at least 3m away. The light in one eye sends an *afferent* impulse along the optic nerve to the midbrain. The afferent anatomical pathway to the midbrain involves the retina, optic nerve, chiasm and optic tract. From the midbrain, a second order neurone travels to the Edinger-Westphal nucleus on both the same and opposite side of the midbrain. From there, *efferent* parasympathetic fibres travel back to the eyes, via the outside of the oculomotor nerve to the ciliary ganglion and to the constrictor sphincter pupillae. If all pathways are working normally, then the pupils in both eyes constrict equally and at the same time in response to light shone in one eye (Fig 12.1A). This represents the normal *light reflex* in the light stimulated eye and the *consensual reflex* (response) in the other eye. A lesion anywhere along that pathway results in a dilated pupil (mydriasis) on the affected side. The resulting defect is called an *afferent pupil defect* if it affects the optic pathway (Fig 12.1C) and an *efferent pupil defect* if it affects the parasympathetic pathway (Fig 12.1 B).

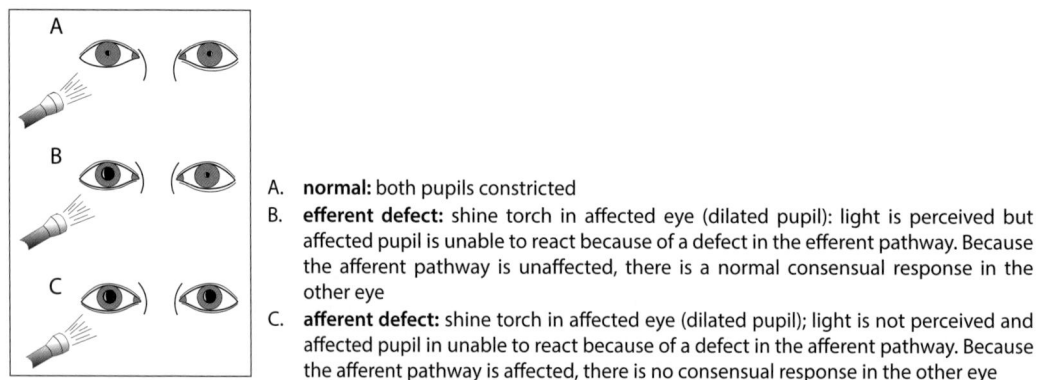

A. **normal:** both pupils constricted
B. **efferent defect:** shine torch in affected eye (dilated pupil): light is perceived but affected pupil is unable to react because of a defect in the efferent pathway. Because the afferent pathway is unaffected, there is a normal consensual response in the other eye
C. **afferent defect:** shine torch in affected eye (dilated pupil); light is not perceived and affected pupil in unable to react because of a defect in the afferent pathway. Because the afferent pathway is affected, there is no consensual response in the other eye

Figure 12.1 Testing for afferent and efferent pupillary disorders

Pathway for pupillary dilatation (sympathetic)

The sympathetic fibres descend on the same side from the hypothalamus via the lateral brain stem to the cervical spinal cord leaving the cord anteriorly at C8, T1. The fibres then ascend on the same side in the sympathetic chain to the superior cervical ganglion and from there on the outside of the wall of the internal carotid artery to the ciliary ganglion and the dilator pupillae in the iris. A lesion anywhere along its path results in a constricted, small pupil *(miosis)*. Because sympathetic nerves also supply fibres to the ipsilateral eyelid (levator palpebrae superioris), the orbit and adjacent skin, a lesion in the sympathetic chain also results in *ptosis, enopthalmos and anhydrosis*. The presence of all four signs together is called *Horner's syndrome,* (Table 12.1).

Swinging torch test

A *relative afferent pupil defect* is a sign of optic neuritis in the eye being examined. It can be demonstrated by the swinging torch test, during which light is repeatedly shone alternatively into the good eye and the affected eye. When light is shone on the non affected good eye, both pupils constrict normally, however, when the light is transferred briskly to the affected or bad eye both pupils dilate (Fig. 12.2). The explanation for this is that the weak direct effect on the bad eye is counterbalanced by the withdrawal of the stimulus from the good eye and the loss of the consensual response. This is a sign of incomplete optic neuropathy and is most commonly seen in optic neuritis.

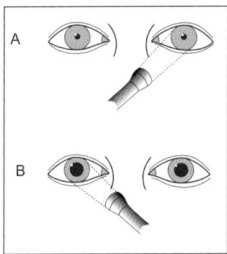

A. Both pupils constrict on shining light in unaffected left eye
B. Both pupils dilate on shining light in affected right eye (relative afferent pupillary defect)

Figure 12.2 Testing for a relative afferent pupillary defect.

THE ACCOMMODATION REFLEX

When using near vision the eyes converge and pupils constrict, this is the *accommodation reflex*. The afferent component of the accommodation reflex is conveyed in the optic nerve and the efferent pathway is less certain but does involve the visual cortex and some of the same pathways as the efferent light reflex. Testing for the presence of the accommodation reflex has become less useful in clinical practice especially with the decrease in the frequency of neurosyphilis worldwide (Chapter 6).

PUPILLARY DISORDERS

Disorders affecting pupils occur at four main sites; *the eye, the afferent or optic pathway*, the efferent or *parasympathetic* pathway and the *sympathetic* pathway (Table 12.1). The main disorders affecting the eye include infection, inflammation and trauma.

Neurological disorders affecting the *afferent pathway* are relatively common in Africa. These are termed optic neuropathies and result in *loss of vision* and *afferent pupil defects* (Fig 12.1C). The main causes are inflammatory (optic neuritis), nutritional and toxic. However, in many cases their cause is unknown.

Disorders affecting the *efferent pathway* (Fig 12.1 B) also occur. If the oculomotor (3rd nerve) is compressed on its path from the brain stem to the eye, then damage to the parasympathetic fibres which travel on the outside will result in a *fixed, dilated pupil* on that side. There may also be features of 3rd nerve palsy depending on the extent of the compression. Important neurological causes include raised intracranial pressure above the tentorium and an aneurysm compressing the nerve.

Disorders affecting the sympathetic pathway can occur anywhere along its pathway from the lateral brainstem to the eye, resulting in *Horner's syndrome*. A *small constricted pupil* and slight ptosis are characteristic. Neurological causes are uncommon and mainly involve lesions in its central pathway. Primary lung cancer involving the apex of the lung is an important cause, although this disorder is still relatively uncommon in Africa.

Other disorders affecting pupils include the *Holmes Adie pupil* which is a benign condition usually affecting one side which is found in women in their 20-40s. The affected pupil is dilated with an impaired response to light but also accommodates slowly. It may be or becomes bilateral and is also associated with absent ankle reflexes (Table 12.1). The *Argyll-Robertson pupil* is a small and irregular pupil that accommodates to near vision but has a reduced or absent light reflex (Table 12.1). It was a well known sign of neurosyphilis but is very uncommon in clinical practice nowadays.

Table 12.1 Characteristics of main pupillary disorders

Disorder/site	Neurological findings	Main Causes
Optic neuritis (optic nerve, afferent)	**pupils dilated,** (afferent pupil defect)	inflammatory, infections, nutritional (vit B def), konzo, TAN* toxic (alcohol, drugs)
Third nerve palsy (parasympathetic, efferent)		
compression	**pupil dilated,** (efferent pupil defect) ptosis (partial or full), eye in down and out position, paralysis of adduction & up/down movements	↑ICP, SOL, aneurysm, cavernous sinus thrombosis
non compression	**pupil not dilated,** otherwise the same as in **compressive lesions**	diabetes, meningitis
Horner's syndrome (sympathetic fibres)	**ptosis** (mild), **miosis** (pupil < other pupil), **enopthalmos** (eye less protruding), **loss of sweating** (may be absent)	cluster headache, apical lung tumours, cervical cord/brain stem lesions, dissecting aneurysms of carotid arteries
Holmes-Adie pupil (iris)	pupil(s) dilated, impaired to light (reacts slowly to near light)	variant of normal, autoimmune
Argyll-Robertson pupil (frontal lobe)	**both pupils small & irregular,** accommodate but no reaction to light	syphilis & diabetes

* tropical ataxic neuropathy

Key points

· pupillary disorders can arise from disorders of the eye, optic, parasympathetic & sympathetic nerves
· commonly found in association with disorders of eyelid (Horner's) and eye movements (3rd N. palsy)
· afferent disorders (optic nerve) are mainly caused by inflammation & toxicity
· efferent disorder (parasympathic) is mainly caused by pressure from the outside on the 3rd nerve
· Horner's syndrome is caused by local compression along the sympathetic nerve pathway

VISUAL ACUITY (VA)

VA is tested using a Snellen chart and the result is expressed as a fraction; the numerator being the distance between the chart and the patient (usually 6 metres depending on the size of the chart) divided by the denominator which is the smallest full line of letters identified correctly by the patient (Chapter 1). 6/6 is normal vision whereas 6/60 represents poor VA, meaning the patient can only read the largest letter on the chart. If the largest letter cannot be read from a distance of 6 metres, then the chart should be brought closer to the patient and VA rechecked. If this still fails, then the patient's ability to correctly count fingers, identify hand movements or perceive light should be checked in each eye respectively. Remember to check patients VA wearing glasses (if the patient uses them) and recheck decreased VA with a pin hole to exclude cataracts and refractive errors as a likely cause. Illustrative charts are available for illiterate patients and hand held reading charts can be used to formally test near vision. Identifying the various sizes of letters from a local newspaper can suffice for a general impression of VA. The main causes of decreased VA are ocular. These include refractive errors in the lens, cataracts and retinal diseases, particularly of the macula. The main neurological causes are disorders affecting the *optic nerve*.

Key points

· first ask if the patient can see, using both eyes or with glasses
· test VA in each eye separately using a Snellen chart or a hand held chart or a newspaper
· if pt is still unable to read large letters check VA by counting fingers, hand movements & light perception
· commonest causes of decreased VA are refractive lens errors & cataracts
· most frequent neurological cause of decreased VA is optic neuropathy

Colour vision

Colour vision is not routinely tested but can be tested using a set of *Ishihara colour plates*. These consist of a series of plates of coloured dots arranged so that persons with normal colour vision can see and identify correctly, a hidden set of numbers or trails arranged in different colours on each plate of dots. The patient must be able to read the first (control) plate before proceeding and each eye should be tested separately. Defective colour vision may be inherited and is a feature of diseases involving the optic nerve in particular optic neuritis.

VISUAL FIELDS

Patient's visual fields are tested by confrontation. The confrontation method is useful for detecting large visual field defects in the visual pathway. In order to interpret and localize the main findings correctly it is important to remember the following three points. The *nasal side of each eye* picks up the *opposite* or *temporal half* of the visual field whilst *the temporal side of the eye* picks up the *opposite* or *nasal half* of the visual field (Fig. 12.3). The optic nerve fibres serving *the nasal sides* of the retina *decussate* to the *opposite side* at the level of the *optic chiasm* (Fig. 12.3). Finally by convention the patient's visual fields are always *described* and *illustrated* from the *patient's own perspective i.e. as if the patient were looking outwards* (Fig. 12.4). The main visual defects, their sites of origin and causes are outlined below (Table 12.2).

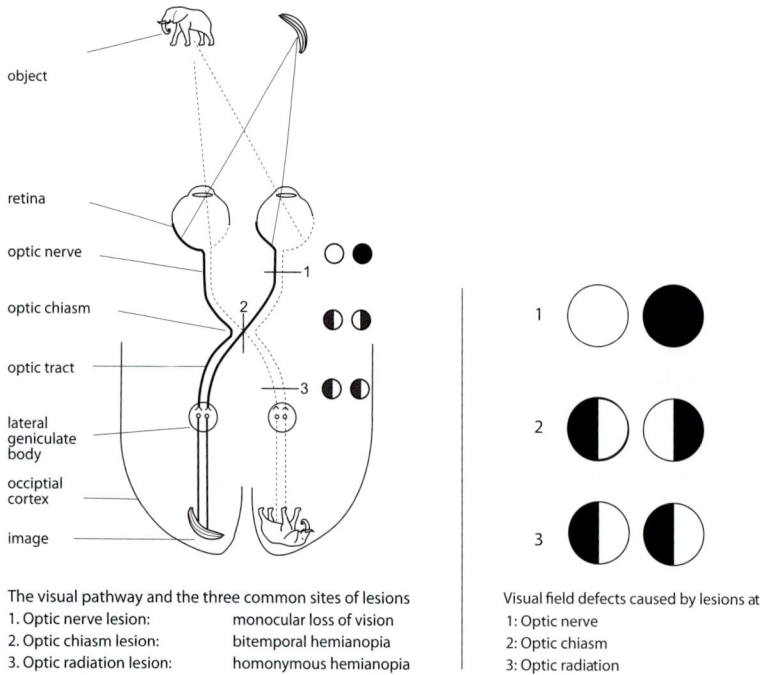

object

retina

optic nerve

optic chiasm

optic tract

lateral geniculate body

occipital cortex

image

The visual pathway and the three common sites of lesions
1. Optic nerve lesion: monocular loss of vision
2. Optic chiasm lesion: bitemporal hemianopia
3. Optic radiation lesion: homonymous hemianopia

Visual field defects caused by lesions at
1: Optic nerve
2: Optic chiasm
3: Optic radiation

Figure 12.3 & 4 The three most common sites of visual field defects

Table 12.2 Visual field defects, sites & causes

Field defect	Site	Main causes
1. monocular	optic nerve	neuritis, vasculitis, **compressive:** *aneurysm, meningioma*
2. bitemporal hemianopia	optic chiasm	pituitary adenoma, craniopharyngioma
3. homonymous hemianopia	optic tract/occipital lobe	stroke, SOL, tumour

Key points

- check for visual field defects in both eyes by confrontation
- if defect is suspected, then test each eye individually
- define the limits or extent of any field defect found
- main sites of origin of visual field defects are optic nerve, chiasm & optic tract/radiation
- most common defect is homonymous hemianopia secondary to a stroke/SOL

FUNDOSCOPY

The technique and details of fundoscopy are described in chapter 1. In summary, it is important to look at and inspect the optic disc, blood vessels and retinal background. An example of a normal fundus is shown in fig 12.5. Disorders affecting the optic nerves may result in swelling of the optic disc, called *papilloedema* or wasting of the optic nerve called *optic atrophy*. Both of these disorders can be easily seen and identified by fundoscopy and are illustrated below (Figs 12.5 & 6). Examples of retinopathy in hypertension and diabetes are included for comparison (Fig 12.7).

Papilloedema

Papilloedema is swelling of the optic disc sometimes with surrounding retinal haemorrhages and exudates. It is nearly always caused by raised intracranial pressure but it may also be due to inflammation of the optic nerves when it is termed *optic neuritis* or *papillitis*. Papilloedema is nearly always bilateral and occurs mostly without visual symptoms. On examination VA is typically normal but the blind spot may be enlarged and the peripheral visual fields constricted. Fundoscopy confirms features of papilloedema, a swollen and sometimes haemorrhagic disc (Fig. 12.5). If the papilloedema is long standing, then VA is lost due to increased pressure around the optic nerve and the optic disc becomes atrophied and pale. The main cause of papilloedema in Africa is raised intracranial pressure secondary to either infections, (cryptococcal and TB meningitis), space occupying lesions (SOL) or malignant hypertension (Table 12.3).

Optic neuritis

Optic neuritis is inflammation of the optic nerve or nerve head. It is usually bilateral but may occasionally be unilateral. It presents with loss of vision and occasionally a dull ache behind the eyes. On examination, VA is decreased or lost and there may be afferent pupil defects, if both eyes are involved. Fundoscopy may show *papilloedema* in the acute stage; however the accompanying loss of VA suggests optic neuritis rather than papilloedema as the true cause. In long standing cases there is *optic atrophy* (Fig. 12.6). The main disorders causing optic neuritis are inflammatory, toxic, nutritional and infections (Table 12.4).

Fundoscopy findings in papilloedema

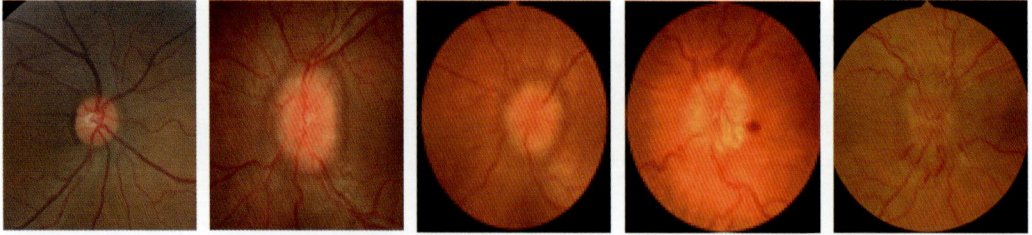

Normal fundus   Loss of optic cup, disc swelling, indistinct & elevated disc margins, haemorrhages
& exudates around the disc

Fundoscopy findings in chronic papilloedema

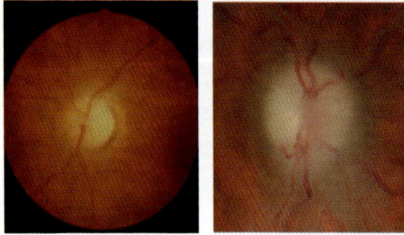

Pallor, loss of optic cup & disc swelling

Figure 12.5 Fundoscopy findings in papilloedema

Table 12.3 Main causes of papilloedema

Disorder	Disease
raised intracranial pressure	cryptococcus/TB, malignant hypertension, SOL
optic nerve lesions	tumours, leukaemia, Drusen
inflammatory	Devic's disease

Optic atrophy

Optic atrophy can be caused by any chronic optic nerve disease process (Table 12.4). The nerve which was swollen acutely in inflammatory optic neuritis and in cases of long standing papilloedema later when chronic becomes *pale* and *atrophic*. Optic atrophy is characterized clinically by a loss of visual acuity coupled with a clearly visible pale/white optic disc with clear margins on fundoscopy (Fig 12.6). The treatment is directed at the underlying disorder. It is important to exclude chronic glaucoma which may present with optic atrophy and painless loss of vision, however it is usually monocular.

Table 12.4 Main causes of optic atrophy

Disorder	Disease
chronic raised intracranial pressure	any cause
post infectious	TB, syphilis, viral
post inflammatory	Devic's disease, autoimmune disorders
toxic	alcohol, methanol, isoniazid, ethambutol, quinine
nutritional	Konzo, TAN*, Vitamin B deficiency
vascular	ischaemia
hereditary	Leber's optic neuropathy

* tropical ataxic neuropathy

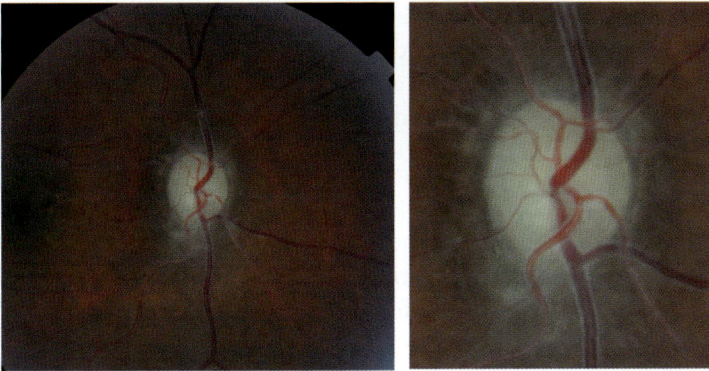

Pale white & atrophic optic disc

Figure 12.6 Fundoscopy findings in optic atrophy

Hypertension

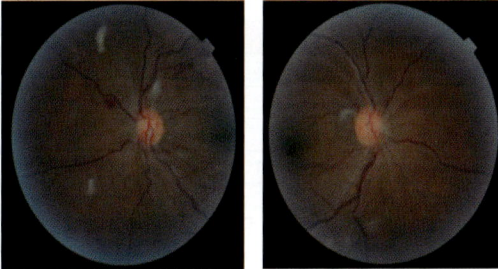

Diabetes

Haemorrhages & cotton wool exudates

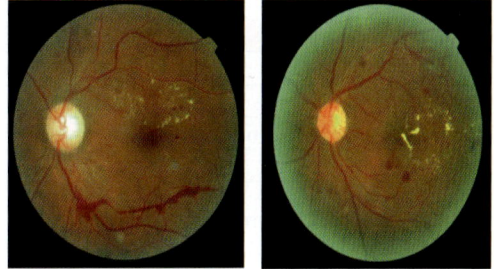

Haemorrhages, perimacular exudates
& new vessel formation

Figure 12.7 Fundoscopy findings in hypertension and diabetes

Key points

· is essential to be able to use the ophthalmoscope
· main disorders are papilloedema & optic atrophy
· in papilloedema the patient sees well but the doctor can't see the disc well
· in optic neuritis the patient can't see well but the doctor can see the disc well
· it is important to be able to distinguish the other main causes of retinopathy

OCULOMOTOR, TROCHLEAR AND ABDUCENS: EYE MOVEMENTS

Disorders affecting eye movements are common. The third, fourth and sixth nerves working together are responsible for normal eye movements. A lesion in any one of these nerves results in a loss of movement in the direction of action of the paralyzed muscles and double vision (diplopia), which is most marked when looking in the direction of action of the paralysed muscles. Eye movements are controlled by two mechanisms: *tracking* and by *voluntary saccades (jumps)*. Tracking or pursuit occurs when we look at and follow a moving object without thinking. This smooth action is controlled automatically in the occipital lobe and brain stem where all eye movements are joined up together into what are termed *conjugate eye* movements. Tracking is tested by asking the patient to follow your finger moving in both vertical and horizontal planes just as you would do when testing for normal eye movements (Chapter 1).

Observe carefully for any impairment, jerkiness (nystagmus) or loss of eye movement (paralysis) in one or more directions and enquire if there is any double vision. *Voluntary saccadic eye movements* originate in the frontal lobe and are tested by asking the patient to look at or fixate between two alternating targets e.g. right fist to left index finger and vice versa. This is an uncommon source of disordered eye movements.

Diplopia

Diplopia or double vision can be either binocular or monocular in origin. Monocular diplopia is distinctly uncommon and is nearly always optical in origin. The majority of *diplopia* occurs when the eyes fail to look together in the same direction and the resulting images no longer correspond with each other. This imbalance between the eyes may occur as a result of disorders at different sites. These sites are at the level of the brain stem, the individual 3rd 4th or 6th cranial nerves, the neuromuscular junction, and the eye muscles. Disorders affecting the individual cranial nerves account for most cases and are the most common cause of diplopia (Table 12.5).

Table 12.5 Main sites & causes of diplopia

Sites	Causes
3rd, 4th & 6th nerves	↑ICP, vascular, trauma, infections, diabetes
brain stem	stroke, inflammation, SOL
neuromuscular junction	myasthenia gravis
muscle	myopathy (thyroid disorders, hereditary)

With disorders affecting individual cranial nerves the double vision is nearly always described by the patient as sudden in onset. The separation of images is described as lying either side by side in the horizontal plane or on top of each other in the vertical plane. In most patients presenting with double vision, the muscle site of origin becomes apparent whilst observing the patient's eyes either at rest or during normal eye movements. If the origin is not readily apparent, then it is necessary to find out the direction in which the diplopia is greatest and in which plane the images are maximally separated. In general the double vision is always maximal in the direction of action of the paralyzed muscle. The false image is always the outermost image, and arises from the affected eye. In order to test for this, each of the patient's eyes is covered in turn and the eye from which the outer image disappears is noted and this is the affected eye. Horizontal diplopia (i.e. images side by side) is due to weakness of the medial rectus (3rd CN) or the lateral rectus (6th CN) and vertical or oblique diplopia (i.e. the images on top/side) is due to weakness of other muscles (3rd or 4th CNs).

Third nerve palsy

In a complete *3rd nerve palsy,* there is full ptosis and the eye (when it is uncovered), is seen to lie in the down and out position as a result of the unopposed action of the 4th and 6th CNs (Fig. 12.8). On attempting to test for normal eye movements, there is paralysis of adduction and up and down movements on the affected side (Figs. 12.8-9). If the parasympathetic fibres which lie on the outside of the 3rd CN (the efferent limb of the light reflex) are compressed, then the pupil on that side is dilated and fixed (non responsive to light). This is frequently termed surgical *3rd nerve palsy* because it indicates mechanical compression from outside the nerve which may require urgent surgical attention. A common cause of painful unilateral 3rd nerve palsy is an aneurysm arising on the posterior communicating artery on the Circle of Willis. If the pupil is spared or is not dilated then this is often termed a medical *3rd nerve palsy* and these may resolve spontaneously over the next 3-4 months. The most common causes of third nerve palsy are tentorial herniation secondary to raised intracranial pressure, aneurysms, DM and infections. Less common causes include granuloma (Tolosa Hunt syndrome) and lesions in the cavernous sinus.

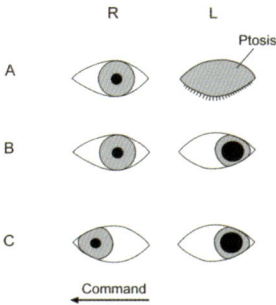

Left occulomotor palsy (compressive type)

A Ptosis
B Pupillary dilatation (with the eyelid held open)
C Failure of adduction of the left eye on looking towards the right

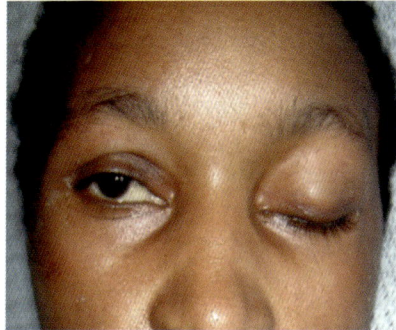

Figure 12.8 Oculomotor palsy (left)

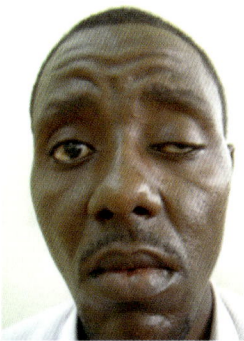

Ptosis & left eye down & out
(looking ahead)

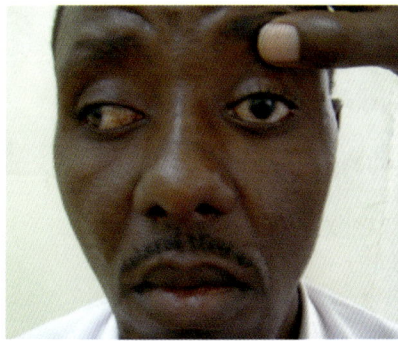

Failure of adduction left eye
(looking right)

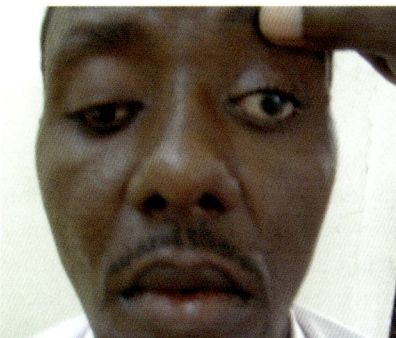

Failure of down gaze left eye
(looking down)

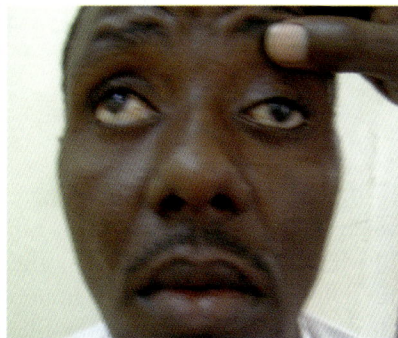

Failure of up gaze left eye
(looking up)

Figure 12.9 Oculomotor palsy (left)

Fourth nerve palsy

In *4ᵗʰ nerve palsy*, there is failure to depress the adducted eye. The diplopia is most noticeable by the patient on walking down steps or stairs and he tries to compensate by tilting the head away from the paralysed eye. Isolated 4ᵗʰ nerve palsies are uncommon but do occur in association with DM, head trauma and cavernous sinus lesions. Uncomplicated 4ᵗʰ nerve palsies usually resolve with time.

Sixth nerve palsy

In *6ᵗʰ nerve palsy*, the patient is unable to abduct the affected eye and has diplopia. The diplopia is most noticeable by looking horizontally in the direction of action of the paralysed muscle (Fig. 12.10). The eye at rest is held in the adducted position because of unopposed action of the medial rectus (Fig. 12.10). It is a common cranial nerve palsy occurring in diabetes and hypertension and usually resolves spontaneously. However it may also be a false localizing sign in raised intracranial pressure, because during its long intracranial course it is vulnerable to increased pressure as it passes over the sphenoid ridge.

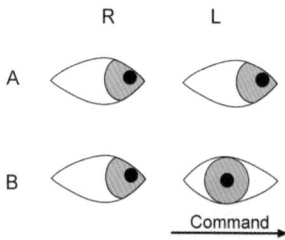

Left sixth nerve palsy
A Normal conjugate eye movement to the left
B Failure of abduction of left eye on looking to the left

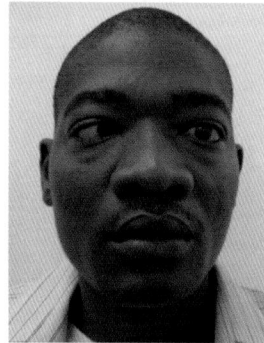

Figure 12.10 Sixth nerve palsy (left sided)

Key points

- diplopia arises from either CN disorders or diseases of neuromuscular junction or muscle
- most common cause are CN disorders, 3rd 4th & 6th
- double vision is maximal in the direction of gaze of the paralysed muscle
- false image is always the outer one
- false image arises in the affected eye

SQUINT

A squint occurs when the visual axes of both eyes are no longer together. It is a common disorder in children when it is usually termed a *non paralytic squint* (NPS). This is in contrast to *paralytic squint* (PS) which mostly affects adults. The main causes of squint in children are refractive lens problems. Diplopia does not occur in non paralytic squint whereas it does occur in paralytic squint. This is because in children the brain gets accustomed over years to false image and suppresses it. If the non paralytic squint continues beyond the age of 6 years, then a permanent lazy eye develops with poor or no vision in that eye.

The diagnostic feature of a *non paralytic squint* is that movements are full in each eye when tested separately. This is in contrast to *paralytic squint* where movement in the affected eye is usually not full. This can be easily demonstrated by testing movements in each eye individually in turn, whilst at the same time covering the other eye. This is termed *the cover test*. In *non paralytic squint* when conjugate eye movements are tested together, a weakness in one or both eyes may become apparent. To test for *non paralytic squint* first ask the patient to look with both eyes at your right eye and cover his left eye. Then uncover his left eye and cover his right eye and look to see if his left eye has to correct in order to look back at your right eye. Repeat the same sequence covering the right eye. The test is positive when the squinting eye immediately moves to fixate when attempting to look at an object, in this case your right eye. This is the basis for correction of a non paralytic squint in childhood. This is achieved by the wearing of a patch over the good eye thereby forcing the bad eye to work fully. If wearing a patch over the good eye fails then corrective surgery may be necessary. Squints are usually classified as non paralytic or paralytic. They may also be classified as congenital or acquired, as affecting one eye or both eyes and as convergent or divergent.

Key points

- NPS is common in children whereas PS is common in adults
- in NPS full movement is preserved in each eye when examined individually
- in NPS the cover test reveals weakness in one or both eyes
- correction of NPS should take place before 6 yrs of age
- treatment includes wearing a patch over the good eye +/- corrective surgery

NYSTAGMUS

Nystagmus is an abnormal rhythmic oscillatory or to and fro movement of the eyes. Characteristically it has a slow drift in one direction with a fast corrective phase in the other direction. By convention, nystagmus is described in the direction of the fast phase. Disorders causing nystagmus are classified as *peripheral* (arising from the vestibular system/nerve), *central* (arising from the brain stem/cerebellum) and *ocular* (arising from the eye, retina/lens). In order to check for the presence of nystagmus, you must first inspect the patient's eyes in the at rest or primary position with the eyes looking ahead and then ask the patient to follow your finger with both eyes, moving vertically and horizontally as if testing for normal eye movements. Be careful not to move the eyes too far laterally (<30 degrees from midline), otherwise a few beats of non sustained physiological nystagmus can occur normally. Note if any nystagmus occurs and whether it is symmetrical or jerky and the direction of the fast phase e.g. horizontal, vertical or rotary and the position of the eyes when the nystagmus occurs and is most marked.

The characteristics of the nystagmus help to localize its site of origin. If it is symmetrical with movements of the same speed in both directions this is called *pendular nystagmus*. Pendular nystagmus is nearly always *ocular* in origin and is seen in persons with longstanding blindness or impaired vision; a major cause is congenital cataracts. If the nystagmus is characterized by a slow phase in one direction followed by a fast corrective phase in the opposite direction this is called *jerk nystagmus*. This is the most common type and is seen in both peripheral and central disorders. Jerk nystagmus occurs only on attempted gaze holding in any direction (up, down, left or right) and is not present in the primary position looking straight ahead. The fast phase determines the direction of the nystagmus i.e. *upbeat or downbeat nystagmus.* Jerk nystagmus is commonly seen in cerebellar disease. The direction of the fast phase is towards the lesion in central disorders of the brain stem and cerebellum, and away from the lesion in peripheral disorders in the vestibular system. The commonest causes of jerk symmetrical horizontal nystagmus with the quick phase in the direction of gaze are drugs or medications e.g. phenytoin and alcohol. *Rotary nystagmus* can occur in both peripheral and central disorders, though mainly in disorders of the peripheral vestibular system. The main distinguishing clinical features between peripheral and central nystagmus are presented below in Table 12.6.

Table 12.6 Key clinical features distinguishing peripheral and central nystagmus

Clinical features	Peripheral (vestibular nerve & labyrinth)	Central (brain stem and cerebellum)
main causes	neuronitis, BPPV* Ménière's disease	vascular, drugs, alcohol, structural
duration of illness	short (3-6 weeks)	long (often years)
duration of nystagmus	<60 secs	continuous
direction	away from lesion, horizontal, unilateral	towards lesion, multidirectional
latency/vertigo/vomiting/worsened by position and fatigues	yes	no
associated neurological signs	no	yes

* benign paroxysmal positional vertigo

Key points

· decide whether nystagmus is present
· describe the type, direction & position it occurs maximally
· determine whether it is peripheral or central
· persistent nystagmus suggests a central origin
· vertigo, vomiting & worsening with change in position suggests a peripheral origin

TRIGEMINAL NERVE

The *fifth nerve* has three branches, *ophthalmic* V1, *maxillary* V2 *and mandibular* V3. It is a mixed motor and sensory nerve (Chapter 1). Power is tested by measuring resistance to jaw opening, closure and side to side movement. *Motor involvement* is rare but occurs clinically in myasthenia gravis and muscular dystrophy (myotonic and fascioscapular). To test sensation touch the face lightly with cotton wool separately in all three divisions (V1-V3) comparing sides. Only very occasionally is it necessary to test for pain and temperature on the face. Disorders affecting the fifth nerve can arise either centrally in the brainstem or peripherally involving the whole nerve or more commonly in one of its main branches. Causes of central brain stem disorders include stroke and mass lesions. In healthy persons the *jaw jerk* is either minimally present or absent. The jaw jerk may be increased in upper motor neurone disorders affecting the upper brain stem and above e.g. motor neurone disease (MND) and stroke. Disorders affecting the peripheral nerve are mostly caused by *herpes zoster* (Fig. 12.11), trigeminal neuralgia and rarely compression by tumours compressing the nerve e.g. acoustic neuroma. The frequency of herpes zoster is increased in HIV disease (Chapter 8). An absent *corneal reflex* in the presence of normal facial movements (7th CN) is a sign of *sensory* 5th CN (V1) *neuropathy.* Patients with trigeminal neuropathies present mostly with pain or impairment or loss of facial sensation, typically without any loss of power of mastication. Trigeminal neuralgia is the most common clinical disorder affecting the 5th CN or its branches (Chapter 15).

Key points

- sensory involvement is more common than motor in 5th CN neuropathy
- jaw jerk is increased in some UMN lesions
- absent corneal reflex indicates a lesion in either the 5th or the 7th CN
- herpes zoster is the commonest infectious cause of trigeminal neuropathy

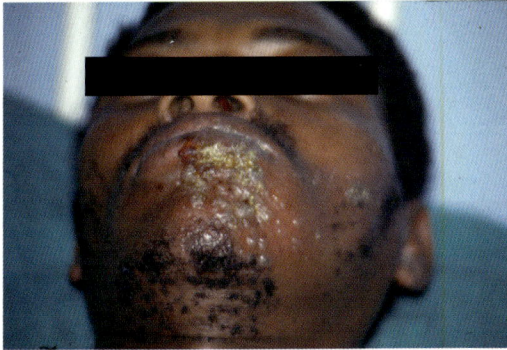

Figure 12.11 Herpes zoster in HIV. Vesicular eruption in V3 division of trigeminal nerve (left).

FACIAL NERVE

Facial nerve paralysis is one of the most common cranial nerve disorders. The examination has already been outlined in chapter 1. In brief first inspect the face for asymmetry, loss of normal wrinkling, eye closure, nasolabial fold and decreased facial movement. To demonstrate the facial nerve ask patient to smile (show teeth), close eyes tightly and look up. Facial nerve paralysis may either be central (upper motor neurone) in origin as occurs in *stroke* or peripheral (lower motor neurone) in origin as occurs in *Bell's palsy*. Peripheral facial nerve disorders arise mainly from inflammation, infiltration or compression of the nerve along its course. The main inflammatory causes are Bell's palsy and infections including herpes zoster i.e. Ramsay-Hunt syndrome. The main infiltrative and compression causes include acoustic neuroma, meningioma and diseases affecting the skull base or parotid gland.

BELL'S PALSY

Bell's palsy is the most common disorder of the facial nerve. It is an acute lower motor neurone disorder (LMNL) which is associated with viral infection and facial nerve swelling within the facial canal although its precise cause is not known. It is associated with asymptomatic HIV infection (Chapter 8). It presents as a painless loss of power on one side of the face over 24 hours; there may be an associated ache around the ear at the start which typically clears. The patient becomes very aware of his facial appearance and may have difficulties smiling, speaking or initiating swallowing and closing the eye on the affected side (Fig. 12.12). It affects all the muscles on one side of the face (Fig. 12.13) which distinguishes it from central causes which affect only the lower half of the face. It may occasionally occur bilaterally when the correct diagnosis can be easily missed (Fig. 12.14) unless it is tested. The main differences between a lower and upper motor neurone lesion are presented in Table 12.7. The weakness usually clears fully without any treatment in the majority >90% of patients within 6 to 12 weeks. However if at onset the paralysis is complete and there is involvement of taste and hearing (increased) then the outlook for a full recovery is worse.

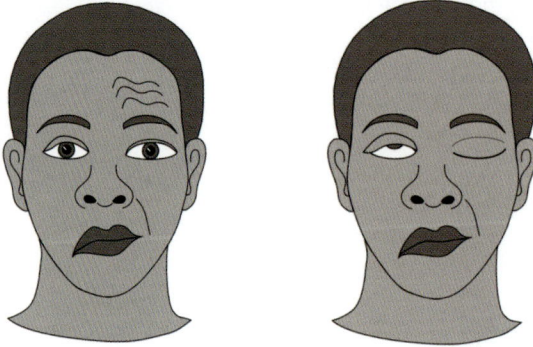

Facial nerve palsy right lower motor neurone lesion

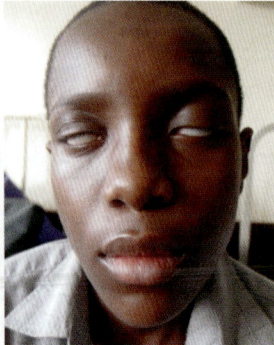

Loss of wrinkling of forehead
Loss of nasolabial fold
Drooping of the mouth

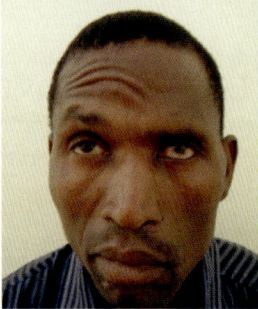

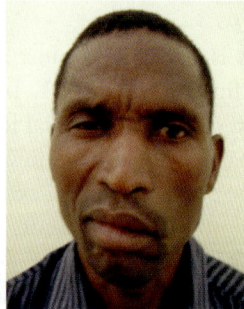

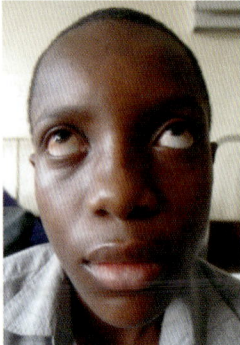

Facial nerve palsy, right sided
(lower motor neurone lesion)
(during eye closure)
Failure to close the eye
Loss of nasolabial fold
Drooping of the mouth.

Figure 12.12 Lower motor neurone facial nerve palsy (right sided)

Loss of wrinkling   **Loss of eye closure**   **Loss of nasolabial fold & drooping mouth**

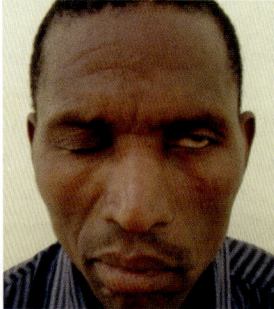

Figure 12.13 Lower motor neurone facial nerve palsy (left sided)

Loss of wrinkling   **Loss of eye closure**   **Loss of smiling**

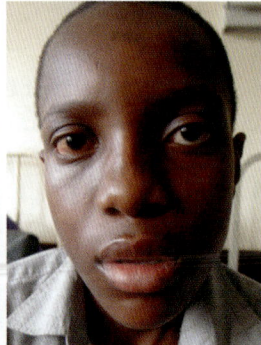

Figure 12.14 Lower motor neurone facial nerve palsies (bilateral)

Table 12.7 Differences between lower and upper motor neurone facial nerve palsy

Main clinical features	Lower motor neurone lesion	Upper motor neurone lesion
Main Cause	Bell's palsy	stroke
Clinical findings*		
forehead wrinkling	absent	spared
eye closure	absent	partially spared
movement lower face	absent	absent/decreased
Outcome	90% recover fully	variable

* may only be partially present in incomplete lesions

Management

If the patient is seen within 48 to 72 hours of onset then a short course of steroids and antiviral drugs may help to improve outcome. This includes prednisolone 60 mg/po/daily and aciclovir 400 mg/po/tds for a total of 7 days. Prevention of corneal damage during recovery is important. The use of artificial tears and application of a cover patch particularly overnight may be sufficient to prevent the cornea from being damaged before recovery. Glasses with side protection and eye covers may help during the day. Severe cases may need a temporary tarsorrhaphy. Physiotherapy with facial exercises may be helpful to the patient.

Key points

- Bell's palsy is the most common cause of LMN facial nerve paralysis
- signs are drooping of the corner of the mouth, loss of eye closure & absence of wrinkling
- loss of eye closure and wrinkling distinguish it from an UMN facial nerve lesion
- frequency of Bell's palsy is increased in HIV infection & patients should have a screening HIV test
- recovery occurs in most patients without treatment

ACOUSTIC NERVE

The eight nerve or acoustic has two divisions: *cochlear* and *vestibular*. Disorders affecting the *cochlear* division result in difficulties with *hearing* whereas disorders affecting the *vestibular* division result in difficulties with *balance*. The main symptoms of the cochlear division are deafness and tinnitus and the vestibular division are vertigo and loss of balance.

HEARING

Details concerning the examination of the cochlear division of the acoustic nerve are presented in chapter 1. Bedside tests include asking and checking the patient's ability to hear by whispering about 1 metre way when the other ear is blocked. If hearing is found to be reduced then do the *Rinne* and *Weber* tests. In the Rinne test the beating tuning fork is held first on the mastoid (bone conduction, BC) and then placed just outside the ear (air conduction, AC). In the Weber test the beating tuning fork is placed on the vertex of the head. The possible results of the tuning fork tests are summarized in Table 12.8. The main causes of *deafness* alone are wax in the outer ear, otitis media in the middle ear, presbycusis in the cochlea and diseases affecting the cochlear nerve in the inner ear. Neurological causes of hearing loss include nerve deafness after meningitis, ototoxic drugs e.g. quinine and streptomycin and rare causes such an acoustic neuroma. Ménière's disease is the most common cause of combined deafness and vestibular dysfunction.

Table 12.8 Possible results of tuning fork tests in deafness

	Rinne (deaf ear)	Weber
Conductive deafness	BC > AC	best in the deaf ear
Sensorineural deafness	AC > BC	best in the non deaf ear

VERTIGO/DIZZINESS

Vertigo is an illusion of a sensation of giddiness or spinning during which the patient or more commonly the world outside the patient appears to move. Dizziness is commonly used to describe the unsteady feeling or sensation of vertigo and care must be taken to distinguish it from true vertigo. Vertigo can be caused by either peripheral or central disorders. Diseases affecting the *peripheral vestibular nerve* causing vertigo include viral infections causing acute labyrinthitis, benign paroxysmal positional vertigo (BPPV) and drugs e.g. quinine and streptomycin. *Centrally,* the main cause of *vestibular dysfunction* is ischaemic or vascular. Vertigo of vestibular origin is characteristically paroxysmal and brought on or aggravated by a change in position. This in contrast to vertigo of central origin which is more continuous and is not usually provoked by change in position. The Hallpike's test (see below) can help to differentiate and distinguish between these two sites. The duration of symptoms depends on the cause and may last from weeks in labyrinthitis to less than a minute in BPPV. Drugs commonly used in the treatment of acute vertigo include betahistine 16 mg/po/tds or prochlorperazine 5 mg/po/tds.

Ménière's disease

This is a disease characterized by intermittent attacks of severe vertigo, tinnitus and deafness. The deafness eventually becomes permanent and the vertigo eventually ceases after years. Management is by decreasing salt intake, thiazide diuretic, and using an antihistamine e.g. betahistine, cinnarizine, cyclizine or prochloperazine.

BENIGN PAROXYSMAL POSITIONAL VERTIGO (BPPV)

BPPV is a benign condition characterized by transient vertigo brought on by head movements. The acute vertigo lasts less than a minute but symptoms may persist for weeks or months and may recur. There may be associated nausea and vomiting in severe persistent attacks. It arises mainly from dislocation of otoliths or debris blocking the posterior semicircular canals. Characteristically, a change of head position particularly rolling over in bed or rising suddenly from the lying or seated position provokes an attack. The diagnosis may be confirmed by bedside techniques including *Hallpike's test. Epley's manoeuvre* can help to disperse the debris.

Hallpike's test

This is a bedside test of vestibular function which is used in patients suspected as having positional vertigo. The test begins with the patient seated upright on the examining couch and is positioned so that when he lies flat his head and neck will extend beyond the examining couch unsupported. Whilst seated the patient is first instructed to turn the head to one side with the eyes looking in the same direction as the head. Whilst maintaining that head position the patient is reassured and instructed to lie flat. The head should now lie about 30 degrees below the horizontal and now be supported by the examiner's hands. In normal persons there is no nystagmus or vertigo. In vestibular disorders nystagmus and vertigo starts after a delay of a few seconds, and then fatigues and resolves after a number of seconds. This is a positive *Hallpike's test*. After sitting upright the test may be repeated on the other side. In central or brain stem disorders there is usually no delay in the onset of symptoms and signs which are not worsened by change in position and any nystagmus which is present persists.

Epley's manoeuvre

This involves lying down sideways in the position in which the Hallpike test brings on the vertigo and then rolling over changing sides and remaining sideways there until symptoms subside followed by sitting upright for 30 seconds and then back to the first position. This manoeuvre should be repeated at least 3-4 times daily until symptoms persistently resolve.

Key points

- disorders of the vestibular division of the 8th CN result in difficulties in balance
- symptoms include dizziness, vertigo, tinnitus, nausea, vomiting & ataxia
- main causes are BPPV, vestibular neuronitis & Ménière's disease
- nystagmus provoked by change in position is characteristic of vestibular origin
- relief with antiemetics, antihistamines & positional manoeuvres

ACCESSORY NERVE

This nerve supplies the *sternomastoid* and *the trapezius muscles* and is responsible for turning and flexing the head and shrugging the shoulders. The clinical examination is done by inspection of the main neck and shoulder muscles for any obvious wasting, fasciculations or hypertrophy and then by opposing each of the main movements, in turn resisting elevation of the shoulders and turning the head (Chapter 1). The main neurological disorders affecting these movements are diseases of muscle and neuromuscular junction including myopathies, polymyositis, dystrophies and myasthenia gravis (Chapter 13). Management is by treatment of the underlying disorder.

GLOSSOPHARYNGEAL, VAGUS AND HYPOGLOSSAL NERVES

These cranial nerves supply the mouth, throat and tongue for the main functions of speech and swallowing. The *glossopharyngeal* is sensory to the posterior one third of tongue and the pharynx and middle ear whereas the *vagus* is motor to the muscles of the palate, pharynx and larynx. Their joint function is tested by inspecting the uvula at rest, getting the patient to say "Aah" and testing the gag reflex. The *hypoglossal* nerve is motor to the muscles of the tongue and is examined by inspecting the tongue at rest, and on repeated protrusion in and out. If an abnormality is still suspected the movements and strength of the tongue can be further assessed by asking the patient to push his tongue into his inside cheek against your thumb outside opposing the movement. The pharynx and larynx can be assessed functionally by checking the patient's ability to generate a normal cough and swallow a cup of water normally. The larynx can be visualized by laryngoscope but this requires an ENT specialist.

The lower cranial nerves are commonly involved together in diseases and their joint impairment results in a significant loss of function in the mouth and bulbar area. If the site of the lesion is a lower motor neurone, then the disorder is termed a bulbar palsy and if the site of the lesion is an upper motor neurone, it is termed a pseudobulbar palsy. The main symptoms common to both types of disorders are difficulty speaking (dysarthria) and swallowing (dysphagia) which is frequently progressive depending on the aetiology. A lower motor neurone lesion results in wasting and fasciculation of the tongue and a reduced or absent gag reflex. There is deviation of the tongue to affected side if it's unilateral. An upper motor neurone lesion results in spasticity with a contracted immobile tongue and an increased gag reflex. The main neurological causes of a bulbar palsy are motor neurone disease (MND) and myasthenia gravis and of pseudobulbar palsy are stroke and MND. The main non neurological cause is local malignancy. Emotional lability is a feature in patients with a pseudobulbar palsy. Management is the treatment of the underlying disorder.

Key points

- disorders of the lower cranial nerves present with difficulties with speaking & swallowing
- they are classified as bulbar (LMNL) or a pseudo bulbar (UMNL)
- main neurological disorders causing these are stroke, MND & myasthenia gravis
- the differential diagnosis includes local malignancy

Selected references

Azonobi IR, Olatunji FO, Addo J. *Prevalence and pattern of strabismus in Ilorin*. West Afr J Med. 2009 Jul-Aug;28(4):253-6.

Bourne RR, Dolin PJ, Mtanda AT, Plant GT, Mohamed AA. *Epidemic optic neuropathy in primary school children in Dar es Salaam, Tanzania*. Br J Ophthalmol. 1998 Mar;82(3):232-4.

Bowman RJ, Wedner S, Bowman RF, Masanja H, Bunce C, Wood ML, et al. *Optic neuropathy endemic in secondary school children in Dar es Salaam, Tanzania*. Br J Ophthalmol. 2010 Feb;94(2):146-9.

Dalmar AA, Hodson KE, Plant GT. *Epidemic optic neuropathy is evident in the Somalian population*. J Neuroophthalmol. 2011 Jun;31(2):127-30.

Dolin PJ, Mohamed AA, Plant GT. *Epidemic of bilateral optic neuropathy in Dar es Salaam, Tanzania*. N Engl J Med. 1998 May 21;338(21):1547-8.

Fuller Geraint, *Neurological examination made easy*, Churchill Livingstone, 3rd edition 2004.

Ginsberg Lionel, *Neurology, Lecture Notes*, Blackwell Publishing 8th edition 2005.

Harrison Michael, Neurological Skills, *A guide to examination and management in Neurology*, Butterworth's 1st edition 1987.

Komolafe MA, Fatusi OA, Alatise OI, Komolafe EO, Amusa YB, Adeolu AA, et al. *The role of human immunodeficiency virus infection in infranuclear facial paralysis*. J Natl Med Assoc. 2009 Apr;101(4):361-6.

Odebode TO, Ologe FE. *Facial nerve palsy after head injury: Case incidence, causes, clinical profile and outcome*. J Trauma. 2006 Aug;61(2):388-91.

Omoti AE, Waziri-Erameh MJ. *Pattern of neuro-ophthalmic disorders in a tertiary eye centre in Nigeria*. Niger J Clin Pract. 2007 Jun;10(2):147-51.

Pokroy R, Modi G, Saffer D. *Optic neuritis in an urban black African community*. Eye (Lond). 2001 Aug;15(Pt 4):469-73.

Turner, Bahra, Cikurel, *Neurology, Crash Course*, Elsevier Mosby 2nd edition 2006.

Tinley C, Grötte R. *Comitant horizontal strabismus in South African black and mixed race children--a clinic-based study*. Ophthalmic Epidemiol. 2012 Apr;19(2):89-94

van Well GT, Paes BF, Terwee CB, Springer P, Roord JJ, Donald PR, et al. *Twenty years of pediatric tuberculous meningitis: a retrospective cohort study in the western cape of South Africa*. Pediatrics. 2009;123(1):e1-8.

PART II – NEUROLOGICAL DISORDERS

CHAPTER 13
MYOPATHIES AND MYASTHENIA GRAVIS

CONTENTS

CHAPTER 13

MYOPATHIES AND MYASTHENIA GRAVIS

Myopathies are classified as either inherited or acquired. The main inherited myopathies are muscular dystrophies and acquired myopathies are inflammatory and non inflammatory. The main disorder which affects the neuromuscular junction is myasthenia gravis (MG). The aim of this chapter is to review the clinical features and management of muscular dystrophy, polymyositis and MG. The student should aim to be able to recognize these main muscle disorders and manage a patient presenting with muscle weakness.

Clinical history

The defining symptom of disorders of muscle and neuromuscular junction is weakness. Muscle weakness in myopathy is usually proximal. Patients typically present with weakness or difficulty elevating their arms above the shoulders, getting out of chairs or rising from the lying position. Other symptoms may include muscle pain and tenderness, muscle cramps on exercise and dysphagia. The history should include age of onset, time course, pattern and distribution of weakness, fatigability and any relevant past, family and drug history. Muscular dystrophies tend to have their onset in childhood or teens and are usually recognizable clinically. Inflammatory myopathies present with proximal muscle weakness, frequently with muscle pain, tenderness and sometimes dysphagia. The diagnostic characteristic of myasthenia gravis is fatigable muscle weakness, worse after exercise and commonly affecting the extra ocular and bulbar muscles.

Physical Examination

The characteristic clinical finding in myopathies and MG is muscle weakness. The weakness affects mainly the trunk and proximal limb muscles, and may also affect the neck muscles and facial expression. Power distally may be maintained in early disease but is lost or decreased later on. Muscle wasting occurs in most myopathies, tone is typically decreased and reflexes are preserved but may be reduced or absent in advanced disease. There are no sensory signs. Patients with muscle disease often have a very characteristic myopathic or "waddling" gait due to hip girdle weakness. The pattern of muscle weakness may indicate the underlying disorder. Muscle psudohypertrophy confined to the calves in boys is diagnostic of dystrophy and contractures may occur in long standing disease. Weakness of the eye muscles suggests myasthenia gravis whereas weakness of the face muscles is more of a feature of facioscapulohumeral dystrophy and myotonic dystrophy. Weakness of the neck muscles is typical of myasthenia gravis and polymyositis. Proximal weakness in combination with a skin rash is characteristic of dermatomyositis.

Key features of myopathy/MG

- proximal weakness
- fatigability
- hypertrophy
- contractures
- myopathic gait

Investigations

Routine bloods tests should include FBC, ESR, HIV, glucose, creatinine, electrolytes, thyroid function tests and serum creatine kinase (CK). CK is the best indicator of muscle disease with very high levels in inflammatory muscle disease and in most dystrophies but can be normal in myotonic dystrophy (MD) and facioscapulohumeral dystrophy (FSHD). It is important to remember that CK may be modestly elevated after strenuous exercise, injections, and viral infections and occasionally in healthy African populations which may sometimes lead to unnecessary investigation. Molecular genetic testing is increasingly important in the diagnosis of inherited muscle disease. An ECG and echocardiogram are indicated in the dystrophies to screen for cardiomyopathy.

Electromyography (EMG)

This measures the electrical activity in a motor unit. In myopathies there is a decrease in the duration and amplitude of motor unit potentials with spontaneous fibrillations. There are also characteristic EMG findings in MG and in myotonic dystrophy.

Muscle biopsy

The biopsy site should be from moderately affected muscle and away from injection sites. This may show evidence of inflammation and dystrophic changes. Immunostaining is also helpful depending on the diagnosis.

Key points

- muscle disorders may be inherited (dystrophies) or acquired (polymyositis)
- proximal weakness is the key clinical finding in muscle disorders
- pattern of weakness points to the underlying disease
- marked elevation in CK is the best lab indicator of muscle disease

INHERITED MYOPATHIES

The main inherited myopathies are the dystrophies, myotonic dystrophy (MD), Duchenne (DMD), Becker (BMD), limb girdle (LGMD) and facioscapulohumeral (FSHD). The main clinical features and genetics are presented below (Table 13.1). DMD and BMD are both X-linked inherited and occur almost exclusively in males. Disease is caused by mutations of the X-linked dystrophin gene which leads to the complete absence of the muscle protein dystrophin in DMD or abnormal dystrophin in BMD. This affects both skeletal and cardiac muscle. The diagnosis of muscular dystrophy is usually based on clinical findings and a markedly elevated CK. A muscle biopsy can confirm the clinical diagnosis and genetic studies identify the causative mutation. Management includes genetic counselling.

Table 13.1 Characteristics of Muscular Dystrophies

Type	Genetics	Sex/age of onset	Clinical features
Myotonic	autosomal dominant	m = f,/birth to adult	proximal & distal limb weakness, facial weakness, myotonia, frontal balding, cataracts DM, cardiomyopathy
Duchenne	X-linked recessive	males/early childhood	proximal limb weakness, Gower's sign, calf pseudohypertrophy, cardiomyopathy
Becker	X-linked recessive	males/in teens or as adult	proximal limb weakness, slow progression, calf pseudohypertrophy, cramps, cardiomyopathy
Facioscapulo-humeral	autosomal dominant	m = f/in teens	facial weakness, winging of scapulae, proximal upper limb weakness, waddling gait, lumbar lordosis
Limb girdle	autosomal recessive autosomal dominant	m = f/in teens/young adult	proximal limb girdle weakness, cardiomyopathy (variable)

MYOTONIC DYSTROPHY

Myotonic dystrophy is an autosomal dominant multisystem disorder characterized by progressive proximal and distal muscle weakness, especially affecting the upper limbs. It gets its name from its characteristic of sustained muscle contraction or myotonia. It is the most common dystrophy with a prevalence of around 1/10,000 in high income countries. The frequency in Africa is not known and although isolated cases have been reported it is considered to be very uncommon in black populations there. It presents most commonly in adults of either sex but can present at any age.

Genetics

It is caused by an unstable expanded trinucleotide repeat (>50 CTG repeats) in the myotonin gene on chromosome 19q. There is a strong correlation between the number of repeats and the age of onset and thus severity of the disorder.

Clinical features

The clinical presentation varies from lethal disease at birth (congenital DM with CTG repeats above 1000) to very mild disease with late onset cataracts (CTG repeats 50-80). The classical or adult form (20-50 yrs; CTG repeats 200-500) presents with myotonia, frontal balding (even in women), bilateral ptosis, facial weakness, wasting and weakness of sternomastoids, proximal and distal weakness of mainly the upper limbs, cataracts, testicular atrophy, diabetes and sometimes cognitive impairment. Myotonia is persistence of muscle contraction, lasting several seconds if the muscle is actively used. It typically occurs during gripping or hand shaking when the affected person is unable to let go for the first few seconds. It is more pronounced during cold weather. Tapping affected muscles repeatedly with a tendon hammer demonstrates a sustained dimple and a typical muscle contraction. Classic myotonic discharges on EMG testing sounding like a dive bomber are diagnostic. The diagnosis can be confirmed by DNA testing.

Management

Management includes genetic counselling especially as the severe congenital form occurs in children of affected females with >100 repeats. Myotonia if disabling may be treated with phenytoin and also mexiletine if ECG QT interval is normal. There is an increased risk of sudden death and anaesthetic complications.

Key points

- MD is an autosomal dominant disorder confirmed by DNA testing
- uncommon in the black population in Africa
- C/Fs: ptosis, facial, sternomastoid &, limb weakness, cataracts, balding and DM
- characterised by sustained muscle contraction & inability to release grip
- increased risk of sudden death & anaesthetic complications
- management includes genetic counselling

DUCHENNE'S MUSCULAR DYSTROPHY

The incidence of DMD in high income countries is about 1 per 3,500 live births. There are few reports of DMD from Africa for comparison but a much lower prevalence of 1/250,000 was reported in one study in South Africa, suggesting that it is much more uncommon there.

Clinical features

DMD almost always presents in early childhood (1-5 yrs) usually presenting early with difficulty or a delay in walking and a characteristic toe walking gait. Other diagnostic features are calf hypertrophy and contractures. Patients may also demonstrate "Gower's sign" which is using the hands to climb up the legs whilst getting up from the squatting or lying position (Fig 13.2). The main complications are scoliosis, cardiomyopathy and immobility with nearly all patients becoming wheelchair bound by the end of the first decade. There is no long term effective drug treatment although the use of steroids is now established practice in some high income countries.

Prognosis

In high income countries most deaths used to occur before or in the early teenage years but now occur in late teens or early twenties. This improved survival is mainly due to intervention with assisted nocturnal ventilation and early management of complications.

BECKER'S MUSCULAR DYSTROPHY

The incidence of BMD in high income countries is around 1/35-40,000. There are few reports from Africa but a very much lower prevalence of <1/750,000 has been reported from South Africa. The range of symptoms is similar to DMD but it is much milder. It frequently has its onset during the first decades at around 10-11 years of age but many are mild and usually go unnoticed in childhood. They present mostly in teens or early adult life with mild limb girdle weakness, cramps and calf hypertrophy. Many are wheelchair bound by their late 20s. Cardiac involvement occurs in around 10% and shortens life expectancy.

Key points

- Duchenne presents with walking difficulties in boys in very early childhood
- most progress to wheelchair dependence by the start of second decade
- death usually occurs before or by early teens in Duchenne in Africa
- Becker is a much milder form affecting males in their early teens
- C/Fs: calf hypertrophy, contractures and Gower manoeuvre
- elevation of CK is a characteristic finding in all dystrophies

OTHER DYSTROPHIES

The other main muscular dystrophies include facioscapulohumeral dystrophy (FSHD)(Fig. 13.1), an autosomal dominant dystrophy caused by a complex genetic defect on chromosome 4q and limb girdle muscular dystrophy (LGMD)(Fig. 13.2). LGMD is genetically very heterogeneous: mostly autosomal recessive with at least 15 genes involved and less frequently autosomal dominant with at least 8 genes involved. These dystrophies are uncommon with a reported incidence rate for FSHD in high income countries of 1-2/100,000. Their frequency in Africa is not known. The pattern of muscle weakness follows the description in their names. Severity is variable from the uncommon rapidly fatal mainly childhood forms, to the more common mild and slowly progressive mainly adult forms.

Incomplete eye closure   **Failure of smiling**   **Winging of scapulae**

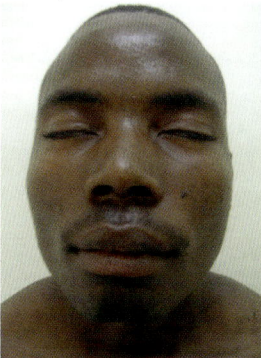

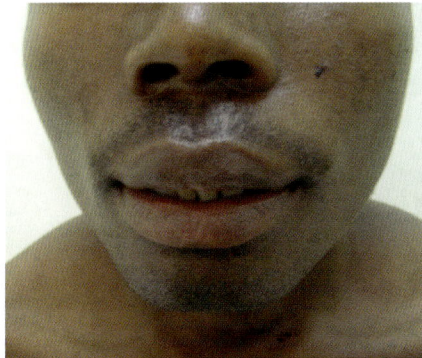

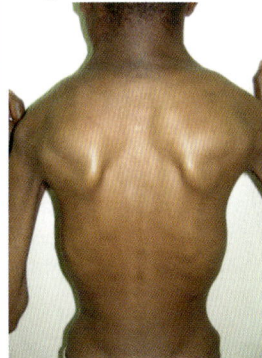

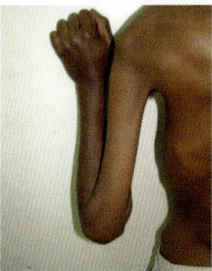

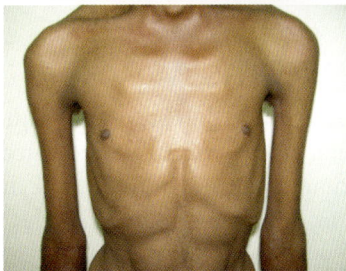

Wasting of proximal (humeral) limb muscles, triceps & biceps

Figure 13. 1 Facioscapulohumeral dystrophy

Wasting of upper limb girdle muscles

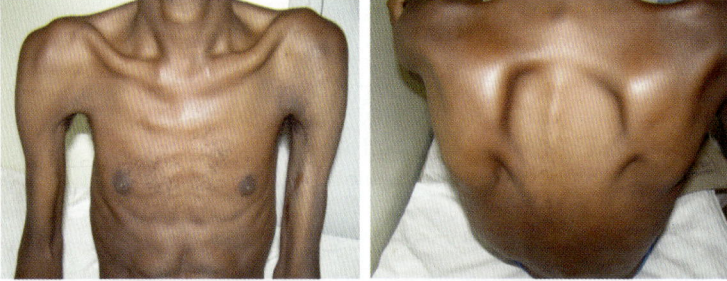

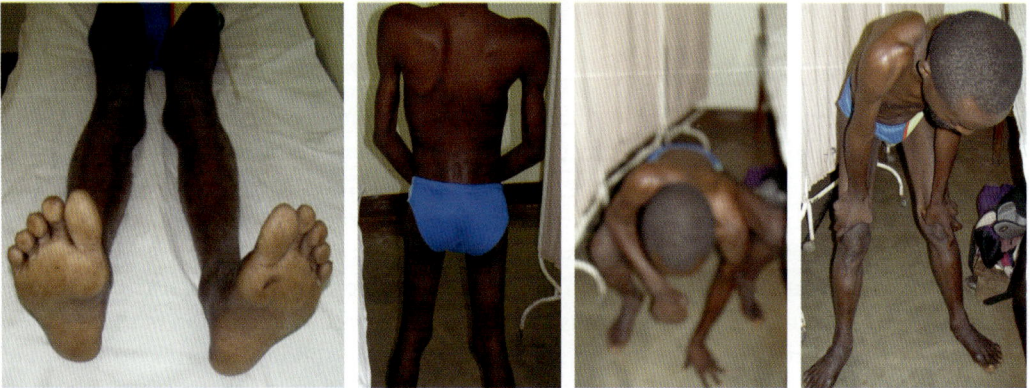

Wasting of proximal lower limb girdle muscles   Gower's manoeuvre

Figure 13. 2 Limb girdle muscular dystrophy

Key points

- muscular dystrophies are uncommon in adults
- two main types, limb girdle and facioscapulohumeral
- the pattern of muscle weakness follows their name
- survival into early and mid adulthood is a feature of both types

INFLAMMATORY MYOPATHIES

DERMATOMYOSITIS AND POLYMYOSITIS

Dermatomyositis and polymyositis are the main inflammatory myopathies. They are defined by inflammation in muscles and their general characteristics are presented below (Table 13.2). Their approximate frequency in high income countries is 5/100,000. In Africa they mostly affect the age group 20-40 yrs but occur in other age groups. Females are more commonly affected than males.

Clinical features

Patients present with sub acute mainly proximal muscle weakness and pain over months but occasionally over weeks. Dysphagia may occur because of involvement of pharyngeal muscles.

In dermatomyositis both skin and muscle are involved. On examination, there is marked symmetrical proximal weakness and signs of muscle atrophy in long standing disease. There is a characteristic blue-purple rash, plus oedema of upper eye lids (heliotrope), erythema over cheeks, knuckles and chest (Fig. 13.3) and dilated capillaries at the base of finger nails.

Table 13.2 Characteristics of inflammatory myopathies

Characteristics	Polymyositis	Dermatomyositis
age group	20-40 yrs	10-50 yrs
female:male ratio	2:1	2:1
onset	months	weeks to months
proximal muscle weakness	yes	yes
skin involvement	no	yes
malignancy	no	slight risk
elevation in ESR & CK	marked	marked
response to steroids	yes	yes

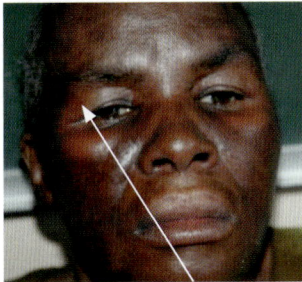

Rash/oedema/heliotrope sign   Rash on neck & chest   Rash/oedema over hands/knuckles

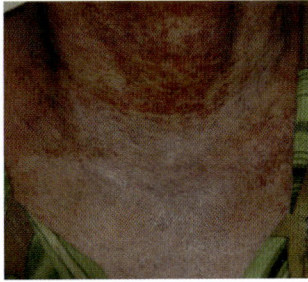

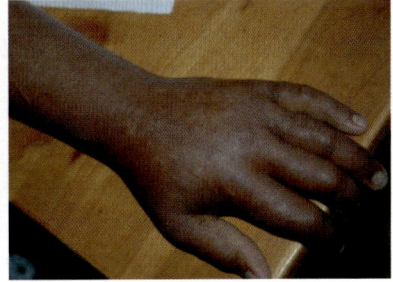

Figure 13.3 Dermatomyositis

Investigations

The ESR and serum CK are markedly elevated in polymyositis. The diagnosis is confirmed by muscle biopsy. Malignancy should be screened for in patients with dermatomyositis.

Management

The management of polymyositis is based on corticosteroids and immunosuppressant drugs. Treatment is with prednisolone 1mg/kg or 60 mg/po/daily. After months, when CK returns to normal and there is clinical improvement, the steroids can be reduced gradually by 5 mg decrements per dose on the alternate day, until the steroids are being administered only on alternate days. If the improvement is maintained, the prednisolone can be further decreased by 10 mg decrements every 4 weeks, until a maintenance dose is found. The usual maintenance dose is 5-10 mg prednisolone on alternate days. This may need to be continued for a further period of 3-6 months. Consider using an immunosuppressant drug from the start with steroids. The drug of choice is azathioprine 2.5 mg/kg/day. Start with 50 mg per day and increase by weekly intervals to 125-150 mg daily in divided doses. The main side effects are bone marrow suppression and hepatic toxicity. A FBC and liver function should be checked at the start and at least every four months during treatment with azathioprine. Alternatives are methotrexate or cyclophosphamide.

Key points

- C/Fs include progressive proximal muscle weakness & pain over weeks/months
- proximal weakness & characteristic skin rash are diagnostic of dermatomyositis
- ESR and CK are both elevated
- diagnosis is confirmed by muscle biopsy
- treatment is with steroids & another immunosuppressant for >6-12 months

INCLUSION BODY MYOSITIS

Inclusion body myositis (IBM) is another form of progressive inflammatory muscle disease which occurs in people >50 yrs. It is relatively common in high income countries but its frequency in Africa is not known. It occurs more frequently in older males and presents with painless proximal weakness with selective involvement of finger flexors and quadriceps muscles and frequently involves swallowing. Diagnosis is established by muscle biopsy and long term treatment is unsatisfactory. The differential diagnosis of inflammatory myopathies includes myasthenia gravis, non inflammatory myopathies and neuropathies.

OTHER MYOPATHIES

There is a large group of acquired non inflammatory myopathies. The main causes are outlined in table 13.3. Patients may range from being relatively asymptomatic with just muscle wasting to having severe weakness of limbs and trunk muscles. Most cases remit once the underlying disorder is treated or the offending drug is withdrawn.

Table 13.3 Causes of acquired non inflammatory myopathies

Classification	Causes
infections	HIV, TB
endocrine	thyroid disorders
	Cushing's disease
neoplastic	any malignancy
metabolic	hyper/hypokalaemia
organ failure	chronic cardiac, respiratory, liver disease
drugs	alcohol, steroids, statins, ARTs (zidovudine)

MYASTHENIA GRAVIS

Myasthenia gravis (MG) is an uncommon autoimmune disease that is caused by acetylcholine receptor antibodies (AChRA) at the neuromuscular junction. The antibody binds to the post synaptic acetylcholine receptor sites which makes them unavailable for the transmission of nerve impulses. It is a worldwide disorder with an incidence in high income countries of around 3-30/1,000,000 per year and with most cases expected to survive, the approximate prevalence rate is much higher at around 10/100,000 with a reported increase over time in age related MG. The incidence rates across Africa are not known, but a detailed study from Cape Town in SA using AChRAs as in indicator of MG reported an incidence rate there of 12.6/1,000,000 which is similar to that in high income countries. MG affects all age groups but mainly females in the age group 20-40 yrs and males in an older age group. It is associated with hyperplasia of the thymus (70%) and less commonly with thymoma (10%).

Clinical features

Symptoms

The most important diagnostic feature of MG is fatigable muscle weakness. In the early stages, weakness may be transient and variable. The busiest muscles at rest are the ones most commonly affected and patients frequently present for the first time with involvement of the extra ocular muscles (diplopia), eyelid (ptosis) and bulbar muscles (dysphagia) (Fig. 13.4). These may be accompanied by proximal weakness of the limbs and involvement of the face, neck, and trunk; typically the weakness worsens after exercise or at the end of the day.

Signs

On examination, fatigable ptosis, diplopia and limitation of eye movement are the main demonstrable eye signs. Bulbar involvement is evident by nasal type speech, difficulty in swallowing and nasal regurgitation of liquids. Facial weakness is demonstrated by bilateral weakness of eye closure and inability to smile normally giving the characteristic "myasthenic snarl" (Fig. 13.4). Fatigability may be demonstrated by asking the patient to look upwards holding the gaze in that position for 1-2 mins or to repeatedly elevate the arms above the head (>20 times) in quick succession without resting. In patients with MG, ptosis or upper limb weakness may appear for the first time or becomes more obvious during these manoeuvres. Reflexes and sensory exam are normal. In about one fifth of cases, the weakness is confined to the eyes only. When this persists without systemic involvement, it is called ocular myasthenia gravis.

Differential diagnosis

The differential diagnosis includes other causes of neuromuscular weakness in Africa, including inflammatory myopathies, motor neurone disease, and other myopathies.

Complications

Involvement of bulbar and respiratory muscles in MG is a neurological emergency (Fig 13.4). The major complication is respiratory failure. It is essential to monitor patients closely who are weak or bedbound and to measure vital capacity regularly. A forced vital capacity level <1.5 litres requires ITU care and urgent assessment for emergency ventilation.

Table 13.4 Symptoms of weakness in myasthenia gravis

eyes	double vision & drooping eye lids
face, mouth	weakness smiling, chewing & swallowing
speech	voice weak & easily tires
limbs	weakness combing hair weak hand grip difficulty arising from chairs or climbing stairs
central muscles	head drop weakness sitting up
respiratory	shortness of breath

Ptosis & ocular paresis (note overactive frontalis)

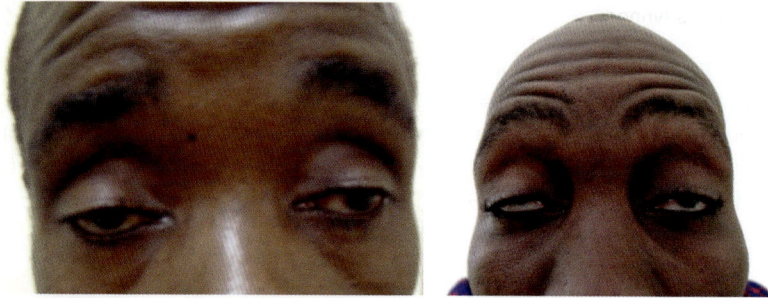

Ptosis & snarl

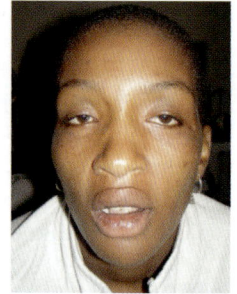

Complications

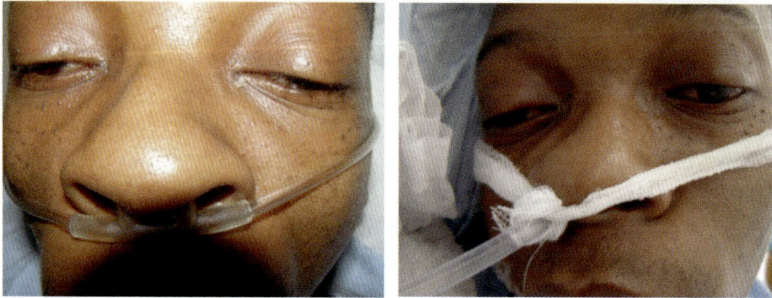

Figure 13.4 Myasthenia gravis

Key points

- key feature of MG is fatigable muscle weakness
- CFs are double vision, ptosis, dysphagia & weakness
- bulbar & respiratory involvement is an emergency
- may require ITU care & possible ventilation

Diagnosis

The diagnosis can be confirmed by a Tensilon (Edrophonium) test (Table 13.5). Edrophonium is a quick acting cholinesterase inhibitor which prevents available acetylcholine being broken down at the neuromuscular junction; this allows the excess acetylcholine to increase neuromuscular transmission and temporarily improve symptoms and signs. In order to carry out the test, two observers should ideally be present and cardiac resuscitation measures should be available. Other investigations are acetylcholine receptor antibodies (AChRA) which are present in 85% of patients with systemic MG. EMG shows a characteristic diagnostic pattern of decreasing amplitude of the compound muscle action potential with repeated stimulation. A CT of chest may show an enlarged thymus or a thymoma.

Table 13.5 Tensilon (edrophonium) test

1. tensilon 10 mg is drawn up into a syringe
2. a test dose of 3 mg is given intravenously as a bolus
3. observe the patient for any improvement in the weakness
4. in MG the weakness improves within a minute and lasts only 5 minutes or less
5. if there is no response then 7 mg is given intravenously
6. the outcome may be difficult to interpret hence the need for a second observer
7. atropine 0.5 to 1.0 mg should always be available for emergency iv use because of potential bradycardia.
8. atropine may also be given prophylactically just before the tensilon is given

Key points

- confirmatory tests are positive tensilon test, AChRA & EMG
- clinical diagnosis is confirmed by response to anticholinesterase drug treatment
- chest X-ray/CT may show thymic enlargement or infrequently a tumour

Management

The management of myasthenia involves the use of cholinesterase inhibitors and immunosuppression (Table 13.6). Treatment is very effective at reducing or abolishing weakness but requires scrupulous attention to detail.

Cholinesterase inhibitors

Pyridostigmine (60 mg tablets) is a long acting anticholinesterase which acts within 1 hour and lasts for 4 hours. The starting dose is 15 mg/po/qds and this is doubled every 2 days until the patient is taking 60 mg/po/qds. The patient's response will determine the dosage needed and the maximum total daily dose is 360 mg. Overdose causes a cholinergic crisis with severe bulbar and respiratory weakness, and patients need to be strictly warned about this possibility. The main side effects are abdominal pain and diarrhoea. Probanthaline 15-30 mg given 15 to 30 minutes before each dose of pyridostigmine is helpful to stop these in particular during the first few weeks of treatment. While anticholinesterases may suppress the symptoms they do not alter the disease and hence the need for immunosuppression.

Immunosuppression

Alternate day steroids are the treatment of choice. These are indicated in most cases. The patient should be admitted to hospital and started on prednisolone 10 mg/po/alternate days increasing slowly by 10 mg increments per dose (every second day) until 1.5 mg/kg or 100 mg is reached whichever is the lower dose. This should be maintained until the patient is stable in remission. Improvement begins after 2-4 weeks and maximises at 6-12 months. Then prednisolone is reduced by 10 mg every 4 weeks until the patient is on 40 mg alternate days, and by 5 mg every 4 weeks until on 20 mg and then by 1 mg every month thereafter. If during this steroid reduction stage there is a relapse, then begin again as at the start of treatment. If there is steroid intolerance or lack of response, azathioprine is started in addition to steroids at a dose of 25 mg/po/bd and increased by 25 mg/daily until the patient is on 2.5 mg/kg/po or 150 mg/po/daily. The main side effect is bone marrow depression. The patient needs a FBC and liver function tests every week for 2 months and then every 3 months.

Intravenous immunoglobulin (IVIG) or plasma exchange and ventilation

These may be needed in myasthenic crisis. The main indications for their use are increasing respiratory and bulbar weakness. However, these treatment options are unavailable at most centres in Africa. Respiratory failure (FVC <1.5 litres) is an urgent indication for consideration for mechanical ventilation.

Thymectomy

This is considered in patients on treatment who are under 45 years or who have the disease for less than 10 years or for suspected thymoma. As many as half the patients will go into complete remission after a thymectomy.

Table 13.6 Summary of management of myasthenia gravis

Treatment	Drugs	Indication
cholinesterase inhibitors	pyridostigmine	any muscle weakness
immunosuppression	prednisolone	inadequate control on pyridostigmine alone
	azathioprine	inadequate control on prednisolone & pyridostigmine
IVIG/plasma exchange		myasthenic crisis, bulbar & respiratory weakness
ventilation		bulbar/respiratory failure
thymectomy		all patients <45 years and suspected thymoma at any age

Key points

- mainstay of management is with pyridostigmine and steroids
- steroids should be introduced slowly under close supervision
- IVIG and plasma exchange are indicated in myasthenic crisis
- ventilation is necessary in respiratory failure
- treatment of MG is very effective but requires scrupulous attention to detail

Selected references

Bateman KJ, Schinkel M, Little F, Liebenberg L, Vincent A, Heckmann JM. *Incidence of seropositive myasthenia gravis in Cape Town and South Africa.* S Afr Med J. 2007 Oct;97(10):959-62.

Bellayou H, Hamzi K, Rafai MA, Karkouri M, Slassi I, Azeddoug H, et al. *Duchenne and Becker muscular dystrophy: contribution of a molecular and immunohistochemical analysis in diagnosis in Morocco.* J Biomed Biotechnol. 2009;2009:325210.

Diallo M, Fall AK, Diallo I, Diedhiou I, Ba PS, Diagne M, et al. *[Dermatomyositis and polymyositis: 21 cases in Senegal].* Med Trop (Mars). 2010 Apr;70(2):166-8.

Dieng MT, Diallo M, Dia D, Sow A, Ndiaye B. *[Dermatomyositis in Senegal. Study of 56 cases].* Dakar Med. 2005;50(3):123-7.

Ekenze OS, Onwuekwe IO, Ezeala Adikaibe BA. *Profile of neurological admissions at the University of Nigeria Teaching Hospital Enugu.* Niger J Med. 2010 Oct-Dec;19(4):419-22.

El-Tallawy HN, Khedr EM, Qayed MH, Helliwell TR, Kamel NF. *Epidemiological study of muscular disorders in Assiut, Egypt.* Neuroepidemiology. 2005;25(4):205-11.

Ginsberg Lionel, *Neurology. Lecture Notes.* Blackwell Publishing 8th edition 2005.

Goldman A, Ramsay M, Jenkins T. *Ethnicity and myotonic dystrophy: a possible explanation for its absence in sub-Saharan Africa.* Ann Hum Genet. 1996 Jan;60(Pt 1):57-65.

Grob D, Brunner N, Namba T, Pagala M. *Lifetime course of myasthenia gravis.* Muscle Nerve. 2008 Feb;37(2):141-9.

Hallwirth Pillay KD, Bill PL, Madurai S, Mubaiwa L, Rapiti P. *Molecular deletion patterns in Duchenne and Becker muscular dystrophy patients from KwaZulu Natal.* J Neurol Sci. 2007 Jan 15;252(1):1-3.

Heckmann JM, Hansen P, Van Toorn R, Lubbe E, Janse van Rensburg E, Wilmshurst JM. *The characteristics of juvenile myasthenia gravis among South Africans.* S Afr Med J. 2012 May 23;102(6):532-6.

Heckmann JM, Owen EP, Little F. *Myasthenia gravis in South Africans: racial differences in clinical manifestations.* Neuromuscul Disord. 2007 Dec;17(11-12):929-34.

Krahe R, Eckhart M, Ogunniyi AO, Osuntokun BO, Siciliano MJ, Ashizawa T. *De novo myotonic dystrophy mutation in a Nigerian kindred.* Am J Hum Genet. 1995 May;56(5):1067-74.

Mafojane NA, Bill PL, Lotz BP. *Problems in the optimal management of myasthenia gravis patients--a prospective clinical survey at Kalafong Hospital.* S Afr Med J. 2002 Mar;92(3):225-30.

Matuja WB, Aris EA, Gabone J, Mgaya EM. *Incidence and characteristics of Myasthenia gravis in Dar Es Salaam, Tanzania.* East Afr Med J. 2001 Sep;78(9):473-6.

Ojini FI, Danesi MA, Ogun SA. *Clinical manifestations of myasthenia gravis - review of cases seen at the Lagos University Teaching Hospital.* Niger Postgrad Med J. 2004 Sep;11(3):193-7.

Onyekwulu FA, Onwuekwe IO. *Critical care of myasthenia gravis in a resource poor setting: a study of South East Nigeria.* Neurologist. 2010 Nov;16(6):368-70

Stubgen JP, Stipp A. *Facioscapulohumeral muscular dystrophy: a prospective study of weakness and functional impairment.* J Neurol. 2010 Sep;257(9):1457-64.

Warlow Charles. *The Lancet Handbook of treatment in Neurology.* Elsevier, 1st edition 2006.

PART II – NEUROLOGICAL DISORDERS

CHAPTER 14
MOVEMENT DISORDERS AND MOTOR NEURONE DISEASE

CONTENTS

CHAPTER 14

MOVEMENT DISORDERS AND MOTOR NEURONE DISEASE

Movement disorders occur mainly because of disease of the basal ganglia and its central connections. Drugs may also cause them. They are characterized as those with too little movement or hypokinetic disorders as occurs in Parkinson's disease or with too much movement or hyperkinetic disorders as occur in tremor, dystonia and chorea. The most common overall movement disorder is tremor and the most common major movement disorder is Parkinson's disease (PD). This chapter outlines the main movement disorders and also motor neurone disease. The student should aim to be familiar with their main clinical features and management.

PARKINSON'S DISEASE (PD)

Parkinson's disease is a progressive neurodegenerative disorder characterized by four key clinical features: tremor, rigidity, poverty of movement also known as bradykinesia or akinesia, and loss of normal posture with a tendency for falls (Figs. 14.1 & 2). PD occurs all over the world affecting >1% of the population >65 years in high income countries. PD also occurs in Africa but may be less frequent there with lower reported age adjusted prevalence rates of 40-67/100,000. Males and females are both equally affected. PD typically begins in the age group 50-60 years and then occurs with increasing frequency in older age groups. PD may also affect a younger age group <40 yrs (5-10%). Juvenile onset PD (<20 yrs) is usually hereditary and may have more dystonic features than the adult onset disorder.

Causes
The underlying cause of most cases of PD is not known and the term idiopathic PD is used to describe the disease. Many of the clinical features of PD can result from a variety of other conditions including vascular disease, drugs, neurodegeneration and rarely encephalitis. When this happens the condition is called parkinsonism rather than PD.

Pathophysiology
The classic features of PD are a result of degeneration of dopamine secreting substantia nigra neurones which project from the brainstem via the striatal neurones to the basal ganglia. This leads to a loss of the characteristic black pigment and the remaining dopamine secreting cells may show Lewy inclusion bodies. Clinical disease starts when the substantia nigra cell loss is >50% and striatal dopamine levels are reduced by >80%. Recent studies have shown however that the pathology in PD is more widespread and occurring much earlier than originally believed.

Clinical Diagnosis

The initial presentation of PD is often mild with up to two thirds of patients presenting at onset with an asymmetrical rest tremor, affecting one limb or difficulty with fine repetitive motor movements e.g. doing buttons or tying shoelaces. If the dominant hand is involved then writing as it crosses the page becomes noticeably smaller. The **tremor** is characteristically coarse, regular, occurs at rest and disappears initially on intent such as holding a cup. The tremor becomes more noticeable when the person is distracted or whilst walking. It mostly affects the limbs but can affect any part of the body including the head, chin and tongue. The typical resting tremor is a rhythmical movement of the thumb on the hand called pill rolling. This is usually accompanied by increasing **bradykinesia** or slowing down of movements e.g. carrying out the activities of daily living (ADL) or walking. There may be a lack of spontaneous movement and facial animation **(expressionless face)**, (Fig. 14.1 & 2) and the blink rate is decreased.

On neurological examination, there is **rigidity** or stiffness of the limbs which results in increased tone throughout the full range of passive movement. This is called lead pipe rigidity or cog wheel rigidity if a tremor intrudes. **Gait disturbances** are usually mild in the first few years. Then posture becomes stooped and the gait is semi-flexed and shuffling with reduced arm swing and difficulty starting or stopping walking and turning (Fig. 14.1). There is a loss of postural righting reflexes which may lead to falls. The patient's voice may become quiet and muffled or hypophonic. Smell has recently been shown to be decreased or absent, sometimes for years before the onset of the other main symptoms.

Table 14.1 Main parkinsonian disorders

Extrapyramidal disorder	Clinical characteristics	Main Causes
Parkinson's disease	rest tremor rigidity akinesia loss of posture	idiopathic neurodegeneration genetic
Parkinsonism	akinesia & rigidity	neuroleptics antiemetics vascular head injury

Diagnosis

The diagnosis of PD is made clinically and laboratory investigations and standard CT/MRI neuroimaging are usually not helpful. The diagnosis is made if there are at least two of the four major clinical features present (Table 14.1) and is supported if there is a rapid clinical response to treatment with dopaminergic drugs.

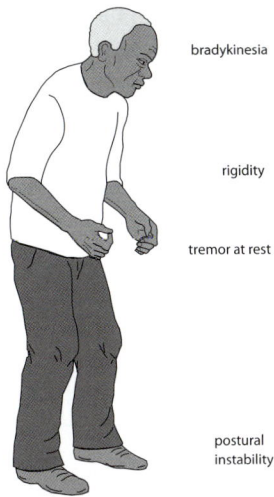

Patient with Parkinson's disease

Figure 14.1 Parkinson's disease

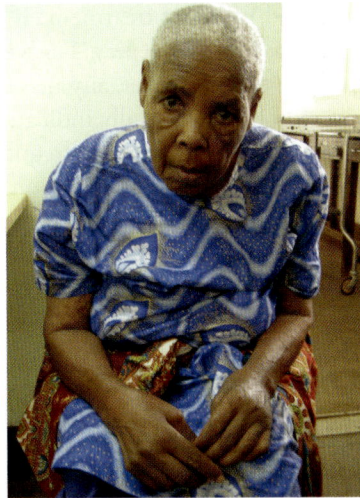

Akinesia & semi flexed posture

Figure 14.2 Parkinson's disease

Key points

- PD is caused by a progressive loss of dopamine secreting cells in substantia nigra
- key features are rest tremor, rigidity, poverty of movement & postural instability
- tremor at rest in one hand /arm is often the earliest clinical sign
- diagnosis is supported by a good response to dopamine treatment

Treatment

Levodopa

Early Parkinson's disease does not require any drug treatment. The main aim of treatment of PD (Table 14.2) is to reduce motor disability. Levodopa (L-dopa) does this by replacing the missing dopamine which helps to relieve the symptoms but does not prevent disease progression. L-dopa is given orally and this is later converted into dopamine in the brain by the enzyme dopa decarboxylase which comes from the remaining substantia nigra neurones. In order to prevent conversion of the inactive L-dopa to dopamine in the peripheral circulation L-dopa is given in combination with a dopa decarboxylase inhibitor, either carbidopa or benserazide. Because the dopa decarboxylase inhibitors do not cross the blood brain barrier, this will result in increased dopamine levels in the brain without similar increases in the peripheral blood. This also reduces the nausea that results from peripheral dopamine. The overall aim is to keep the daily maintenance dose of L-dopa as low as possible in order to maintain good motor function and yet reduce any long term motor complications.

Generic preparations of these are available as carbidopa/levodopa and benserazide/levodopa. Treatment is started slowly with gradual increases in dosages. The usual starting dose is in **25/100 mg tabs,** either ½ or 1 tab taken three times daily taken initially with meals. The main acute side effects are nausea, vomiting, hypotension, confusion and hallucinations. These often resolve spontaneously or with concurrent administration of an antiemetic e.g. domperidone

10-20 mg tds for the first 4 weeks of treatment. If the initial response is inadequate, then the L-dopa dose can be increased slowly every **4-6 weeks** by **½ tab tds** to a usual maintenance dose of **25/250 mg tabs 1 tds**. However, any necessary increases in dosage (½ tab tds) can be brought forward to **weekly** if it is clinically indicated and the patient tolerates it. Later, usually after years L-dopa may have to be given more frequently (changing from 8 to 6 to 4 to 3 hourly as necessary). A controlled release (CR) preparation may be helpful to be taken at night because of a longer duration of effect. Most patients respond very well initially but larger doses are required as the disease progresses.

In the later stages, the duration of response to each dose may shorten (the wearing off effect) and motor fluctuations may occur (the on–off phenomenon) and involuntary motor movements or dyskinesia are likely. The response to treatment may then become unpredictable and any sudden reduction or withdrawal of L-dopa is associated with deterioration.

Table 14.2 Levodopa treatment of Parkinson's disease

Medication	Class	Initial dose	Maintenance dose	When to use	Main side effects
carbidopa/levodopa *or* **benserazide/levodopa**	levodopa	(25/100 mg tab) ½-1 tab tds	(25/250 mg tab) 1 tab tds	early and throughout illness (effect good)	nausea, vomiting, hypotension, confusion, hallucinations, dyskinesia

Other drug treatments

The L-dopa/decarboxylase inhibitor combinations are the most effective symptomatic treatment for PD. Other treatments include dopamine agonists, catechol-O-methyltransferase inhibitors (COMT), NMDA antagonists, monoamine oxidase B inhibitors (MOB) and anticholinergics (Table 14.3). In general, these treatments are added on when the response to L-dopa preparations has decreased or failed. The dopamine agonists may be used early on either as first line treatment alone or in combination with L-dopa especially in younger onset PD patients. The use of dopamine agonists is associated with less dyskinesia after 3-5 years of therapy. They act postsynaptically and therefore mimic the effects of dopamine in the basal ganglia. The dopamine agonists fall into two main groups: the ergot derived group which includes bromocriptine and cabergoline and the non ergot derived group which includes ropinirole among others.

The side effect profiles are similar to dopamine except that ergotism may occur in the first group. Ergotism is a serious limitation to their long-term use as up to 3% of treated patients develop pulmonary or less frequently retroperitoneal fibrosis. The newer non-ergot agonists have been associated with hypersomnolence and impulse control disorders, including, overeating, excessive shopping, gambling and hypersexuality. Their use is contraindicated in pre-existing vascular, heart and lung disease. Amantadine is considered a useful drug to start treatment for the first 6-12 months. It has relatively few side effects but only a modest effect on motor symptoms and a limited duration of action. It is effective however, for the dyskinesia seen as a side effect of levodopa. Other useful add on drugs include the COMT inhibitor entacapone and the MOB inhibitor selegiline. These inhibit the breakdown of dopamine and prolong its activity. Their use is mainly indicated in late disease for motor fluctuations and decreasing response to L-dopa. The side effects are largely similar to levodopa. The use of anticholinergics (benzhexol) may be helpful mainly in tremor dominant disease in younger patients. The drug treatment of PD is summarised in the table below.

Table 14.3 Other drug treatments of Parkinson's disease

Medication	Class	Initial dose	Maintenance dose	When to use	Main side effects
amantadine	NMDA antagonist	100 mg/day	100 mg/bid/tds	*early* (effect modest), dyskinesia	restlessness, confusion
bromocriptine	dopamine agonists (ergot)	2.5 mg/day	5-10 mg/tds	*early* delays need for L-dopa	as in levodopa *ergotism
cabergoline	(ergot)	0.5-1 mg/day	2-6 mg/day	*late* motor symptoms, fluctuations	as in levodopa *ergotism
ropinerole	(non ergot)	0.25 mg/tds	2-6 mg/tds	*early or late*	as in levodopa somnolence, impulse control disorders
entacapone	COMT inhibitor	200 mg tab with each dose levodopa	max 2000 mg/day	*late* motor symptoms & fluctuations	as in levodopa, dyskinesia, diarrhoea
selegiline	MOB inhibitor	5 mg/bd	5 mg/bd	*late* motor symptoms & fluctuations	confusion, insomnia
benzhexol	anticholinergic	1-2 mg/bd	2-5 mg/tds	*early* for tremor (effect modest)	confusion, cognitive impairment, dry mouth, constipation urinary retention

Ergotism: 3% of patients develop pulmonary or less commonly retroperitoneal fibrosis

Non drug treatments

Physiotherapy is helpful to many patients with PD and their quality of life can be helped by the provision of simple aids to the activities of daily living. Surgical treatment is helpful when drug treatment has failed or is intolerable usually in selected younger patients. Surgery usually involves either a thalamotomy or pallidotomy or deep brain stimulation of the globus pallidus or subthalamic nucleus and accounts of these are available in larger textbooks.

Course

PD progresses slowly over many years. There is no cure and progression is variable with many patients functioning well despite the presence of the disease for years. Drug treatment is necessary for patients with motor disability and can be effective and long-lasting. As the disease progresses immobility, pain, sleep disturbance, depression and dementia (40-50%) are all very common and these may require separate management and treatment. The deterioration is slow and variable with death occurring on average 10-15 years after onset.

Key points

- early PD does not usually require drug treatment
- Levodopa is the most effective drug treatment for PD
- side effects are nausea, vomiting , hypotension, confusion, hallucinations & dyskinesia
- drug treatments are started at a lower dosage & slowly increased over weeks
- PD typically progresses slowly over years with death following after 10-15 yrs

OTHER EXTRAPYRAMIDAL SYNDROMES

Parkinson plus syndromes

There are other uncommon or rare neurological disorders with features of parkinsonism which are briefly mentioned here. These are all disorders characterized by clinical features of parkinsonism in addition to other neurological findings more typical of the specific underlying neurological disorder. These are **multiple system atrophy (MSA), progressive supranuclear palsy (PSP), corticobasal degeneration (CBD), vascular parkinsonism** and **dementia with Lewy bodies**. MSA is characterized by parkinsonism coupled with cerebellar and/or autonomic dysfunction (hypotension) and partial initial response to L-dopa. PSP is characterized by akinetic rigidity, late onset dementia and a slowing or failure of voluntary vertical and eventually all eye movements. CBD is characterized by asymmetric bradykinesia, rigidity and limb apraxia. Vascular parkinsonism involves mainly the lower half of the body with a prominent gait disorder. Dementia with Lewy bodies is characterized by dementia, rigidity and hallucinations. A characteristic of all these disorders is either a reduced, nonsustained or absent response to levodopa treatment. Management is mostly symptomatic and supportive.

Key points

- Parkinson plus syndromes are uncommon
- characterized by akinesia & other distinguishing neurological features
- they can be separated clinically from PD
- response to L-dopa treatment is generally poor
- prognosis is determined by the underlying condition

PARKINSONISM

Drug induced parkinsonism

The neuroleptic drugs, phenothiazines (e.g. chlorpromazine) and the butyrophenones (e.g. haloperidol) are one of the main causes of drug induced parkinsonism in Africa where they are mostly used in the treatment of schizophrenia and chronic confusional states. This is particularly the case with the use of long acting depot or intramuscular preparations. The long term use of some antiemetics including metoclopramide and prochloperazine may also cause parkinsonism. These drugs cause parkinsonism by blocking the effect of dopamine centrally in the brain. Drug induced parkinsonism is characterized by generalized slowness and rigidity without any tremor.

Management is to lower the dose or stop the offending drug. The parkinsonism usually remits within days or weeks of stopping the drug. However if the preparations have been used long term it may take a year or two to recover or there may be no recovery at all. The anticholinergics benzhexol or benztropine prescribed in adequate doses are the drugs of choice in the treatment of drug induced parkinsonism (Table 14.3).

Key points

- long-term use of antipsychotic & antiemetics can cause drug induced parkinsonism
- management is to stop the offending drug and use anticholinergic drugs

Neuroleptic malignant syndrome

This is an important syndrome because of the widespread use of neuroleptics and in particular the use of depot preparations for sedation of confused or aggressive patients. The main causes are phenothiazines and haloperidol. The symptoms usually start within days or weeks or months of starting the offending drug and is commonly misdiagnosed as meningitis because of neck rigidity and fever. It is characterized by generalised rigidity, altered level of consciousness and autonomic instability and high fever. The disorder is life threatening and the patient needs intensive medical care. Management is to stop the neuroleptic and to add a dopaminergic drug e.g. bromocriptine. Anticholinergics and muscle relaxants may also be used.

Key points

- neuroleptic syndrome is characterized by fever, rigidity & history of recent drug exposure
- Rx: withdraw offending drug, use dopamine agonist & anticholinergic & muscle relaxants

Akinetic-rigid syndrome

Decreased or absent movement (akinesia) can be the outcome of all causes of parkinsonism. It is characterized by generalised rigidity and immobility with the patient eventually confined to bed. The main causes are summarized in Table 14.4. It is a life threatening condition which frequently requires urgent medical attention. Complications include dehydration, pneumonia and pressure sores. The differential diagnosis in Africa includes other causes of increasing immobility including stroke, subdural haematoma, SOL, dementia and chronic psychosis. Management includes the use of parenteral anticholinergics and muscle relaxants and treating the underlying cause and complications.

Table 14.4 Causes of akinetic-rigid syndrome

Parkinson's disease **parkinsonism** **parkinson plus syndromes**
Drugs neuroleptics antiemetics
Vascular strokes (multiple lacunar) subdural haematoma (chronic)

continues

| **Trauma** |
| traumatic brain injury |
| **Chronic psychosis** |
| schizophrenia |
| **Other causes** |
| dementia |
| post encephalitic/inflammatory |
| toxins, chronic carbon monoxide, manganese |
| Wilson's disease |

Key points

- akinetic-rigid syndrome is characterized by immobility & rigidity
- management includes anticholinergics & muscle relaxants
- treat the underlying cause & complications

INVOLUNTARY MOVEMENTS

The main involuntary movement disorders are tremor, dystonia, chorea, athetosis, hemiballismus, myoclonic jerks and tics (Table 14.5 & 6).

Tremor

Tremor is an involuntary repetitive, rhythmical shaking movement of a part of the body, most commonly seen in the fingers, hands and arms. Tremors are categorized as either fine or coarse and according to the position in which the tremor occurs maximally. In order to demonstrate this, the hands are examined in three main positions: at rest, with the arms and hands outstretched and on action. The common tremors in these positions are outlined in Table 14.5.

Rest

This is a coarse, regular tremor which mainly affects the limbs, occurs at rest and improves initially on action such as holding a cup or newspaper. It can affect any part of the body including the fingers, toes hands, feet, limbs, chin, tongue, head and trunk. The main causes are Parkinson's disease and parkinsonism.

Postural

This is a fine regular tremor and is the most common type of tremor. This occurs on posture e.g. when holding the hands outstretched and affects the fingers and hands. It may also affect the lower limbs, head, and trunk. The two most common types are physiological and benign essential tremor.

Action

This is a regular coarse tremor which occurs on action and mainly affects the limbs but may involve the trunk. It is most evident when testing for finger nose or heel shin co-ordination during neurological examination of the limbs. The main causes are cerebellar disease and benign essential tremor.

Table 14.5 Common Tremors

Position	Cause	Clinical features	Treatment
Rest	Parkinson's disease	regular, coarse, slow	anticholinergics levodopa
Postural	physiological, benign essential tremor, anxiety, hyperthyroidism beta agonists, alcohol, HIV	regular, fine, medium, fast	treat the cause beta-blockers
Action	cerebellar, essential	regular, coarse, slow	no effective treatment beta-blockers or primidone (essential tremor)

BENIGN ESSENTIAL TREMOR

Benign essential tremor (BET) or familial tremor is one of the more common neurological disorders and is a very recognizable tremor. There are few studies on its frequency in Africa but its reported frequency there ranges widely from 5-81/100,000. It is frequently inherited as autosomal dominant, so there is often a positive family history. It occurs in all age groups including teenagers and young adults but with increasing frequency in advancing age, hence is more common in older age groups. The tremor affects the hands and/or the head but usually spares the legs. It is most apparent during posture such as holding a cup or newspaper and may persist throughout the action as evident on finger nose testing. The tremor is usually helped by a small amount of alcohol, made worse by anxiety and worsens slowly but over many years.

Many patients require only reassurance and no further treatment. If treatment is required beta-blockers are the drugs of first choice. Propranolol is prescribed initially in a low dose of 10 mg twice daily increasing slowly over months to a maximum dose of 80 mg twice or three times daily. The dose should be titrated against response or may be taken only on an as required basis at times when the tremor is likely to be very disabling. Adverse effects of beta blockers include fatigue, hypotension and bronchospasm. Primidone may also be used. The initial dose is 25-50 mg daily increasing slowly by 50 mg every 2 weeks to a maximum of 250 mg twice or three times daily. A dose of 100-150 mg three times daily may be effective. Adverse effects are drowsiness, fatigue and occasionally idiosyncratic reaction.

Key points

- BET is a mainly postural tremor with a strong family history
- occurs in teenagers and young adults but is more common in old age
- worsens slowly over years but usually does not cause disability
- patients may need reassurance because of anxiety & embarrassment
- drug treatment is with propranolol or primidone

DYSTONIA

Dystonia is a complex disorder of motor control characterized by prolonged muscular contraction that gives rise to abnormal postures and involuntary movements. These are most apparent during voluntary action but may also occur at rest. Dystonia may be focal affecting one part of the body e.g. Meige syndrome (Fig. 14.3) or generalised affecting more than one part (Fig. 14.4). It may occur at any age and clinical pattern, age of onset, and systemic features may point to the underlying cause. The focal dystonias are fairly common and the main examples in clinical practice are torticollis, blepharospasm and writer's cramp. The generalized dystonias are uncommon and these tend to occur in childhood or in young adults.

The main causes of dystonia are idiopathic, genetic or secondary to a systemic disease such as stroke, drugs or Wilson's disease. In a typical severe generalized dystonia the head may be tilted or retracted, the back rotated or twisted (Fig. 14. 4). and the limbs extended with inverted feet or cramping of the hand. This posture may be maintained or be triggered by movement or a specific action. The main causes of drug induced dystonias are levodopa, chlorpromazine, metoclopramide and haloperidol. A more complex involuntary chewing and grimacing movement, associated with the use of long term neuroleptics is called tardive dyskinesia.

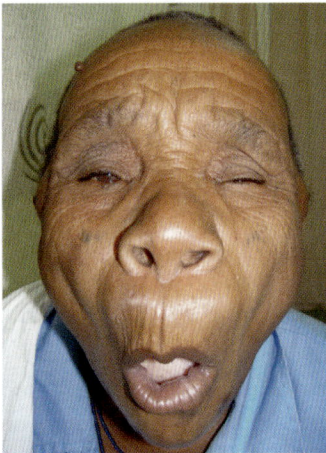

Orofacial dyskinesia & blepharospasm

Figure 14.3 Dystonia (Meige syndrome)

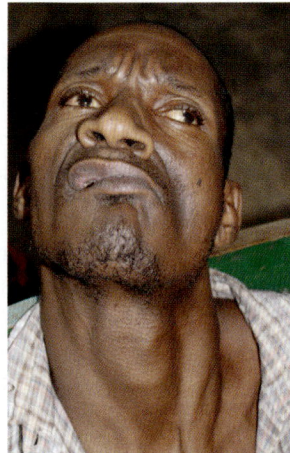

Torticollis & hemifacial dystonia

Figure 14.4 Dystonia generalised

Management of drug related dystonia includes the withdrawal of suspected drugs and the use of benzodiazepines. Management of persisting dystonia is generally disappointing but all patients under 40 years should first have a trial of levodopa. Other treatments include high dose anticholinergics (Benzhexol 5-10 mg three to four times daily or tetrabenazine used either alone or together in combination with a dopamine agonist e.g. bromocriptine). Focal dystonias e.g., torticollis, blepharospasm and laryngospasm respond well but temporarily to local botulinum toxin injections. Deep brain stem stimulation targeting the globus pallidus can be effective in some generalized dystonias.

Acute dystonic reactions

These occur typically within 24 hours after a single dose of neuroleptics or antiemetics, in particular metoclopramide. These may be focal or generalised and are usually self limiting. They are recognizable by the characteristic writhing movement of the tongue, mouth, face and neck and occasionally limbs and trunk. If the eyes roll up involuntarily, this is called an oculogyric crisis. The treatment of choice is parenteral benztropine 1-2 mgs iv/im and repeated within 30 mins, if the first dose is not effective. Oral anticholinergic therapy should be continued for the next 5-7 days. The patient should be advised to avoid the offending drug in the future.

Chorea

Chorea is an irregular dance-like, semi-purposeful, non repetitive, movement involving flexion and extension of the limbs and trunk. The movement is unpredictable, jerky, chaotic and fidgeting in nature. The main causes are streptococcal infection in Sydenham's chorea and genetic in the case of Huntington's disease (Chapter 18). It occurs very occasionally in HIV disease secondary to an opportunistic process involving the basal ganglia and as a long-term side effect of dopaminergic drugs. Unilateral chorea can result from a stroke affecting the basal ganglia. Sydenham's chorea is typically self limiting after a few days or weeks or occasionally months and does not require treatment. Huntington's chorea may respond initially to low dose haloperidol, tetrabenazine and also benzodiazepine if there is a disability or anxiety. However over time it usually becomes resistant to symptomatic treatment.

Athetosis

This is a characteristic slow writhing movement that mainly affects trunk muscles. The main causes are cerebral palsy and basal ganglia disease. It may occur in combination with chorea and dystonia and these can be difficult to distinguish from each other. Treatment is similar to that of chorea.

Hemiballismus

This is a sudden irregular explosive flinging movement of the limbs on one side. The main cause is vascular or a stroke affecting the contralateral subthalamic nucleus and it may occur after head injury in young persons. Opportunistic processes in HIV disease in particular toxoplasmosis affecting the area of the basal ganglia are also a known cause. Hemiballismus may remit spontaneously or with treatment of the underlying cause. Haloperidol or tetrabenazine may be helpful if it becomes disabling.

Myoclonus

Myoclonus is a sudden shock movement or jerk that may occur normally in children and in adults on falling asleep. It is only pathological if it persists such as occurs in myoclonic epilepsy, organ failure, dementia and occasionally with the use of the SSRI drugs in the treatment of depression. It arises in the CNS from cortical, sub cortical and spinal cord levels and can be stimulus sensitive or elicited by noise or touch, disappearing in sleep. The management is the treatment of the underlying disease. Myoclonus may respond to benzodiazepines such as clonazepam or to the anticonvulsants sodium valproate or levetiracetam.

Tics

A tic is a brief stereotyped irresistible repetitive purposeful movement. It differs from chorea in that it can be voluntarily suppressed at will for a short while. Simple tics like blinking, grimacing or shoulder shrugging are common in children and are usually outgrown. A wider range of tics causing vocalizations, noises and sometimes expletives is very suggestive of **Gilles de la Tourette syndrome**. This responds to dopamine antagonists e.g. haloperidol but the drug needs to be continued long term.

Asterixis

This is a characteristic sudden flapping of the outstretched dorsiflexed hands. It is an important clinical bedside sign suggestive of metabolic encephalopathy. It occurs in association with organ failure characteristically liver, renal and respiratory failure. Treatment is management of the underlying disorder.

Hiccups

Hiccups are caused by a sudden spontaneous contraction of the diaphragm. They are usually transient and are a normal phenomenon but may be a complication of renal failure. In rare cases hiccups can persist for days or even months. In this case a local source of irritation of the diaphragm, either from above or below, should be excluded. Management of persistent hiccups is not easy. The usual drug of choice is chlorpromazine initially 25 mg twice or three times daily increasing to 50 mg as needed. Baclofen and gabapentin have been used with variable success.

Table 14.6 Main characteristics of other involuntary movements

Type	Clinical features	Causes
Dystonia generalized	abnormal posture, involuntary movements	neuroleptics: phenothiazines, haloperidol, levodopa, Wilson's disease, idiopathic
focal	localised abnormal posture **(e.g. torticollis, blepharospasm, writer's cramp)**	
Chorea	irregular, dance-like, non repetitive, semi purposeful	Sydenham's, Huntington's, HIV, stroke
Athetosis	slow, writhing, purposeless	cerebral palsy
Hemiballismus	explosive, unilateral	stroke, head injury, HIV
Myoclonus	sudden jerk	encephalopathy, epilepsy
Tics	movement, brief, stereotyped, suppressible **(e.g. blinking, sniffing, shrugging)**	psychological, basal ganglia disorder

Key points

- tremor is a rhythmical alternating movement of part of the body
- dystonia is an abnormal posturing & involuntary movement
- chorea is a brief dance-like semi purposeful non repetitive movement
- myoclonus is a sudden jerk like movement
- a tic is a brief stereotyped irresistible repetitive purposeful movement

MOTOR NEURONE DISEASE

Motor neurone disease (MND) is a progressive neurodegenerative disease that affects upper and lower motor neurones in the brain and spinal cord. The cause is not known. It is an uncommon worldwide disorder with an incidence rate of 2 per 100,000 reported in high income countries with most cases occurring in >60 year age groups. However MND can affect all age groups and around 5% of reported cases are familial; these occur mostly in a younger age group. The frequency of MND in Africa in not known but may be less frequent there because of the lower overall life expectancy. An association between MND and HIV has been reported in some high income countries.

The pathogenesis of MND is not known but may involve a form of neuroexcitatory cell death mediated by free radicals. MND is exclusively a motor disease without any clinical sensory, bladder or ocular involvement. It is made up of four clinical subtypes; amyotrophic lateral sclerosis, progressive bulbar palsy, progressive muscular atrophy and primary lateral sclerosis.

CLINICAL SUBTYPES

Amyotrophic lateral sclerosis (ALS)

ALS is the most common clinical presentation of MND accounting for approximately three quarters of all cases. ALS is an alternative name which is frequently used to describe MND. Patients with ALS present typically with slow but progressive weakness and wasting involving the limbs occurring usually over months. The upper limbs are more commonly involved earlier on than the lower limbs and limb involvement can be asymmetrical early on (Fig. 14.5).

On examination, there is a mixture of upper and lower motor neurone signs in the limbs. Typically there is marked wasting and hyperreflexia in the upper limbs combined with increased tone, hyperreflexia in the legs and extensor plantar reflexes. Fasciculation is frequently widespread involving limbs and trunk muscles and may involve the tongue. There are no sensory signs. Emotional lability is a feature in some patients. All four limbs and the brain stem become involved later on (Fig. 14.6). Clinical presentation in Africa is typically late with most patients at the time of clinical presentation having a mixture of quadriplegia and a bulbar/pseudobulbar palsy. The average survival time from the onset of first symptoms is 2-3 years.

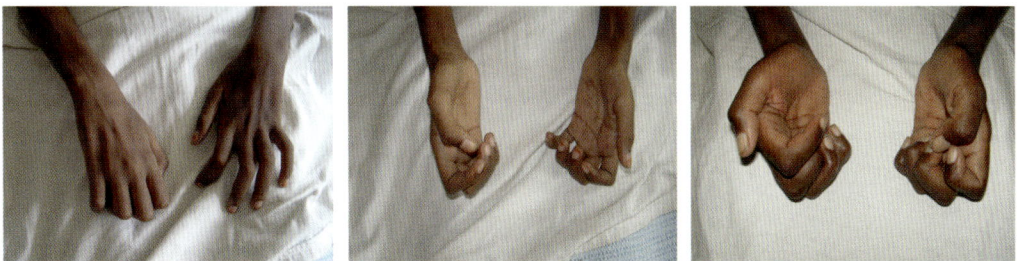

Wasting of the hand muscles & clawing of the hands in advanced MND

Figure 14.5 Amyotrophic lateral sclerosis affecting the hands

Progressive bulbar/pseudobulbarpalsy (PBP/PSP)

PBP/PSP is the main form of clinical presentation of MND in 10-20% of patients. It occurs more commonly in the elderly. Dysarthria and dysphagia progressing over months are the main presenting complaints. Signs of mixed bulbar and pseudobulbar palsy are always present. The main neurological findings are those of a spastic, immobile and fasciculating tongue (Fig 14.6) coupled with either an increased or absent gag reflex. The jaw jerk is usually brisk. Isolated signs of limb involvement including spasticity and hyperreflexia and occasionally fasciculation may already be apparent on neurological examination or more typically develop later on. Survival times are usually shorter than in ALS.

Spastic & ridged tongue in ALS

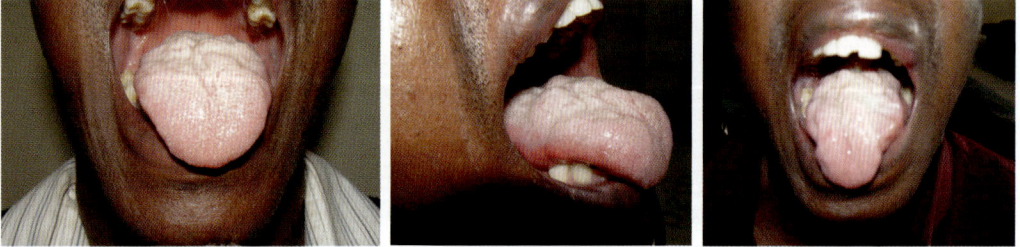

Spastic immobile tongue & wasted hands in ALS

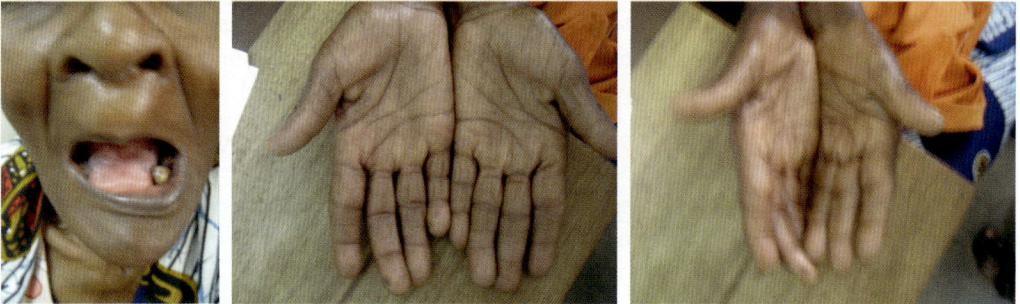

Figure 14.6 Bulbar/pseudobulbar palsy

Progressive muscular atrophy (PMA)

PMA accounts for about 5% of cases. PMA presents as progressive lower motor neurone weakness in the limbs (Fig. 14.7). The neurological findings are weakness, wasting, fasciculation and absent reflexes. Bulbar involvement may follow. Survival times are 4-5 years.

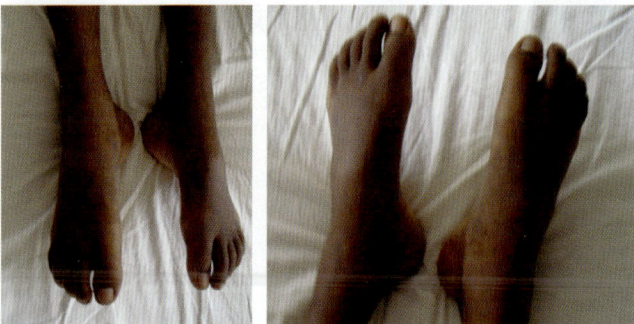

Figure 14.7 Progressive muscular atrophy. Foot drop (bilateral) in MND

Primary lateral sclerosis (PLS)

PLS accounts for 1% of cases. PLS presents as a very slowly progressive upper motor neurone type weakness affecting the limbs. There are no lower motor neurone findings and survival times are 15-20 years.

Other rarer clinical presentations of MND include flail arm, man in the barrel syndrome, head drop and dementia. Cognitive & behavioural changes may precede, accompany or follow the development of clinical MND/ALS. Cognitive changes in MND are much commoner than is generally appreciated and although in most patients these are subtle, a minority may develop a frank dementia or aphasia, usually of a frontotemporal dementia type (FTD). In some familial cases the same gene mutation can cause FTD, MND, or both.

Differential diagnosis

The main differential diagnosis includes cervical spondylosis, syringomyelia, post polio syndrome and lead poisoning. Uncommonly or rarely some genetic or inherited muscle and nerve disorders need to be considered in the differential diagnosis. These include limb girdle muscular dystrophy (LGMD), spinal muscular atrophy (childhood or adolescent onset), affecting mainly the proximal limbs and slowly progressive and may mimic LGMD), and Kennedy's syndrome (twitching movements of chin & tongue fasciculations, tremor hands, proximal weakness, gynecomastia, diabetes and neuropathy, slowly progressive).

Investigations

Laboratory investigations in MND are usually normal apart from an occasional elevated creatinine phosphokinase and/or infrequently isolated elevation in CSF protein. X-ray of the neck excludes cervical spondylosis and neuroimaging of the brain may occasionally be necessary to exclude other possible causes.

Diagnosis

The diagnosis in MND is mostly a clinical one and clinical diagnostic criteria for MND have been established by the World Federation of Neurology according to the degree of clinical certainty. The definite diagnosis of MND requires the presence of upper and lower motor signs in at least two spinal regions (cervical, thoracic and lumbosacral) and also involving the bulbar region. The diagnostic criteria are set out in Table 14.7

Table 14.7 El Escorial criteria for diagnosis of MND*

Diagnostic certainty	Clinical features
Definite	upper & lower motor neurone signs in the bulbar and two spinal regions or in three spinal regions
Probable	upper & lower motor neurone signs in two or more regions; the regions may differ but some UMN signs must be proximal to LMN signs
Possible	upper & lower motor neurone signs in only one region or UMN signs alone in two or more regions or LMN signs proximal to UMN signs
Suspected	LMN (not UMN) signs in at least 2 regions

* criteria of the World Federation of Neurology

Management

The management of MND involves explaining to the patient and family the nature of the illness. It is important to emphasise the practical approach in caring for the patient. Most drug treatment is symptomatic. The anticholinergic drug benzhexol is used for reducing saliva secretions and baclofen and diazepam for spasticity and anxiety. Other medications include paracetamol for pain, quinine sulphate for cramps and opiates as required for palliative care. The antiglutamate drug Riluzole 50 mg bd has been shown to increase life expectancy but only by about 3-6 months in some patients.

Prognosis
Survival with MND from onset is on average 3-5 years with around 10% surviving 5 years or longer. The cause of death is most frequently respiratory infection.

Key points

- MND is an uncommon neurodegenerative disease
- characterized by a mixture of upper & lower motor neurone signs
- common presentations are limb weakness & bulbar palsy
- treatment is largely symptomatic & supportive
- survival on average ranges 3-5 years from onset

Selected references

Abdulla MN, Sokrab TE, el Tahir A, Siddig HE, Ali ME. *Motor neurone disease in the tropics: findings from Sudan.* East Afr Med J. 1997 Jan;74(1):46-8.

Adam AM. *Unusual form of motor neurone disease in Kenya.* East Afr Med J. 1992 Feb;69(2):55-7.

Bower JH, Teshome M, Melaku Z, Zenebe G. *Frequency of movement disorders in an Ethiopian university practice.* Mov Disord. 2005 Sep;20(9):1209-13.

Carr J, Kies B, Fine J; *Movement Disorders Group of South Africa. Guideline for the treatment of Parkinson's disease.* S Afr Med J. 2009 Oct;99(10):755-6, 758.

Cosnett JE, Bill PL. *Parkinson's disease in blacks. Observations on epidemiology in Natal.* S Afr Med J. 1988 Mar 5;73(5):281-3.

Cosnett JE, Bill PL, Bhigjee AI. *Motor neurone disease in blacks. Epidemiological observations in Natal.* S Afr Med J. 1989 Aug 19;76(4):155-7.

Dean G, Elian M. *Motor neurone disease and multiple sclerosis mortality in Australia, New Zealand and South Africa compared with England and Wales.* J Neurol Neurosurg Psychiatry. 1993 Jun;56(6):633-7.

Dotchin C, Jusabani A, Walker R. *Three year follow up of levodopa plus carbidopa treatment in a prevalent cohort of patients with Parkinson's disease in Hai, Tanzania.* J Neurol. 2011 Mar 26.

Dotchin C, Msuya O, Kissima J, Massawe J, Mhina A, Moshy A, et al. *The prevalence of Parkinson's disease in rural Tanzania.* Mov Disord. 2008 Aug 15;23(11):1567-672.

Dotchin CL, Walker RW. *The prevalence of essential tremor in rural northern Tanzania.* J Neurol Neurosurg Psychiatry. 2008 Oct;79(10):1107-9.

Haimanot RT. *Parkinson's disease in Ethiopia: a prospective study of 70 patients.* East Afr Med J. 1985 Aug;62(8):571-9.

Leigh PN, Ray-Chaudhuri K. *Motor neurone disease.* J Neurol Neurosurg Psychiatry. 1994 Aug;57(8):886-96.

Marin B, Kacem I, Diagana M, Boulesteix M, Gouider R, Preux PM, Couratier P. *Juvenile and adult-onset ALS/MND among Africans: incidence, phenotype, survival: a review.* Amyotroph Lateral Scler. 2012 May;13(3):276-83.

Matuja WB, Aris EA. *Motor and non-motor features of Parkinson's disease.* East Afr Med J. 2008 Jan;85(1):3-9.

McInerney-Leo A, Gwinn-Hardy K, Nussbaum RL. *Prevalence of Parkinson's disease in populations of African ancestry: a review.* J Natl Med Assoc. 2004 Jul;96(7):974-9.

Moulignier A, Moulonguet A, Pialoux G, Rozenbaum W. *Reversible ALS-like disorder in HIV infection.* Neurology. 2001 Sep 25;57(6):995-1001.

Okubadejo NU, Bower JH, Rocca WA, Maraganore DM. *Parkinson's disease in Africa: A systematic review of epidemiologic and genetic studies.* Mov Disord. 2006 Dec;21(12):2150-6.

Okubadejo NU, Ojo OO, Oshinaike OO. *Clinical profile of parkinsonism and Parkinson's disease in Lagos, Southwestern Nigeria.* BMC Neurol. 2010 Jan 5;10:1

Schoenberg BS, Osuntokun BO, Adeuja AO, Bademosi O, Nottidge V, Anderson DW, et al. *Comparison of the prevalence of Parkinson's disease in black populations in the rural United States and in rural Nigeria: door-to-door community studies.* Neurology. 1988 Apr;38(4):645-6.

Tolosa E, Wenning G, Poewe W. *The diagnosis of Parkinson's disease.* Lancet Neurol. 2006 Jan;5(1):75-86.

Verma A, Berger JR. *ALS syndrome in patients with HIV-1 infection.* J Neurol Sci. 2006 Jan 15;240(1-2):59-64.

Winkler AS, Tutuncu E, Trendafilova A, Meindl M, Kaaya J, Schmutzhard E, et al. *Parkinsonism in a population of northern Tanzania: a community-based door-to-door study in combination with a prospective hospital-based evaluation.* J Neurol. 2010 May;257(5):799-805.

PART II – NEUROLOGICAL DISORDERS

CHAPTER 15
HEADACHE AND FACIAL PAIN

CONTENTS

CHAPTER 15

HEADACHE AND FACIAL PAIN

Headache is a very common problem which affects most persons at some point during their lives. The vast majority are due to tension headache, migraine and analgesic overuse. These are termed primary headaches and are mostly benign, but for some they are very debilitating disorders. The diagnosis of **primary headache** is made entirely from the history as there are no abnormal signs or investigations. A much smaller group consists of **secondary** or **medically serious headaches**. These headaches are caused by an underlying disease or disorder. This group includes infections, space occupying lesions, intracranial haemorrhage and usually have signs and abnormal investigations. It is important to separate these two groups clinically as they obviously have different implications for the patient. This chapter reviews the main headache disorders and facial pain and their investigation and treatment. After reading it the student should aim to be able to recognise and distinguish the medically serious headaches and the main primary headache disorders and also facial pain.

Pain

The brain itself is a painless organ. The source of the pain in headache arises from the structures overlying the brain; these include the scalp, skull, meninges and blood vessels. The dura and blood vessels are the most pain sensitive structures in the head. The site of the headache may sometimes be a guide to the origin of the headache. In general pain arising from the anterior and middle cranial fossa is referred to the forehead and front of the head whereas pain arising in the posterior fossa and upper cervical area is referred to the back of the head and neck. Pain arising from the surface of the brain tends to be diffuse, "all over" or occipital or nuchal as in meningitis or spread more focally over the overlying vertex or parietal and temporal areas as in tumours. Pain in the head may also be referred to the face, neck, ears, eyes, teeth and sinuses.

Classification

Headaches can be broadly classified into primary and secondary. The main causes are outlined below in Tables 15.1 & 15.4.

The history

A good history based on the temporal pattern of symptoms is essential in determining the cause of headache. This will include the time course, (onset, duration etc), site, severity, pattern and factors which alter or affect it. It is important to check specifically whether this is the first attack, the onset was sudden or gradual, continuous (daily) or intermittent (periodic), increasing or decreasing and whether the time course is acute (hours and days), sub acute (days and weeks) or chronic (months years). Determine the main site of the pain, whether it is unilateral or bilateral, frontal, temporal or occipital and its radiation. The character of the pain is also important, whether it is sharp or dull or throbbing in nature. Severity can be scored by the patient and recorded on a scale of 1-10, with 10 being the worst pain ever experienced and 1 the least. There may be some specific exacerbating factors e.g. movement, coughing, bending and relieving factors such as rest and analgesics. Check for any other associated symptoms and in particular whether there is any previous history of a similar headache or chronic analgesia intake.

Examination

Carefully record the vital signs including BP and check particularly for signs of raised intracranial pressure, meningism, tenderness of the temporal arteries, and focal neurological signs. Fundoscopy is essential as papilloedema may indicate raised intracranial pressure. Examine for local causes in the head and neck.

Key points

- headache is a common medical disorder
- vast majority of headaches are primary
- only a small minority are medically serious
- history is the most important part of evaluation of headache
- fundoscopy should be performed in all patients with persistent headaches

PRIMARY HEADACHES

The main primary headaches are tension, migraine, analgesic overuse, and cluster (Table 15.1).

Table 15.1 Main primary headaches

Primary	Frequency*	Site	Clinical Features	Treatment
Tension *(Chronic > 6/12)*	2-3%	bilateral, frontal, temporal, occipital, neck	dull, chronic, band like, scalp tenderness, episodic	reassurance, relaxation amitriptyline 10-25 mg/nocte 6-12 weeks
Migraine	5-10%	unilateral, frontal, bifrontal holocephalic, vertex, occipital	throbbing, moderate/severe, periodic, nausea or vomiting, photophobia, familial	avoid precipitants, regular sleep, aspirin, paracetamol, NSAIDs, ergotamine, triptans
Analgesic overuse	2%	bilateral, generalised	mild, bilateral, daily, migraine or tension like	stop all analgesics
Cluster headache	0.1%	unilateral, retro-orbital	very severe, redness & tearing, Horner's syndrome, mostly in men	100% oxygen, steroids, verapamil

based on studies in high income countries

TENSION HEADACHE

This is the most common form of headache experienced by most people during their lives. Tension headache is characterized by recurring daily attacks of mild to moderate bilateral headaches that may last from hours to weeks. The tension headache becomes chronic when it persists on >15 days per month and lasts for >6 consecutive months. Chronic tension headache affects 2-3% of adults in high income countries at any one time. A lower prevalence (0.4%) was reported in one study in Tanzania. The pain in tension headache is bilateral mostly occipital, also frontal or temporal in site and often described as a tight band around the head, starting within an hour or so of waking and increasing in severity throughout the day. It frequently radiates to the back of the neck. The severity may fluctuate with the patient going for days or weeks without noticing it. It is distinguished from migraine by its bilaterality, a lack of nausea and lack of discrete episodic attacks. The source of the pain is considered to be secondary to chronic muscle contraction of the scalp, neck and face although this may in itself be a secondary phenomenon. The scalp may be painful and tender on palpation and this may provide a useful clue to the diagnosis. There may be a background of anxiety and worry and a lack of response to ordinary analgesics.

Management

Management is by reassurance, regular exercise, relaxation and local measures. The dose of analgesics may need to be reduced and finally discontinued. Low dose amitriptyline 10-25 mg/po/nocte for 3-6 months may help to break the cycle in chronic tension headache but can take at least 4-6 weeks to work. Benzodiazepines although effective in the short term should be avoided because of the danger of habituation.

Key points

- tension, migraine & analgesic overuse are the main primary headaches
- tension headache is the most common & may persist for months or years
- frequently described as dull "like a tight band around my head"
- scalp may be tender to touch
- treatment includes stopping analgesics, increasing exercise & relaxation
- specific measures include low dose amitriptyline at night for 3-6 months

MIGRAINE

Migraine is a primary headache disorder characterized by periodic attacks that are variably associated with nausea, vomiting, and neurological symptoms. Pain is typically associated with increased sensitivity to light and noise. The attacks last 4-72 hours and their frequency is variable. The majority of patients have one attack or less per week which lasts <24 hours Migraine affects >10% of the world's population and its frequency is reported to be >5% in Africa. A family history of migraine is present in most patients and people usually suffer their first attack in their teens or early twenties, or before the age of 40 yrs. Women are affected twice as often as men. There are a number of well known triggers for individual attacks of migraine; these include stress, relaxation, fatigue, hunger, exercise, menstruation and specific foods including cheese, chocolate, red wine, citrus fruits, food additives and caffeine. Spontaneous remission may occur during pregnancy and after the menopause.

Clinical features

In over half of patients with migraine, the onset of headache is preceded in the first 24 hours by a prodrome of warning mood changes, cravings or hunger feelings. A typical migraine may begin with an aura in 10-20% of patients. It occurs characteristically during the hour before the onset of headache. The commonest aura is visual with bright zig zag lines and blurring or loss of vision. Less commonly, there may be tingling in one limb spreading to ipsilateral tongue and face and dysphasia. Rarely there is a temporary hemiplegia or even complete aphasia. The aura typically lasts a few minutes but sometimes may last longer. These symptoms precede the headache and mostly resolve as the headache starts. When these are present, it is called **classical migraine** or migraine with aura and when absent is called **common migraine**.

The next phase is the headache itself. The headache of migraine is characteristically dull at onset and later becomes throbbing, severe, usually unilateral, frontal, radiating to the neck. It may be bilateral in one third of patients. The headaches last between 4 hours and 3 days with most attacks lasting <24 hours. Normal physical activity usually makes the headache worse. The headache is often accompanied by pallor, nausea or vomiting and the need to lie in a quiet and darkened room. A period of sleep early on may abort the attack. The patient feels completely normal between the attacks but they can recur at variable intervals. Investigations are generally not necessary

Key points

- migraine affects >5% adults in Africa, females >males and clusters in families
- aura is characterized by bright zig zag lines and blurring or loss of vision
- headaches are periodic, mostly unilateral & throbbing lasting 4-72 hours
- associated with nausea/vomiting & visual/neurological disturbance

PATHOGENESIS

This involves abnormal nerve impulses originating mainly from the brain stem in the distribution of the trigeminal nerve and spreading to the cortex causing release of inflammatory substances and neuropeptides that stimulate pain fibres on meningeal arterioles. The symptoms of migraine have been attributed to an initial spreading occipital wave of vasoconstriction of cortical blood vessels with decreased blood flow (the aura phase) followed later by regional cortical vasodilatation (the headache phase). Serotonergic neurones occur extensively in the brain and brain stem and their involvement in migraine is suggested by the effectiveness of the 5–hydroxytryptamine (5-HT1) agonists e.g. the triptans in treating the headache phase of an acute attack.

Treatment

Identification of trigger factor(s) and avoiding them should be the first line of treatment. Attacks are often infrequent and mild, and resolve with simple analgesics such as aspirin, paracetamol or ibuprofen taken either alone or in combination with an antiemetic, like metoclopramide. Failing that the triptans are of great benefit (Table 15.2).The triptans are the drugs of first choice but are contraindicated in pregnancy, coronary artery disease, vascular disease, and uncontrolled hypertension. They are not recommended in hemiplegic migraine or in migraine with complex auras (sensory, motor or speech disturbances). They are recommended to be taken at the onset of the headache but not before. The main route is oral but if vomiting is a problem then triptans can be given either by nasal spray or subcutaneous injection. A second dose is usually effective for relapse within the first 6-48 hours. The side effects of triptans include chest discomfort and nausea and are more common with parenteral administration. Information on sumatriptan is outlined below, but any of the other triptans are equally efficacious.

An alternative cheaper treatment regime is ergotamine, however it should never be used in pregnancy and regular repeated usage is not recommended because of the danger of ergotism, gangrene, and rarely pulmonary fibrosis. Ergotamine is also contraindicated in peripheral and cardiovascular disease. It is important to note that the combined use together of a triptan and ergotamine is also contraindicated. If the patient is not responding to the combination of analgesics and antiemetics then triptans may be helpful

Table 15.2 Treatment of migraine

Acute treatment	Dose/range/frequency	Main side effects
Non specific treatment		
aspirin	300 mg tab, 2-3 tab/po/12 hourly	bleeding
paracetamol	500 mg tab, 2 tab/po/6 hourly	nausea
ibuprofen	2-400 mg tab, 1-2 tab/po/6-8 hourly	bleeding
metoclopramide/domperidone	10 mg tab, 1 tab/po/6-8 hourly	dyskinesia
Specific treatment		
Ergot derivatives		
ergotamine tartrate	1 mg tab, 2 tab/po or suppositories/at onset followed by 1 tab every 30 mins, (max 24 hours dose 6 mg, the total max weekly dose is 10 mg)	nausea, vomiting, ergotism
dihydroergotamine*	0.5-1mg/iv/8 hourly as required, (max total dose 10 mg, supervised)	
Triptans		
sumatriptan**	50 mg tabs, 1 or 2 tab/po/at onset, repeat in 2 hours, (max 24 hour dose 200 mg) *or* 6 mg/sc/at onset, repeat in 2 hours, (max 24 hour dose 12 mg) *or* 5-20 mg/nasal spray at onset, repeat in 2 hours, (max 24 hour dose 40 mg)	chest tightness, paraesthesiae, fatigue

used only in intractable migraine in specialist headache units
***other triptans are equally effective*

PROPHYLAXIS

Dietary triggers for migraine should be avoided and oestrogen containing contraceptives used with caution. Preventative treatment reduces the frequency, severity and duration of the attacks (Table 15.3). If the frequency is weekly or greater or the attacks are disabling, then those patients may benefit from daily prophylaxis. Medications used in prophylaxis and their dosages and main side effects are outlined below, and the initial treatment duration is for 3-6 months. The most commonly used options include amitriptyline, beta-blockers and sodium valproate. The anticonvulsant topiramate can also be very effective in cases resistant to other medications, but it is more expensive.

Table 15.3 Prophylaxis of Migraine

Medication	Dosage/range/frequency	Main side effects
Beta blockers		
propranolol	10-80 (160) mg/po/bid	postural hypotension, fatigue
atenolol	50-200 mg/po/daily	
Tricyclics		
amitriptyline	10-100 mg nocte	dry mouth, sedation, urinary retention
Anticonvulsants		
sodium valproate	250-750 mg/po/bid	nausea, weight gain, alopecia, tremor, liver dysfunction
topiramate	25–50 mg bid	renal stones, paraesthesia, weight loss
Calcium channel blockers		
verapamil	40-160 mg/po/tid	constipation, fatigue, oedema
5-HT2 antagonists		
pizotifen	0.5-3 mg/po/daily	weight gain

Key points

- majority do not require treatment or respond to simple analgesics & antiemetics
- triptans are the treatment of choice but are expensive and have contraindications
- ergotamine preparations may also be used at onset but have contraindications
- if attacks are severe or >1 per week then daily prophylaxis is recommended
- main prophylaxis includes beta blockers or anticonvulsants in adequate doses

ANALGESIC OVERUSE HEADACHE

These are a group of headaches lasting longer than 4 hours a day which persist for at least 15 days every month for at least 3 months. The term chronic daily headache (CDH) is also used to describe them. These are usually cases of transformed migraine or chronic tension headaches and may affect over 2% of the population in high income countries, most commonly females. These occur mostly as a result of prolonged use of analgesics including simple analgesics, non steroidal anti-inflammatory drugs (NSAIDs), opiates, ergotamine and triptans. Patients typically complain of daily throbbing bilateral headaches which are only transiently and incompletely relieved by increasing doses of medications. Neurological examination is entirely normal.

Management

The management aim is to decrease the frequency, severity and duration of the headaches by complete withdrawal of medication. The patient will need to be encouraged to have a regular life style and avoid caffeine and be specifically educated about the overuse of analgesics. In particular they will need to understand that there will be persisting symptoms including headaches, nausea, agitation and insomnia, particularly during the first two weeks after stopping. Withdrawal for ordinary analgesics, ergotamine and triptans should be carried out abruptly over a period of 24-48 hours. Withdrawal of opioids may take a period of 2-4 weeks. Remission occurs 2-12 weeks after withdrawal. The patient may need interim symptomatic treatment with an antiemetic, NSAIDs and occasionally a brief course of steroids. Underlying anxiety and depression may also need to be treated. Preventive medications include amitriptyline 10-50 mg/po/nocte.

Key points

- analgesic overuse is a cause of chronic daily headache
- most common sources of CDH are chronic tension headaches & transformed migraine
- management is abrupt withdrawal of all non opioid medication over 24-48 hours
- opioids may take 2-4 weeks to withdraw

CLUSTER HEADACHE

This is an excruciatingly severe, unilateral, headache located around one eye and accompanied by local autonomic dysfunction, redness, swelling and watering of the eye. It occurs in high income countries with a frequency of approximately 1/1000. It has its onset mostly in the 3rd and 4th decade and the male female ratio is about 5:1. It receives its name from its tendency to cluster usually 1-3 times daily (can be up to 8 times) for periods of 3-6 weeks or longer at a time with long intervals, sometimes years completely free of attacks. The attacks are brief, lasting between 30-120 minutes, in contrast to migraine which persists for 4-72 hours. Cluster headaches typically occur at the same time in the 24 hour cycle often waking the patient from sleep.

Management

Stopping the acute attacks of pain quickly is critical. These can be well controlled by inhalation via a mask of 100% oxygen @ 7-10 litres/min for 15-20 minutes. Triptans can be successful if used by injections (e.g. sumatriptan 6 mg/sc) or intranasally (sumatriptan 20 mg). Alternatives include zolmitriptan 5 mg orally. They can be repeated once in 24 hours but should be avoided in patients with multiple attacks because of the danger of overuse. Concomitant use of ergot drugs is absolutely contraindicated because of the danger of a stroke. Prophylaxis during a cluster can be helpful with high dose steroids, prednisolone 60 mg/po/daily for 5 days decreasing by 10 mg every 3 days. Long term prevention is indicated for chronic cluster headaches. This includes verapamil 80 mg bd for 2 weeks increasing by 80 mg every 2 weeks to a maximum of 320 mg bd or tds. Avoiding tobacco and alcohol is also important.

Key points

- cluster headache is severe, unilateral with redness and tearing of the eye
- recognised by its distinctive pain, recurrence and male preponderance
- acute attack can be treated with 100% oxygen inhalation or as for migraine
- prophylaxis is with high dose steroids or verapamil for 1-2 months

SECONDARY HEADACHES

The main causes of secondary headaches are intracranial tumours, infections, intracranial haemorrhage, temporal arteritis and benign intracranial hypertension (Table 15.4). Other causes to be considered include hypertension, arterial dissection, head injury, brain abscess, subdural haematoma and medications. Secondary headaches may lead to serious consequences if the underlying cause is not identified and treated.

Table 15.4 Secondary headaches

Main Causes	Onset	Type	Clinical features
Tumour	sub acute	severe, generalised, worse on waking, aggravated by coughing & straining	↑ICP & FNDs*
Meningitis	acute/sub acute	severe, generalised & meningism	fever, neck stiffness & Kernig's sign
Subarachnoid haemorrhage	acute	explosive, thunderclap & meningism	neck stiffness, Kernig's sign, ± FNDs*
Temporal arteritis	sub acute	non specific/uni/bilateral	tender temporal arteries, blindness, age >50-60 yrs, ESR>60
Benign intracranial hypertension	sub acute	throbbing, visual obscurations & loss)	female, young, overweight, visual loss, papilloedema, 6th nerve palsy, gait ataxia

focal neurological disorders/deficits

INTRACRANIAL TUMOUR

The majority of patients presenting with brain tumour do not have headaches. The headache of an expanding intracranial tumour is produced by raised intracranial pressure and is often described as bursting and severe in nature. The pain is typically continuous and increases in severity over weeks or months. Characteristically it is present on waking in the morning or may wake the patient at night and improves during the day. It is aggravated by measures that increase intracranial pressure; these include lifting, bending, lying down, coughing, sneezing and straining. The distribution of the pain is either generalized or referred to the fronto/temporal area, or vertex/occipital area depending on the site of origin of the tumour. The presence of nausea, vomiting, visual disturbances, altered level of consciousness all suggest raised intracranial pressure.

Neurological examination should check carefully for papilloedema (Chapter 12) and focal neurological findings. A CT scan of the head is indicated in patients when a SOL is suspected. Details on brain tumours, abscess, subdural haematoma and other space occupying lesions are presented elsewhere in this textbook (Chapters 6, 7, 16 & 19).

Key points

- majority of patients with headache do not have an intracranial tumour
- clinical features include bursting pain on waking, increasing over time, worse on coughing/straining
- tumours rarely present with headache alone & usually have FNDs or ↑ICP
- head CT scan is indicated in patients with suspected SOL

MENINGISM

Meningism results from inflammation or irritation of the meninges. The two major causes are meningitis and subarachnoid haemorrhage (Chapters 5 & 6). The headache in meningitis is usually severe, generalised and associated with fever, photophobia and signs of meningism including neck stiffness and Kernig's sign. In subarachnoid haemorrhage the headache is typically sudden or explosive in onset with vomiting and meningism. Diagnosis is confirmed by lumbar puncture. Headaches frequently occur with other CNS infections including encephalitis.

Key points

- headache in meningitis is severe & generalised
- headache in SAH is sudden and explosive
- both result in symptoms and signs of meningism

TEMPORAL ARTERITIS (TA)

In persons >50 yrs old the extra cranial vessels may become inflamed with an arteritis. The arteritis causes a new onset, severe, throbbing, mostly bilateral headache and exquisite local scalp tenderness. The headache may be non specific at onset later localizing to the temples. Exacerbation of headache with chewing suggests the diagnosis. On palpation, the superficial temporal artery may be hot, tender, swollen and non pulsatile. Other arteries may be similarly affected and blockage of the ophthalmic artery may result in transient blindness which can become permanent in about 25% of cases. Strokes are not uncommon. Females are affected more frequently than males and temporal arteritis is associated with polymyalgia rheumatica. The ESR is characteristically elevated >60 mm/hr. The age of onset is usually >60 yrs. Diagnosis is confirmed by a temporal artery biopsy which ideally should be performed early on but this may not always be practical.

Management is with immediate high dose steroids as soon as the diagnosis is suspected without waiting for investigation results. Prednisolone 60 mg/po/daily is prescribed for a total of 2-3 months and then tapering to a maintenance dose of 5-10 mg on alternate days. The response to steroids is usually dramatic, often within the first 24-48 hours. Steroids may be needed for a total of 18-24 months or until symptoms fully clear. Treatment is guided by monitoring the ESR.

Key points

- headache in TA is intense, focal & localised to the temples
- temporal arteries may be tender on palpation
- blindness and strokes are major complications
- both patient's age and the ESR are generally >60
- treatment: high dose daily steroids for 2-3/12 & maintenance dose for 18-24/12

BENIGN INTRACRANIAL HYPERTENSION (BIH)

It is an uncommon disorder characterized by headaches with elevated intracranial pressure without any evident cause. It is more widely known in Africa as pseudotumour cerebri. This occurs mostly in young, overweight females in their 20s and 30s. The oral contraceptive pill is a risk factor. Patients typically present with a severe morning throbbing type headache often associated with nausea, vomiting and sometimes visual disturbances. Visual disturbances include transient often postural episodes of loss of vision lasting seconds, as well as more sustained blurring and sometimes permanent loss of vision. The characteristic finding is **bilateral papilloedema**. Neurological examination is otherwise normal apart from occasional isolated 6th nerve palsy and a mild gait ataxia. The differential diagnosis includes the other causes of medically serious headaches including cerebral venous sinus thrombosis. Brain imaging with a CT is always normal but should be carried out in order to exclude another organic cause. The diagnosis is confirmed by finding an elevated CSF opening pressure of >250 mm on lumbar puncture.

Management

Acute treatment measures include repeated lumbar punctures in combination with high dose steroids used over 3-5 days. The main long term management includes weight loss, stopping the contraceptive pill and a diuretic, **acetazolamide tablets 250 mg tid**. Furosemide is an alternative diuretic. BIH remits spontaneously after these measures in many patients but the measures, in particular **weight loss**, have to be vigorously adhered to. If there is visual loss, (decreased visual acuity, and constricted visual fields) then a lumboperitoneal CSF shunt or optic nerve sheath fenestration should be considered to prevent permanent blindness.

Key points

- BIH presents as headaches, visual disturbances & papilloedema
- typically occurs in young overweight females taking the contraceptive pill
- neurological investigations are normal including neuroimaging
- acute measures include steroids over first 3-5 days and repeated lumbar punctures
- long-term management includes weight loss, diuretics & stopping the pill

Other causes of headache

Other primary headaches include trigeminal neuralgia (see below under facial pain), exertional and coital headaches. These latter headache types are precipitated by exercise or sexual activity. These are benign but can mimic a SAH and this may need to be excluded.

FACIAL PAIN

Facial pain has many local causes including diseases of the eyes, ears, nose, sinuses, throat, teeth and temporomandibular joints and referred pain. Neurologic causes of facial pain need to be distinguished from local causes. Many of the neurological disorders which cause headache may also cause facial pain; these include cluster headache, temporal arteritis and occasionally migraine. However there are some neurological disorders where the pain is restricted to the face, these include trigeminal neuralgia, post herpetic neuralgia and atypical facial pain. The local causes of facial pain are usually determined clinically by their site and associated clinical findings.

TRIGEMINAL NEURALGIA (TN)

This is a very painful disorder affecting the trigeminal nerve. It affects persons of all age groups but mostly those over the age of 40 yrs. It is more common in females than males. Previously no cause was found in most patients with trigeminal neuralgia and these were termed idiopathic. However many of what were previously termed to be idiopathic causes have been shown by MRI to be due to compression of the trigeminal sensory nerve root near the brain stem by an aberrant arterial branch. Secondary causes include herpetic infection and a cerebellopontine angle tumour compressing the trigeminal nerve during its intracranial course.

Clinical features

Patients with trigeminal neuralgia typically present with unilateral facial pain in the distribution of one or more divisions of the trigeminal nerve. The pains are characteristically sudden, severe, brief, shooting, electric shock like, lancinating or knife like stabs in the distribution of one or more branches of the trigeminal nerve. The attack lasts less than a second usually affecting only one side of the face, typically the corner of the mouth or nose. There are frequently trigger areas on the face where any stimulus however gentle may produce pain. The pain may be triggered by touching, talking, eating, drinking cold or hot liquids or cleaning teeth. The stabs of pains can recur continuously many times per day. Between the stabs there may be a lingering continuous background pain but it is usually much less severe.

The natural history is one of remission but only after weeks or months of facial pain and the neuralgia typically recurs again after a few months. Spontaneous remission can occur. The differential diagnosis includes local causes of facial pain including dental infections, sinusitis, disease of the temporomandibular joint and other atypical forms of facial pain

Management

The pain does not respond to simple analgesics and requires adequate doses of anticonvulsants for control. Carbamazepine is the drug of first choice and a favourable response to treatment is diagnostic of TN. The standard starting dose is 100 mg/po/bd increased as needed over the next few days or weeks. A usual therapeutic and maintenance dose of carbamazepine is 200 to 400 mg twice or three times daily. This may be continued for a period of one or two months depending on the duration of the episode of facial pain and the patient's tolerance of the drug side effects. Drowsiness and ataxia are the main limiting side effects. Second line drugs include gabapentin, pregabalin, phenytoin and sodium valproate. If the pain becomes intractable or intolerable and an adequate trial of drug treatment fails then the nerve can be considered for interruption either temporarily with an injection of alcohol or more permanently with phenol, glycerol or a destructive procedure.

Key points

- trigeminal neuralgia is very painful & affects branches of trigeminal nerve
- recurring shooting facial pains lasting less than a second are diagnostic
- pain is triggered by touching, eating, hot & cold, cleaning teeth & talking
- natural history is remission but both attacks and remissions last months
- carbamazepine taken in adequate doses daily is the treatment of choice

Selected references

Dent W, Stelzhammer B, Meindl M, Matuja WB, Schmutzhard E, Winkler AS. *Migraine attack frequency, duration, and pain intensity: disease burden derived from a community-based survey in northern Tanzania*. Headache. 2011 Nov-Dec;51(10):1483-92.

Ginsberg Lionel. *Neurology, Lecture Notes*. Blackwell Publishing 8th edition 2005.

Goadsby PJ. *Headache (chronic tension-type)*. Clin Evid. 2003 Dec(10):1538-46.

Manji Hadi, Connolly Sean, Dorward Neil, Kitchen Neil, Metha Amrish, & Wills Adrian. *Oxford*

Handbook of Neurology. Oxford University Press 1st edition 2007

Ofovwe GE, Ofili AN. *Prevalence and impact of headache and migraine among secondary school students in Nigeria.* Headache. 2010 Nov;50(10):1570-5.

Ojini FI, Okubadejo NU, Danesi MA. *Prevalence and clinical characteristics of headache in medical students of the University of Lagos, Nigeria.* Cephalalgia. 2009 Apr;29(4):472-7.

Silberstein SD. *Migraine.* Lancet. 2004 Jan 31;363(9406):381-91.

Steiner TJ, Fontebasso M. *Headache.* BMJ. 2002 Oct 19;325(7369):881-6.

Takele GM, Tekle Haimanot R, Martelletti P. *Prevalence and burden of primary headache in Akaki textile mill workers, Ethiopia.* J Headache Pain. 2008 Apr;9(2):119-28.

Wahab KW, Ugheoke AJ. Migraine: *prevalence and associated disability among Nigerian undergraduates.* Can J Neurol Sci. 2009 Mar;36(2):216-21.

Warlow Charles. *The Lancet Handbook of treatment in Neurology.* Elsevier, 1st edition 2006.

Winkler A, Stelzhammer B, Kerschbaumsteiner K, Meindl M, Dent W, Kaaya J, et al. *The prevalence of headache with emphasis on tension-type headache in rural Tanzania: a community-based study.* Cephalalgia. 2009 Dec;29(12):1317-25.

Winkler AS, Dent W, Stelzhammer B, Kerschbaumsteiner K, Meindl M, Kaaya J, et al. *Prevalence of migraine headache in a rural area of northern Tanzania: a community-based door-to-door survey.* Cephalalgia. 2010 May;30(5):582-92.

CHAPTER 16
INTRACRANIAL TUMOURS

CONTENTS

CHAPTER 16

INTRACRANIAL TUMOURS

Intracranial tumours (ICT) include tumours arising from the brain or surrounding tissues. They are classified as either primary or secondary and as malignant or benign. Other classifications include tissue type, grade of malignancy and the main site affected. Primary intracranial tumours originate mostly from brain or meninges whereas secondary or metastatic tumours originate mostly elsewhere in the body. The most common primary tumours are gliomas accounting for between 30-50% of all adult intracranial tumours. Gliomas are malignant tumours which arise from glial support cells rather than neuronal cells and are termed astrocytoma, oligodendroglioma, ependymoma and pinealoma.

The most common primary benign tumours are meningiomas. These arise from the meninges covering the brain and cranial nerves accounting for 20-30% of all adult intracranial tumours. Other benign intracranial tumours are pituitary adenoma, craniopharyngioma, colloid cyst and acoustic neuroma. The aim of this chapter is to present an overview of the main intracranial tumours. The student should aim to know the main types of tumour, their clinical presentation, diagnosis and management.

EPIDEMIOLOGY

The incidence of primary intracranial tumours in high income countries is 1-2/10,000 per year. The incidence in Africa is not known but some studies suggest they may be less frequent there. The cause of most brain tumours is not known but some are related to genetic factors, radiation exposure and possibly environment. Primary intracranial tumours account for the majority, 70-80% of all intracranial tumours, with metastatic tumours accounting for the remaining 20-30% (Table 16.1). The frequency of intracranial tumour increases with age and metastatic tumours are most common in older age groups.

Table 16.1 Estimated intracranial tumour type (%) in Africa

Most common		Uncommon	
Glioma	30-50%	Craniopharyngioma	2-5%
Metastases	20-30%	Lymphoma	1%
Meningioma	20-30%	Acoustic neuroma	<1%
Pituitary adenoma	10-15%	Pinealoma	<1%
		Colloid cyst	<1%

CLINICAL FEATURES

Intracranial tumours in Africa are characterised by late presentation with on average a 2 year delay before diagnosis and a high mortality of >80% at 1-2 years follow up. They can exist for long periods with no or few symptoms and when symptoms do occur the tumours may be advanced. Headache is the most common complaint though occurring only in <50% of cases. Pain is variable, ranging from being dull, low grade and intermittent to being severe, continuous, deep, nocturnal, present on waking and often associated with vomiting. Intracranial tumours have three recognizable main modes of clinical presentation (Table 16.2): (1) focal neurological deficits (FND), (2) seizures, and (3) raised intracranial pressure (↑ICP). These can occur either alone or together depending on type, stage and site of tumour. The pathogenic mechanisms underlying these presentations include tumour mass effect, brain irritation and blocked CSF flow. Highly malignant or fast growing tumours tend to present with combinations of all three main modes of presentation occurring over weeks or months whereas low grade or slow growing tumours tend to present with isolated seizures and/or neurological deficits occurring over months or years. The age of the patient, speed of onset of symptoms and neurological findings all help to determine the site and the probable type of tumour.

Table 16.2 Main presenting clinical features of intracranial tumours

Neurological finding	Symptoms/Signs
focal neurological deficits	hemiparesis, dysphasia, visual loss, field defect, ataxia, cranial nerve palsies
raised intracranial pressure	headaches vomiting, papilloedema, LOC
seizures	simple or complex partial, secondary GTC

Focal neurological deficits

FND are the most common neurological presentation of brain tumour. The type of FND is very variable and reflects the cell type, grade of malignancy and the site affected (Chapter 2). These include hemiparesis, dysphasia, visual loss, field defects, cognitive impairment, personality change, cranial nerve palsies and ataxia. The combination of ataxia and cranial nerve palsies occurs more frequently with tumours arising in the posterior fossa.

Seizures

Seizures are the presenting complaint in approximately a quarter of patients and occur as a complication in about another quarter (Chapter 4). Seizures arise mostly from tumours affecting the temporal lobes and occur most commonly in association with malignant tumours. The seizures are mostly generalised tonic clonic-type seizures with a focal origin.

Raised intracranial pressure (↑ICP)

The symptoms and signs of ↑ICP are headache, vomiting, papilloedema and altered level of consciousness; these occur because of either mass effect or hydrocephalus. Hydrocephalus arises because of mechanical blockage to CSF flow through the ventricles. Headache is the most common symptom being typically severe in advanced tumours, often waking the person from sleep during the night or early morning and frequently associated with vomiting (Chapter 15). The site of the headache is mostly frontal in supratentorial tumours and occipital in posterior fossa tumours, however the site may not necessarily be localising. Mass lesions arising from above the tentorium, and affecting both the hemispheres frequently give rise to combinations of features of FNDs and ↑ICP. The most common neurological deficits include hemiparesis and 3rd, 4th and 6th nerve palsies. These may be false localising signs, if they occur as a result of remote compression at a site away from the tumour. Space occupying lesions (SOL) arising below the tentorium within the posterior fossa cause cranial nerve palsies, ataxia, and long track signs and raised ICP secondary to obstructive hydrocephalus. A history of visual disturbances and the presence of papilloedema are usually late clinical findings. Eventually, the expanding tumour results in herniation either through the tentorium or foramen magnum leading to death.

Key points

- most common malignant ICTs are gliomas & metastases
- most common benign ICTs are meningiomas & pituitary adenomas
- main presentations include progressive FNDs, seizures & ↑ICP
- other presentations are headaches, visual failure, cranial nerve signs & seizures
- most patients presenting with headaches do not have brain tumours

MAIN SITES

The site and types of intracranial tumour determine the presenting symptoms and signs and the main ones are outlined below (Chapter 2).

Frontal lobe

Tumours involving the frontal lobe typically present late because the frontal lobe has a large silent area. Contralateral hemiparesis occurs if the motor strip is involved. Tumours involving the anterior frontal lobe may present with personality changes and a loss of initiative, inhibition and cognitive function. There may also be focal motor seizures, urinary incontinence and loss of smell. An expressive aphasia occurs if Broca's area in the dominant hemisphere is involved.

Parietal lobe

Tumours of the parietal lobe result in difficulties or inability to recognise sensory and proprioceptive input from the opposite side of the body. This may show itself as tending to ignore the contralateral side visuospatially (hemineglect) or as difficulties recognizing familiar shapes, textures or numbers when placed in the opposite hand (astereognosia). If the dominant hemisphere is involved, there may be difficulties particularly with understanding speech, numbers, reading and writing and carrying out motor tasks (apraxia). Patients with non dominant hemisphere involvement may present with or develop hemineglect. Patients may also have a visual field defect involving the lower quadrant from the opposite side.

Temporal lobe

Tumours involving the dominant temporal lobe (usually left sided) may result in aphasia which is receptive in type and also memory impairment. Tumours on either side may result in recent onset temporal lobe seizures and visual field loss in the contralateral upper quadrant.

Occipital lobe

Tumours involving the occipital lobe present with visual disturbances, hallucinations, and a loss of vision from the opposite side of the body, a contralateral homonymous hemianopia.

Brain stem and cerebellum

Tumours of the brain stem present with a combination of ipsilateral cranial nerve palsies and cerebellar ataxia, and contralateral long tract signs. These may be associated with hydrocephalus and ↑ICP depending on the tumour type and site. Tumours involving this area of the brain are more common in children.

GLIOMA

Gliomas account for up to half of all brain tumours and occur most commonly in older age groups >50-60 years. Glioma is the generic name for brain tumours of neuroepithelial cell origin. These are the support cells in the brain and the main ones are astrocytes and oligodendrocytes. Astrocytic tumours are separated histologically into grades I & II which are low grade, well differentiated and relatively benign and into grades III & IV which are high grade, poorly differentiated and highly malignant. Glioblastoma multiforme represents the most malignant stage of glioma. Oligodendrogliomas on the whole tend to be lower grade tumours characterized by a capsule and the presence of cysts and calcium with a good prognosis, but after years about one third may evolve into more malignant tumours.

Other forms of glioma include ependymomas which are derived from cells which line the ventricles and choroid plexus. Medulloblastomas are gliomas of the cerebellum and the roof of the 4th ventricle occurring mostly in young children aged 4-8 years (Fig. 16.1).

Clinical features

Gliomas present clinically with increasing symptoms usually over weeks or months or years depending on the grade of malignancy. Presentations include headache and combinations of focal neurological deficit, seizures, and signs of ↑ICP. Diagnosis is confirmed by neuroimaging, most commonly a CT of the head. It typically shows a unifocal enhancing mass with surrounding oedema and mass effect (Fig. 16.1).

Management

Management where there are full resources includes a combination of surgery, chemotherapy and radiotherapy. Surgery is indicated for biopsy to establish a tissue diagnosis and for partial tumour resection to relieve symptoms. Chemotherapy is used in high grade malignant gliomas and usually involves the alkylating drug temozolomide in combination with other drugs. However temozolomide is expensive, used mostly but not exclusively in younger patients and only available in some specialized oncology units. Radiation is indicated for most high grade gliomas but this is only palliative at this stage.

Prognosis

The prognosis in low grade gliomas is good with a median survival of 8-10 years. However in patients with higher grade malignancy the prognosis even with treatment is poor with survival of usually <12 months.

Key points

- gliomas account for almost half of all ICTs
- presentations include ↑ICP, FNDs & seizures over weeks & months
- diagnosis is by neuroimaging, CT or MRI
- management is mainly with combination of surgery, chemotherapy & radiotherapy
- prognosis for high grade gliomas is poor

CT (with contrast)

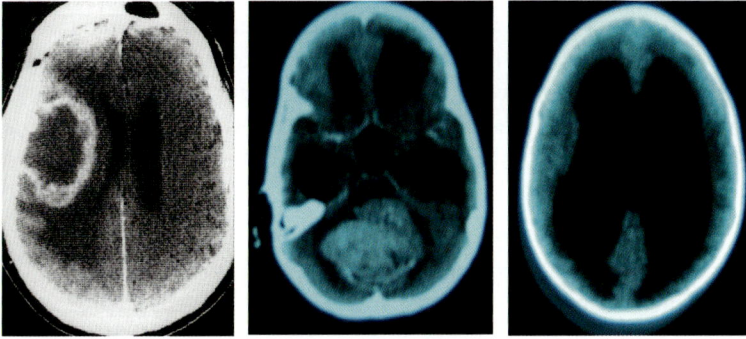

Right frontal glioma   Medulloblastoma & hydrocephalus in a child

MRI T1 & T2 (enhanced)

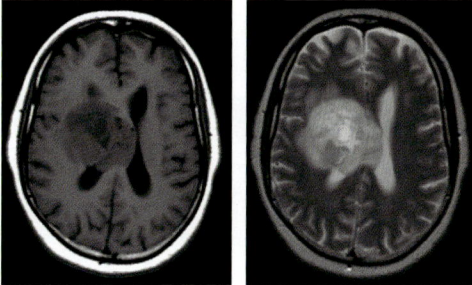

Right sided glioma with midline extension/shift

Figure 16.1 Gliomas

MENINGIOMA

These account for about 20-30% of all intracranial tumours. They occur mostly in the middle and older age groups, >50 years and more commonly in females 2:1. They arise from either the dural or arachnoid meninges, overlying the surface of the brain, cranial nerves, falx and tentorium and are nearly always benign. Less than 1% of meningiomas are malignant. Small meningiomas <2 cm are usually asymptomatic and tumours only become symptomatic when they reach a size sufficient to affect function. Most tumours arise on the convexities of the brain, as these are the largest surface areas.

Clinical features

Meningiomas tend to present clinically with focal neurological signs that reflect the site and size of the tumour in much the same way as malignant tumours but over a much longer time course usually months or years. Focal seizures are an early symptom of tumours that overlie the cortex. ↑ICP may also be a late feature of large meningiomas. Meningiomas affecting certain areas have specific modes of presentation. Parasagittal meningiomas present with spastic paraparesis, olfactory groove meningiomas with anosmia and papilloedema and sphenoid wing and frontal meningiomas with Foster-Kennedy syndrome: unilateral optic atrophy with contralateral papilloedema.

Diagnosis & management

Diagnosis is made by neuroimaging with CT or MRI scans. CT typically shows a meningioma as a uniformly homogenously enhancing extra axial mass which may be partially calcified or eroding adjacent bone (Fig.16.2). The majority of accessible meningiomas can be cured by resection and large symptomatic tumours are an indication for surgery. Convexity lesions are usually completely removed without any residual neurological deficit and the longer term prognosis for these is generally good. However recurrence is likely if surgical removal is incomplete as is frequently the case with very large or relatively inaccessible tumours. If the patient is clinically asymptomatic, then yearly follow up CT scans may be sufficient.

Key points

- meningioma is the most common benign ICT & occurs mostly in older persons
- symptoms can be similar to malignant tumours but occurring over a longer time period
- clinical presentations tend to reflect the site of the tumour
- diagnosis is confirmed by neuroimaging CT/MRI
- management for large, symptomatic meningiomas is surgical removal

CT (with contrast)

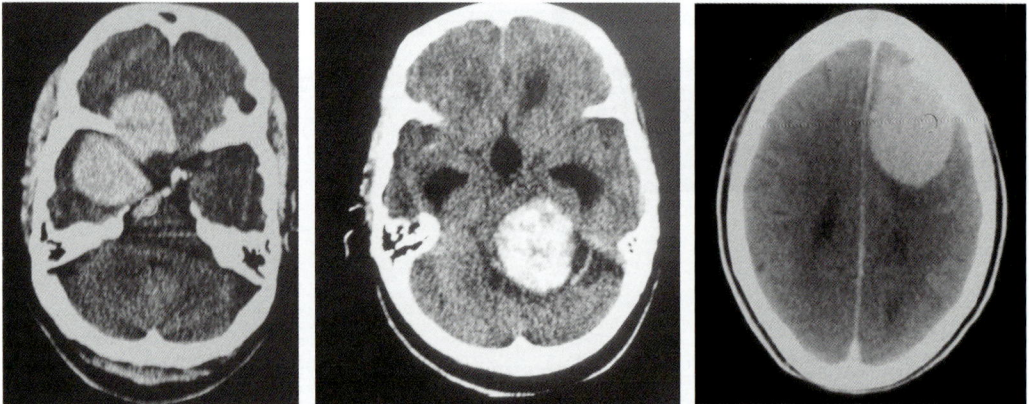

Right sphenoid wing   Left cerebellar tentorium (hydrocephalus)   Left frontal

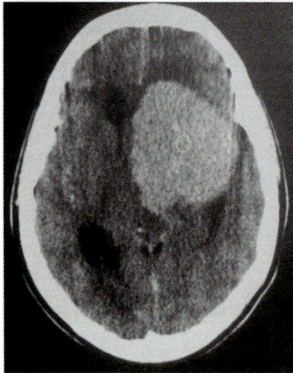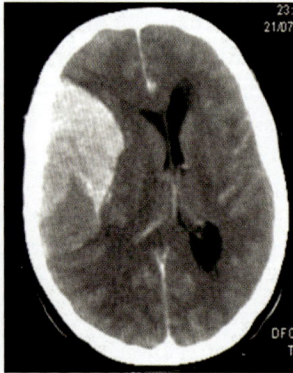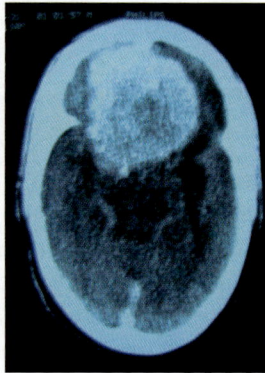

Left frontal   Right frontal   Midline

Figure 16.2 Meningiomas

PITUITARY TUMOURS

Pituitary adenomas account for about a tenth of all intracranial tumours.

Clinical features

These are benign intracranial tumours occurring outside the brain which present with headache, local pressure and also endocrine effects. Expansion of the adenoma upwards leads to compression of the optic chiasm which results in a visual field defect, most commonly bitemporal hemianopia, initially involving the upper quadrants. The endocrine effects may vary from being clinically asymptomatic in non functioning adenomas, to prolactinomas causing amenorrhoea/galactorrhoea and to micro or macro adenomas secreting growth hormone in acromegaly or microadenoma secreting ACTH in Cushing's disease. Infrequently, pituitary tumours undergo infarction and patients then present with sudden headache, vomiting and features of acute hypopituitarism. The differential diagnosis of pituitary tumours includes other mass lesions that may compress the optic chiasm including craniopharyngioma, meningioma and internal carotid aneurysm.

Diagnosis

Diagnosis is confirmed by endocrine and imaging studies. Endocrine studies should measure prolactin, TSH (thyroid stimulating hormone), free T4, morning cortisol and growth hormone levels if available. A plain skull X-ray may show an enlarged pituitary fossa and neuroimaging with a CT or preferably an MRI may show a pituitary tumour (Fig.16.3).

Skull X-ray (lateral view)

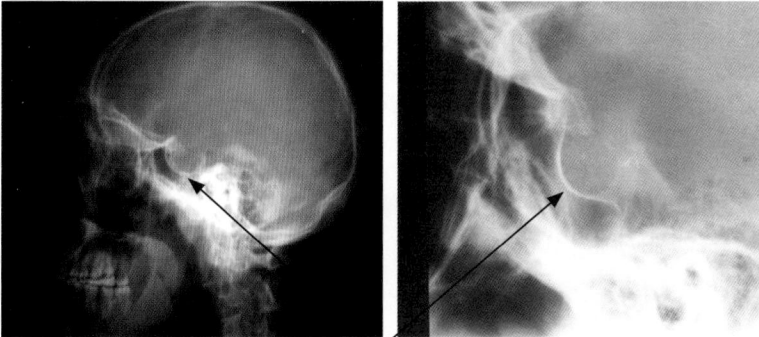

Widened sella turcica

CT (with contrast)   **MRI T1**

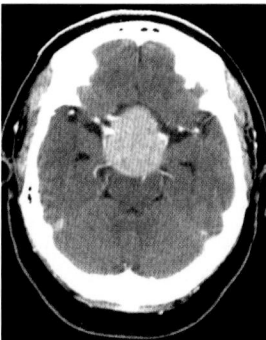

Pituitary tumour

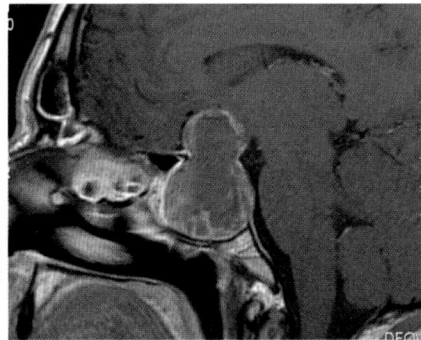

Figure 16.3 Pituitary tumours

Management

Management is either medical or surgical. Surgery via the transphenoidal route is usually the management of choice, if the tumour is intrasellar except in prolactin secreting adenomas which can often be managed medically with dopamine receptor agonists such as bromocriptine up to 20-40 mg daily. Growth hormone secreting tumours can also sometimes be managed medically as well with dopamine agonists or a somatostatin analogue (e.g. octreotide). Larger pituitary tumours extending above the sella may require a transfrontal craniotomy.

Key points

- pituitary tumours are benign and account for about 10% of ICTs
- symptoms are caused by local pressure effects, hormone secretion & pituitary failure
- CFs include headache, visual failure, visual field defect & endocrine disease
- treatment involves hormone replacement, dopamine agonists & surgery

METASTASES

These account for about a quarter of all intracranial tumours and are usually the most common intracranial tumour in the older age groups >60 yrs. They arise mostly by haematogenous spread from cancers occurring outside the brain. The main sources are breast, lung, renal, gastrointestinal cancers and melanoma. Very rarely local metastases can arise within the brain; the usual source is a glioblastoma, the most malignant type of brain tumour. The history in metastatic brain tumour is usually short, involving day or weeks of progressive neurological symptoms of raised intracranial pressure, seizures and focal neurological deficits. Diagnosis is confirmed by neuroimaging usually a CT of the head. Metastases show as multiple ring or solid enhancing lesions anywhere in the brain with surrounding oedema and mass effect (Fig. 16.4). In about 10% of cases the metastases may be solitary.

CT (with contrast)

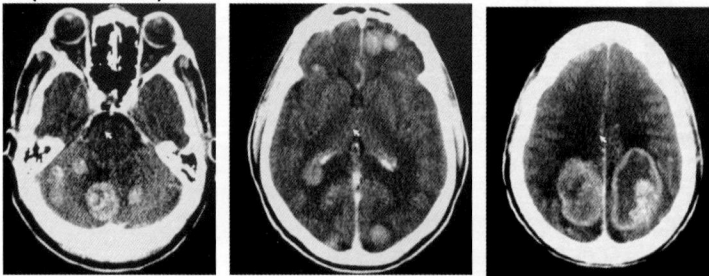

Multiple metastases

Figure 16.4 Metastases

Differential diagnosis

The differential diagnosis of intracranial tumour includes other causes of mass or space occupying lesions (SOL). In Africa these are mostly infections. The most common infectious causes are HIV related and include toxoplasma encephalitis and tuberculoma. Other infectious causes include pyogenic and parasitic infections. The main parasitic infections are hydatid cysts, cysticercosis and very occasionally schistosomiasis. While there may be some difficulty separating a tumour from these causes clinically, the history and signs of systemic illness and typical neuroimaging findings should suggest an infectious origin. The non infectious causes are mostly vascular and include large aneurysms and arteriovenous malformations. These can usually be differentiated from metastatic brain tumours by their typical history, vascular risk factors and appearances on CT scan. A chronic subdural haematoma particularly in the elderly without a history of head trauma may sometimes mimic a brain tumour in clinical presentation and require a CT scan of the head to confirm the correct diagnosis. Other neurological disorders to be considered include hydrocephalus and benign intracranial hypertension.

Investigations

Baseline haematological and biochemical investigations should be carried out in suspected cases. X-rays involving the chest and skull can be helpful. The chest X-ray may show evidence of metastases or a primary lung tumour. The skull X-ray may show enlargement of the pituitary fossa, erosion of bone or other signs of chronic raised intracranial pressure. A lumbar puncture is relatively contraindicated in patients with suspected intracranial tumours and possible ↑ICP as any sudden decrease in intracranial pressure can result in death due to coning. Neuroimaging using computerized tomography (CT) or magnetic resonance imaging (MRI) is the method of choice in the detection of brain tumours. CT is now available in most specialised centres. In patients with a suspected brain tumour having neuroimaging, intravenous contrast is given unless there is a contraindication; a pattern of increased enhancement points to brain tumours.

Management

Management is mostly symptomatic and aimed mainly at palliation. Dexamethasone 4-6 mg 3-4 times daily temporarily reduces cerebral oedema and symptoms. Chemotherapy is usually not indicated and excision surgery is reserved for isolated single accessible metastases. Prognosis is poor anywhere in the world with most untreated patients surviving less than a month after diagnosis.

Key points

- metastases account for about 25% of all ICTs & occur mostly in older age groups
- main sites of origin are breast, lung, kidney, GIT and melanoma
- CFs are similar to gliomas but occurring over a faster time course
- differential diagnosis includes brain abscess, parasitic cysts & vascular causes
- diagnosis confirmed by (CT/MRI) & evidence of primary tumour elsewhere

OTHER TUMOURS

Craniopharyngioma

These are uncommon benign tumours that arise from primitive cells in Rathke's pouch which lies just above the pituitary gland and below the floor of the third ventricle. They represent 2-5% of all intracranial tumours in high income countries and mainly affect children but are also seen in usually younger adults. They present clinically with pressure effects including headache, visual field defect, and occasionally diabetes insipidus and hydrocephalus. Neuroimaging using CT or MRI is diagnostic showing a non enhancing suprasellar cystic mass usually with irregular calcification (Fig. 16.5). The tumours can be quite large at the time of clinical presentation. Management is surgical and by irradiation; however the outcome is often unfavourable because of a high likelihood of recurrence.

CT (without contrast)

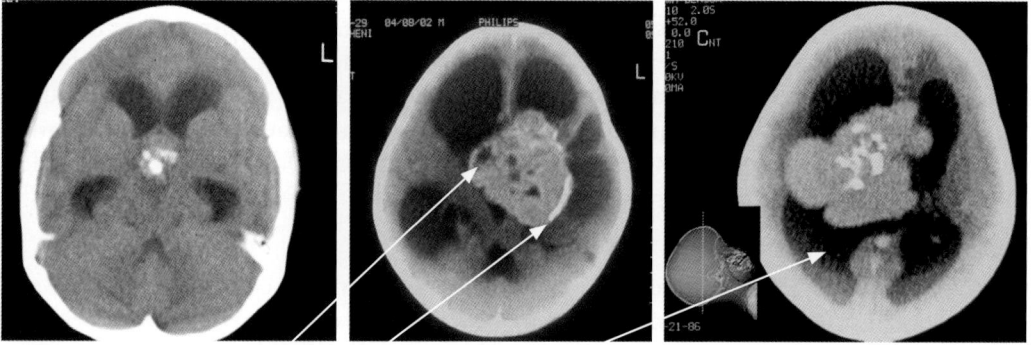

Large suprasellar tumour with cysts, calcification & severe hydrocephalus

Figure 16.5 Craniopharyngioma

Key points

- craniopharyngioma are benign ICTs mainly in children and young adults
- arise from primitive rest cells in Rathke's pouch above pituitary gland
- symptoms are caused by local pressure effects & occasionally diabetes insipidus
- diagnosis is by CT/MRI showing a suprasellar cystic mass usually with calcification
- treatment involves surgical resection & radiotherapy but recurrence is common

Primary CNS Lymphoma (PCNSL)

This is a primary B cell lymphoma that arises within the brain. It is a sporadic tumour affecting mostly older adults and accounts for around 1% of all primary intracranial tumours. PCNSL also occurs in HIV where it affects a mainly younger age group, occurring in <1% of AIDS patients in Africa. It presents in a similar manner to other brain tumours although seizures are less common and meningeal and spinal cord involvement may occur. The diagnosis is suspected when the CT of the head shows a deep seated enhancing periventricular mass lesion with surrounding oedema (Fig. 16.6). The tumour may also occur at more than one intracranial site in HIV disease. The main differential diagnosis in HIV disease in Africa is with a brain abscess secondary to toxoplasmosis or tuberculosis (Chapter 8). Appropriate management is with methotrexate, corticosteroids and whole brain deep X-ray therapy (DXT) which can prolong survival rates to up to 3 years in non HIV patients. The prognosis is very poor in HIV disease and survival is usually <3 months.

CT (with contrast)

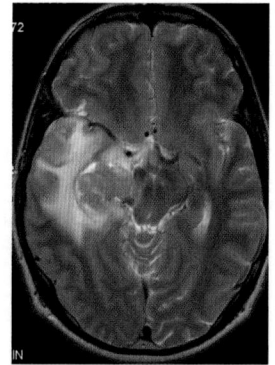

Tumour right temporal lobe with mass effect

Figure 16.6 Lymphoma

Colloid cyst

Colloid cyst is uncommon and accounts for <1% of primary intracranial tumours. It is a benign cystic tumour which arises from the roof of the 3rd ventricle and may block CSF flow initially intermittently. Patients with a colloid cyst present with intermittent headaches which may be sometimes severe, recurrent and related to posture. Affected patients are prone to drop attacks, leg weakness and hydrocephalus and also sudden death if the flow to CSF is completely blocked. CT may show a well demarcated rounded cyst arising within the 3rd ventricle with or without obstructive hydrocephalus (Fig. 16.7). The differential diagnosis includes other causes of intraventricular cysts including neurocysticercosis where cysts are usually multiple. Management is by surgical removal or destruction of the cyst.

Acoustic neuroma (Schwannoma)

These are rare benign slow growing tumours that arise from Schwann cells of the vestibular nerve with an incidence rate of 1 per 100,000 in high income countries. The corresponding incidence reported in a black population in SA is reported to be very low, (0.01/100,000). They arise sporadically on one side but may occur bilaterally in neurofibromatosis type 2 when they usually occur before the age of 21 years (Chapter 18). The principal sites are the internal auditory canal (IAC) and the cerebellopontine angle (CPA). The distinguishing clinical features are unilateral deafness coupled with tinnitus, vertigo, ipsilateral unsteadiness and facial weakness and numbness. Hydrocephalus and raised ICP are a late complication. Diagnosis is by showing high frequency hearing loss either clinically or by audiograph and by demonstrating an expanding lesion in the IAC or in the CPA by either CT or MRI (Fig. 16.8). The main differential diagnosis is between a meningioma and epidermoid cyst. Management is by deep X-ray therapy and by surgical resection, though resection is technically difficult with significant morbidity.

MRI T1

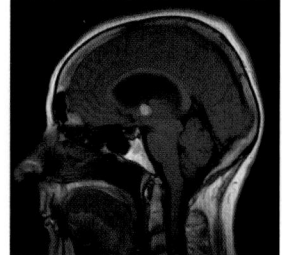

Colloid cyst blocking foramen of Monro with dilatation of lateral ventricle

Figure 16.7 Colloid cyst

MRI T1 (with contrast)

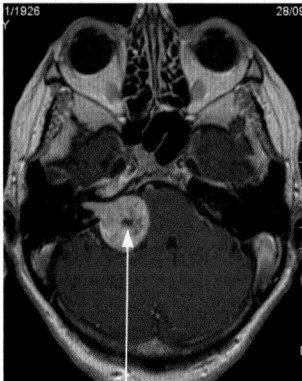

Acoustic neuroma extending into right auditory canal

CT (with contrast)

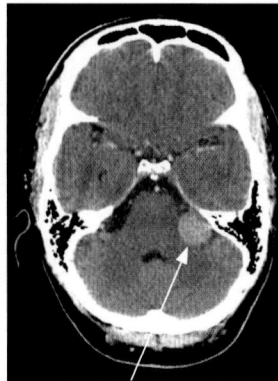

Acoustic neuroma (left sided)

Figure 16.8 Acoustic neuroma

Pinealoma

Tumours may arise from the pineal gland and are uncommon. These are classified as germinomas, pinealomas, teratomas and gliomas. They are uncommon slow growing tumours and occur mostly in children and young adults <30 years. Patients present clinically with disorders of eye movement, mainly up gaze paralysis and symptoms of raised ICP. These symptoms are explained by the local effects of the tumour invading the upper midbrain and blocking the aqueduct of Sylvius causing hydrocephalus (Fig.16.9). The diagnosis is confirmed by neuroimaging, CT or MRI and management is neurosurgical.

MRI T1 (with contrast)   **CT head**

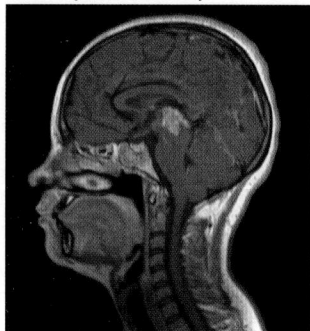

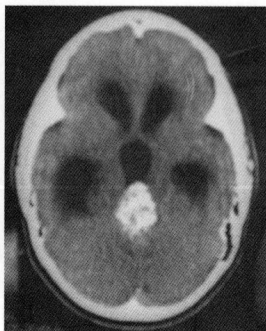

Pinealoma enhancing   Pinealoma with calcification & hydrocephalus

Figure 16.9 Pinealoma

MANAGEMENT OF TUMOURS

The management of intracranial tumours involves confirming the diagnosis histologically, grading the tumour when indicated and treating the patient medically and surgically.

Medical

General measures are aimed at controlling symptoms including pain and anxiety and reducing intracranial pressure. These measures include treating the symptoms and ensuring adequate cerebral perfusion by maintaining hydration, oxygen saturation and blood pressure. The use of osmotic therapy can be effective in reducing acute elevations of intracranial pressure but is only effective for a few days. The drug of choice in ↑ICP is mannitol 20% solution in boluses of 0.25-0.75 g/kg every 4-6 hours. Corticosteroids are useful for patients with cerebral oedema secondary to mass lesions. Dexamethasone is the most commonly used steroid in a dose 4-8 mg/po or iv/three to four times daily. This often provides significant symptomatic relief and can be maintained at the lowest dose that provides relief which is usually 4 mg twice daily. Opiates and anxiolytics may be necessary to control pain and anxiety.

Surgical

Meningiomas, pituitary tumours, acoustic neuromas are among the benign ICTs that can be successfully removed if not too advanced at presentation. Primary malignant brain tumours that are at or near the surface of the brain may be partially removed by debulking operations. The main aim is to palliate symptoms by removing as much tissue as is safely possible. Biopsy of the tumour is also important as the histological findings help to determine the type and grade of tumour and the subsequent management and prognosis. Patients presenting with resectable primary brain tumours should be referred to a national centre with neurosurgical facilities.

Radiotherapy

Middle grade gliomas, acoustic neuromas, incompletely removed pituitary adenomas and some other tumours are often radiosensitive. Tumours of childhood in the posterior fossa of the brain, medulloblastoma and lymphoma are sensitive to radiotherapy.

Chemotherapy

Chemotherapy is sometimes given as adjunctive treatment for some high grade gliomas but the response is usually poor.

Anticonvulsants

Control of epilepsy is an important part of the management of brain tumour. Phenytoin 3-400 mg daily is the drug of choice.

Prognosis

The majority of brain tumours are either malignant gliomas or metastases and carry a poor prognosis with few patients surviving longer than one year. However benign tumours such as meningiomas have a much better prognosis although they frequently present late in Africa.

Key points

- resources in Africa are limited for investigation & management of ICTs
- if ICT suspected then refer to centre with scanning & neurosurgical facilities
- symptomatic treatment of ICTs is very important
- patient & family are helped by being informed of clinical diagnosis & prognosis
- prognosis for most benign ICTs is good & for most malignant ICTs is poor

Selected references

Adeloye A, Odeku EL. *Metastatic neoplasms of the brain in Nigeria*. Br J Cancer. 1969 Jun;23(2):340-8.

Eyenga VC, Ngah JE, Atangana R, Etom E, Ngowe MN, Bassong Y, Oyono JL, et al. *Central nervous system tumours in Cameroon: histopathology and demography*. Sante. 2008 Jan-Mar;18(1):39-42. French

Froman C, Lipschitz R. *Demography of tumors of the central nervous system among the Bantu (African) population of the Transvaal, South Africa*. J Neurosurg. 1970 Jun;32(6):660-4.

Gurney JG, Kadan-Lottick N. *Brain and other central nervous system tumors*: rates, trends, and epidemiology. Curr Opin Oncol. 2001 May;13(3):160-6.

Idowu OE, Apemiye RA. *Delay in presentation and diagnosis of adult primary intracranial neoplasms in a tropical teaching hospital: a pilot study*. Int J Surg. 2009 Aug;7(4):396-8.

Maier D, Doppler M, Gasser A, Zellner H, Dharsee J, Schmutzhard E, et al. *Imaging-based disease pattern in a consecutive series of cranial CTs and MRIs in a rural and an urban Tanzanian hospital: a comparative, retrospective, neuroradiological analysis*. Wien Klin Wochenschr. 2010 Oct;122 Suppl 3:40-6

McKinney PA. *Brain tumours: incidence, survival, and aetiology*. J Neurol Neurosurg Psychiatry. 2004 Jun;75 Suppl 2:ii12-7.

Mwang'ombe NJ, Ombachi RB. *Brain tumours at the Kenyatta National Hospital, Nairobi*. East Afr Med J. 2000 Aug;77(8):444-7.

Odeku EL, Osuntokun BO, Adeloye A, Williams AO. *Tumors of the brain and its coverings. An African series*. Int Surg. 1972 Oct;57(10):798-801.

Olasode BJ. *A pathological review of intracranial tumours seen at the University College Hospital, Ibadan between 1980 and 1990.* Niger Postgrad Med J. 2002 Mar;9(1):23-8.

Seedat RY, Claassen AJ, Mol DA. *Incidence and management of acoustic neuromas in South Africa. Otol Neurotol.* 2002 Nov;23(6):996-8.

Surawicz TS, McCarthy BJ, Kupelian V, Jukich PJ, Bruner JM, Davis FG. *Descriptive epidemiology of primary brain and CNS tumors: results from the Central Brain Tumor Registry of the United States, 1990-1994.* Neuro Oncol. 1999 Jan;1(1):14-25.

Yaari L, Paltiel O, Barchana M, Liphshiz I, Shoshan Y. *Low incidence of brain tumors among Ethiopian immigrants in Israel.* J Neurooncol. 2011 Jan;101(2):279-85.

CHAPTER 17
DEMENTIA

CONTENTS

CHAPTER 17

DEMENTIA

Dementia is a general term for any disorder in which there is progressive loss of higher cortical functions. These higher functions include memory, language production and understanding, visuospatial function, and "executive" or frontal lobe function e.g. planning and judgement. Dementia is not a diagnosis in itself, it is simply a consequence of a wide variety of underlying conditions, such as: degenerative brain disease e.g. Alzheimer's disease (AD), cerebrovascular disease, cerebral infections e.g. HIV infection, deficiency states e.g. B-12, metabolic disorders e.g. hypothyroidism and substance misuse e.g. alcohol. The core features of dementia are impairment in at least two areas of higher cortical function, usually memory plus one other. There is a decline from a previous level of functioning severe enough to interfere with activities of daily living such as work, family or social activities and there is a progression over time. The aim of this chapter is to present a brief overview of dementia. The student should aim for an overall understanding of dementia including definition, aetiology, main clinical features, diagnosis and management.

Key points

- dementia is a loss of memory & at least one other cognitive function
- loss is sufficient to interfere with the activities of daily living
- loss of higher cortical functions is progressive
- need to exclude treatable causes of dementia

EPIDEMIOLOGY

Dementia affects >2% of the population in high income countries at the age of 65 years, with the prevalence doubling every five years thereafter. Thus by the age of 85 years approximately one third of the population there have a dementia of some type. However because of population distribution most persons with dementia now live in low or middle income countries and as life expectancy lengthens that burden is set to increase. There are few studies on dementia from Africa, but age adjusted studies from there in whole populations aged 65 years and over suggest a lower overall burden of 1-3%, this is in comparison to rates of 5-10% in similar age groups in other low and middle income parts of the world. However, the current HIV epidemic in Africa is increasing the overall burden of dementia there but in a mainly younger population.

AETIOLOGY

The main causes of dementia are Alzheimer's disease, cerebrovascular disease and HIV disease. Less common degenerative causes include frontotemporal dementia (FTD) or Pick's disease, dementia with Lewy bodies (DLB), Parkinson's disease with dementia (PDD) and Huntington's disease (Table 17.1). Treatable causes of dementia include HIV, B-12 deficiency, hypothyroidism, alcoholism and rarely syphilis. The differential diagnosis of dementia in Africa includes chronic confusional and psychiatric states, chronic brain disorders, tumours and subdural haematoma.

Main causes of dementia in Africa

- Alzheimer's disease
- cerebrovascular disease
- HIV
- alcohol

Risk factors

The main known risk factors are old age, genetic predisposition (e.g. APO-E genotype) and vascular risk factors such as hypertension, hypercholesterolaemia and diabetes. Diet, lifestyle and lower level of education may also be risk factors. At present there are no known specific preventatives or curative measures for most forms of dementia.

Table 17.1 Classification and main features of dementia

Dementia type	Frequency*	Overall %	Main clinical features
Dementia (all causes)	2 % @ 65 yrs 33% >85 yrs	100%	progressive loss of two or more intellectual functions (e.g. memory, language), sufficient to disrupt daily life
Alzheimer's disease	1.5% @ 65 yrs commonest cause of dementia in later life	60%	core feature is usually poor day-to-day memory, language and visuospatial function
Vascular dementia	0.5% @ 65 yrs	20-30%	usually a history of stroke with physical signs such as limb weakness & dysarthria: cognitive impairment may take many forms
Frontotemporal dementia	less common than AD but an important cause of young-onset dementia: accounts for up to 20% of patients with dementia aged 45-65 years (HIV excluded)	<10%	*frontal:* insidious changes in personality and behaviour, other domains often intact *temporal:* progressive aphasia, fluent or non-fluent
HIV associated dementia	10-20% of patients with advanced HIV	not-known	non-specific: generalised cognitive and motor slowing with poor day-to-day memory
Dementia with Lewy bodies	less common	<1%	parkinsonism, fluctuations, visual hallucinations

* based on high income countries

General course and prognosis in dementia

By definition, dementia is a progressive disorder. Consciousness is not altered, but with time impairments of higher function extend into all cognitive areas (see appendix 1). The level of functioning declines until patients are entirely dependent on others for their care. Death follows either directly from the failure of core brain systems or more often as a secondary consequence of complications such as pneumonia, untreated pressure sores and venous thrombosis. The duration and course of dementia depends on the cause but typically lasts for years. Life expectancy in Alzheimer's disease is about 6-7 years from onset in high income countries.

ALZHEIMER'S DISEASE

Alzheimer's disease is the commonest cause of dementia worldwide (Table 17.1). It is reported to be less common in Africa as compared to similar aged populations in high income countries, including Afro-Americans. However studies from Africa suggest that it still accounts for >60% of all cases of dementia there. Its main cause is unknown. It is rare under 45 years of age but thereafter its prevalence rises exponentially with age and increasingly after 65 years of age. It is associated with a positive family history of dementia and affects females more than males.

Genetics

Alzheimer's is usually a sporadic disease, but can occasionally be familial when it is autosomal dominant, due to mutations in the genes for presenilin 1 & 2 (PS1 & 2) or amyloid precursor protein (APP) on chromosome 21. The majority of familial AD is caused by mutations in PS1, which usually results in very early onset disease (under 45 years) with rapid progression and additional physical signs. Apolipoprotein E (APOE e4), a lipid transport protein which has been identified as an independent risk factor for AD appears not to influence AD progression in SSA.

Pathophysiology

It is due to loss of neurones from the cerebral cortex and is associated with characteristic deposition of beta-amyloid plaques and neurofibrillary tangles in the neurones. This results in decreased acetylcholine synthesis in the brain.

Clinical features

The clinical features range from mild cognitive impairment with an isolated difficulty in day-to-day memory or forgetfulness, followed by slow progression over years to a severe loss of other cognitive functions, including recognition, language and visuospatial awareness. Loss of memory for recent events and recent personal experiences are typical. Behaviour and personality are often well preserved to begin with, and the diagnosis can be overlooked in the early stages. Physical signs appear later in the disease, when patients may develop parkinsonism, myoclonus and incontinence.

Diagnosis

The diagnosis is made by a careful history from the patient and an informant, supported by objective evidence of cognitive impairment on bedside tests. A Mini Mental State Examination (MMSE) (see appendix 2) score of 24/30 or less is supportive of a diagnosis of dementia, having excluded other secondary causes of dementia with appropriate blood tests and brain imaging.

Investigations

The main investigations in dementia are outlined in Table 17.2. The main aim is to exclude a treatable cause e.g. B-12 deficiency or HIV.

Table 17.2 Main investigations in dementia

Investigation	Aetiology
Haematology FBC & ESR	all causes
Chemistry blood sugar renal & liver function tests serum calcium	metabolic causes
Serology & others HIV, VDRL, TPHA T4 B-12 CSF examination	infection: HIV, syphilis, hypothyroidism, vitamin deficiencies, neurodegenerative
X-rays chest CT head	CVD, infection, TB, malignancy brain atrophy, stroke, vascular changes, infection, tumours, subdural haematoma
Others EEG, genetic testing	CJD, APO-E genotype

Management

There is no cure at present for Alzheimer's disease. Non drug interventions are the mainstay of management. This includes the provision of information and support for the carer's family and the community. One aspect of the disease is a deficiency of acetylcholine synthesis in the brain, and centrally acting cholinesterase inhibitors that raise levels of acetylcholine in the brain may result in temporary symptomatic benefit. In high income countries, the cholinesterase inhibitors are recommended for patients with mild to moderate dementia (MMSE range 12-24/30). Patients may derive some limited benefit in cognitive function for 1-2 years but there is no effect on the eventual progression of the disease. These are stopped if the MMSE score is <12/30.

Drug options include the cholinesterase inhibitors donepezil 5-10 mg daily or rivastigmine 1.5–3 mg bid, or galantamine 4-6 mg bd. The main side effects are related to increased peripheral cholinergic activity and include nausea, abdominal colic and diarrhoea. However the high cost of the regular use of these drugs prohibits their widespread use in AD in Africa. For behavioural and psychiatric disorders, it may be necessary to use an antipsychotic medication. These include haloperidol 0.5-1.5 mg twice daily. Alternatives include risperidone 0.5 mg or olanzapine 2.5 mg/po daily initially. Valproic acid may decrease agitation and help as a mood stabilizer and be better tolerated than the antipsychotics. It is wise to start with low doses and adjust any increases in dosages slowly.

Key points

- Alzheimer's is the most common form of dementia worldwide and in Africa
- associated with increasing age >65 yrs & a positive family history
- first symptom is often forgetfulness
- progresses to involve language, recognition, self-care & continence
- there is no cure & death occurs after approximately 6-7 years

VASCULAR DEMENTIA

Cerebrovascular disease is considered to be the second most common cause of dementia worldwide accounting for 20-30% of all cases. Patients are usually >40 years and have a known risk factor for vascular disease including hypertension, diabetes, atrial fibrillation, hyperlipidaemia and smoking.

Clinical features

Vascular disease may cause cognitive impairment by different mechanisms. Firstly, a small (strategic) stroke in an eloquent area or secondly by the cumulative effects of repeated large-vessel strokes. This is associated with the classical "step-wise" deterioration of vascular dementia. Thirdly, due to hypertension affecting the small penetrating arteries supplying the sub cortical white matter, causing multiple lacunar infarcts. This leads to a more insidiously progressive sub cortical dementia with motor findings. Clinically there will usually be physical signs including pyramidal tract signs and often gait disturbance or pseudo-parkinsonism and frequently urinary incontinence.

Diagnosis and management

Neuroimaging of the brain, in particular MRI shows widespread white matter changes particularly around the ventricles or areas of frank infarction. The management is unsatisfactory but involves the reduction and treatment of the usual vascular risk factors.

FRONTOTEMPORAL DEMENTIA

Frontotemporal dementia (FTD), or Pick's disease, is a neurodegenerative disorder characterised by progressive deterioration of behaviour, personality and language abilities together with prominent atrophy of the frontal and temporal lobes. It accounts for <10% of cases of dementia in high income countries and also occurs in Africa but its frequency there is not known. FTD is typically of younger onset, with age of onset between 45 and 65 years, although cases with older onset are well recognised.

Genetics

Up to 40% of patients with FTD have a positive family history of early-onset dementia with an autosomal dominant inheritance pattern. A number of causative genes on chromosome 17 have been identified, including tau & progranulin.

Clinical features

In the frontal or behavioural variant of FTD, typical presenting problems include disinhibition, loss of empathy, changes in eating patterns, ritualized or stereotypical behaviours and apathy. In the language variants of FTD problems include loss of word meaning (semantic dementia) or nonfluent speech (progressive non-fluent aphasia). However, it must be emphasized that there is a good deal of overlap between these variants of FTD. Patients with a predominantly frontal presentation may also show language impairments, and equally patients with a predominantly language presentation may show behavioural disturbance. Physical signs are not usual but there is an overlap with motor neurone disease. A core feature is a lack of insight and patients with behavioural disturbance can be very challenging to manage. Eventually all patients progress to a global dementia.

Diagnosis and management

Neuroimaging reveals a very characteristic selective atrophy of frontal and temporal lobes (Fig 17.1). There is no specific treatment.

CT (without contrast)

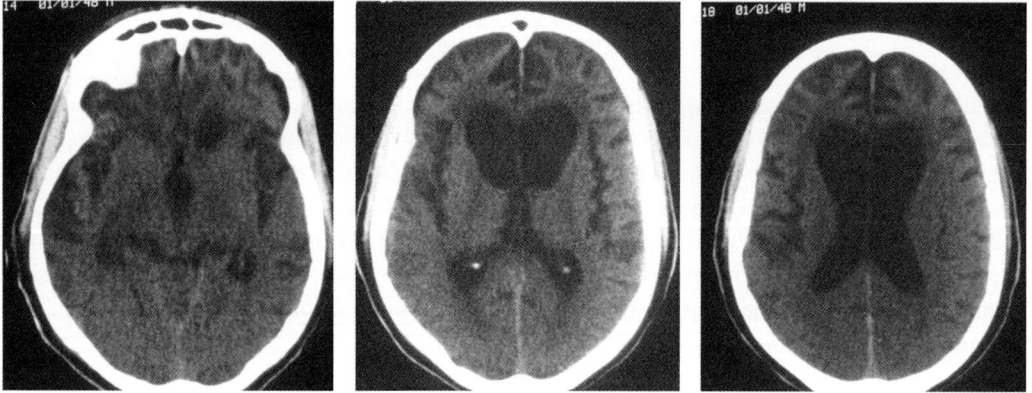

Selective atrophy of frontal & temporal lobes with ventricular dilatation

Figure 17.1 Frontotemporal Dementia

HIV-ASSOCIATED DEMENTIA (HAD)

Chronic HIV infection of the brain leads to a dementia in at least 10-20% of patients in Africa, affecting a younger population than is usual for dementia (Chapter 8). HAD occurs increasingly with advancing levels of immunosuppression and in particular with CD4 counts <100/cm^3. HAD presents with abnormalities of cognition, memory and motor function. The dementia is characterized early on by apathy, disinterest and loss of attention with a characteristic slowing of both mental and motor function (HIV associated neurocognitive dysfunction or HAND). Later, it leads to a global loss of cognitive function, with immobility and incontinence in end stage disease. However, most patients in Africa never reach this advanced stage, dying beforehand mainly of opportunistic processes, mostly infections. Associated neurological findings include frontal lobe release signs (FLRSs), absent ankle reflexes (distal sensory neuropathy) and frequently isolated brisk knee reflexes and extensor plantar responses (vacuolar myelopathy). The FLRSs, the snout reflex and the palmomental reflex, (Chapter 8), are found in the majority (70-90%) of patients with HAD. CT of the head usually demonstrates cerebral atrophy and excludes other confounding causes. The frequency of HAD has been shown in Africa to decrease significantly six months after starting ART.

DEMENTIA WITH LEWY BODIES

This occurs most commonly in the elderly and without a positive family history. This is a degenerative disorder characterized by the presence of Lewy bodies in the neurones of the cerebral cortex, brain atrophy and loss of pigment in the substantia nigra. Clinically, patients present with a dementia, coupled with mild dopamine sensitive parkinsonism, visual hallucinations, delusions and fluctuating cognition. CT of head reveals mild generalised brain atrophy. Patients may benefit from the cholinesterase inhibitors, perhaps even more so than patients with AD. However, caution should be taken with antipsychotic drugs as they may cause a dramatic worsening of the parkinsonism and precipitate the neuroleptic malignant syndrome. Patients with Parkinson's disease may develop a similar dementia later in the course of their illness and the situations are probably just two ends of a spectrum.

Key points

- main causes of dementia are Alzheimer's disease, cerebrovascular disease & HIV disease
- there is no treatment that reverses the decline in Alzheimer's & cerebrovascular disease dementia management involves care of patient in general & treatment of specific symptoms
- care involves practical advice & support to patients, carers & families
- drug treatment generally involves use of anticholinesterases & neuroleptics

APPENDIX 1 SUMMARY BEDSIDE COGNITIVE TESTING*

Higher cerebral function	Clinical testing method	Measurement
Alertness	level of wakefulness	record level e.g. fully awake
Orientation	time, person and place	score out of 10
Attention and concentration	count back from 20 or repeat string of increasing numbers (max 6)	record best result after two trials
Memory		
Antegrade/short term	fictitious name/address or four to seven numbers	assess immediate recall and again after 5 min noting mistakes
Retrograde/long-term	dates/places of schooling, work or marriage or country events	assess accuracy of recall (check with relatives)
Executive function (frontal lobe)		
Word fluency	name as many animals or fruits in one minute	>20 normal <10 abnormal
Abstract thought	proverb interpretation e.g. "a rolling stone catches no moss"	interpretation
Cognitive estimates	how many people in Tanzania	accuracy
Alternating hand movements	open and close right and left fists alternatively	ability to replicate examiner
Dominant hemisphere function		
Aphasia	speech content understanding expression reading/writing	assess spontaneous speech for fluency, content and errors. to simple commands to naming objects to read/write a sentence
Calculation	arithmetic	simple addition/subtraction
Praxia	"wave goodbye" or "hammer a nail"	ability to follow instruction or replicate examiner
Non dominant hemispheric function		
Neglect	ignores all stimuli from one side hemispatial neglect	ignores stimulus on neglected side when bilateral stimuli presented (extinction) when drawing clock face one side is left out

done only on a patient who is awake and cooperative

APPENDIX 2 THE MINI MENTAL STATE EXAMINATION

The Mini-Mental state examination (MMSE)	Maximum test score
Orientation time, date, day, month, year ward, hospital, district, town, country *(score one point for each correct answer)*	5 5
Registration examiner names three familiar objects (e.g. ball, pen, key) patient asked to repeat the three names *(score one point for each correct answer)*	3
Attention and calculation ask patient to subtract 7 from 100, stop after five subtractions, 93, 86, 79, 72, 65 *or* spell a five letter word backwards e.g. world *(score one point for each correct answer)*	5
Recall ask patient to name the three objects that you previously named *(score one point for each correct answer)*	3
Language naming: point to two objects e.g. watch and pen and ask the patient to name them *(score one point for each correct answer)*	2
Repetition ask patient to repeat sentence ("no ifs, ands or buts") no repeated attempt *(score one point for correct answer)*	1
3-Stage command e.g. "take this piece of paper in your right hand, fold it in half, and place it on the table *(score one point for each stage done correctly)*	3
Reading ask patient to read and obey a written command on a piece of paper e.g. close your eyes *(score one point)*	1
Writing ask patient to write a sentence sentence should be sensible and contain a noun and a verb *(score one point)*	1
Copying ask patient to copy picture of two intersecting pentagons *(score one point if all ten angles are present and the two must intersect)*	1
Total	30

Score: > 24/30 = normal, < 24/30 = cognitive impairment

Selected references

Cooper S, Greene JD. *The clinical assessment of the patient with early dementia.* J Neurol Neurosurg Psychiatry. 2005 Dec;76 Suppl 5:v15-24.

Ferri CP, Ames D, Prince M. *Behavioral and psychological symptoms of dementia in developing countries.* Int Psychogeriatr. 2004 Dec;16(4):441-59.

Ferri CP, Prince M, Brayne C, Brodaty H, Fratiglioni L, Ganguli M, et al. *Global prevalence of dementia: a Delphi consensus study.* Lancet. 2005 Dec 17;366(9503):2112-7.

Guerchet M, M'Belesso P, Mouanga AM, Bandzouzi B, Tabo A, Houinato DS, et al. *Prevalence of dementia in elderly living in two cities of Central Africa: the EDAC survey.* Dement Geriatr Cogn Disord. 2010;30(3):261-8.

Guerchet M, Mouanga AM, M'belesso P, Tabo A, Bandzouzi B, Paraïso MN, et al. *Factors associated with dementia among elderly people living in two cities in Central Africa: the EDAC multicenter study.* J Alzheimers Dis. 2012 Jan 1;29(1):15-24.

Gureje O, Ogunniyi A, Kola L, Abiona T. *Incidence of and risk factors for dementia in the Ibadan study of aging.* J Am Geriatr Soc. 2011 May;59(5):869-74.

Kanmogne GD, Kuate CT, Cysique LA, Fonsah JY, Eta S, Doh R, et al. *HIV-associated neurocognitive disorders in sub-Saharan Africa: a pilot study in Cameroon.* BMC Neurol. 2010;10:60.

Kalaria RN, Maestre GE, Arizaga R, Friedland RP, Galasko D, Hall K, et al. *Alzheimer's disease and vascular dementia in developing countries: prevalence, management, and risk factors.* Lancet Neurol. 2008 Sep;7(9):812-26.

Kengne AP, Dzudie A, Dongmo L. *Epidemiological features of degenerative brain diseases as they occurred in Yaounde referral hospitals over a 9-year period.* Neuroepidemiology. 2006;27(4):208-11.

Lawler K, Mosepele M, Ratcliffe S, Seloilwe E, Steele K, Nthobatsang R, et al. *Neurocognitive impairment among HIV-positive individuals in Botswana: a pilot study.* J Int AIDS Soc. 2010;13:15.

Njamnshi AK, Bissek AC, Ongolo-Zogo P, Tabah EN, Lekoubou AZ, Yepnjio FN, et al. *Risk factors for HIV-associated neurocognitive disorders (HAND) in sub-Saharan Africa: the case of Yaounde-Cameroon.* J Neurol Sci. 2009 Oct 15;285(1-2):149-53.

Ogunniyi A, Hall KS, Baiyewu O, Gureje O, Unverzagt FW, Gao S, et al. *Caring for individuals with dementia: the Nigerian experience.* West Afr J Med. 2005 Jul-Sep;24(3):259-62.

Robertson K, Kumwenda J, Supparatpinyo K, Jiang JH, Evans S, Campbell TB et al. *A multinational study of neurological performance in antiretroviral therapy-naïve HIV-1-infected persons in diverse resource-constrained settings.* J Neurovirol. 2011 Oct;17(5):438-47

Sacktor NC, Wong M, Nakasujja N, Skolasky RL, Selnes OA, Musisi S, et al. *The International HIV Dementia Scale: a new rapid screening test for HIV dementia.* AIDS. 2005 Sep 2;19(13):1367-74.

Wong MH, Robertson K, Nakasujja N, Skolasky R, Musisi S, Katabira E, et al. *Frequency of and risk factors for HIV dementia in an HIV clinic in sub-Saharan Africa.* Neurology. 2007 Jan 30;68(5):350-5.

PART II – NEUROLOGICAL DISORDERS

CHAPTER 18
INHERITED NEUROLOGICAL DISORDERS

CONTENTS

CHAPTER 18

INHERITED NEUROLOGICAL DISORDERS

Inherited neurological disorders are generally relatively uncommon (Table 18.1). Their frequency in Africa is largely unknown. Inheritance follows the basic Mendelian laws for autosomal dominant, autosomal recessive and X-linked recessive inheritance. An example of an autosomal dominant disorder is neurofibromatosis and of an autosomal recessive disorder is Friedreich's ataxia. Duchenne's and Becker's muscular dystrophy (Chapter 13) are both X-linked disorders. Huntington's disease is an example of an autosomal dominant and a trinucleotide repeat disorder. A positive family history can usually be elicited in the autosomal dominant and X-linked disorders, underlining the importance of the family history. The aim of this chapter is to review the more commonly encountered hereditary neurological disorders. The student should aim to recognize and be familiar with the main ones.

Table 18.1 Characteristics of the main inherited neurological disorders

Disorder	Genetics	Age of onset	Frequency*	Main clinical features
Neurofibromatosis type 1	autosomal dominant	children & adults	1/4000	neurofibroma on nerves, café-au-lait spots >5, axillary freckling
Neurofibromatosis type 2	autosomal dominant	adults	1/50,000	deafness, bilateral acoustic neuromas
Tuberous Sclerosis	autosomal dominant	children & young adults	1/15,000	epilepsy, adenoma sebaceum on face, hamartoma
Friedreich's ataxia	autosomal recessive	teens	1/50,000	cerebellar signs, progressive gait ataxia, upper motor neurone signs, absent ankle jerks
Charcot-Marie-Tooth disease	autosomal dominant	young adults	1/3,000	peripheral neuropathy, marked lower limb distal wasting, high arched feet (pes cavus)
Huntington's disease	autosomal dominant	middle aged adults	1/10,000	choreaform movements, progressive dementia, psychiatric symptoms

frequencies based on studies in high income countries

NEUROFIBROMATOSIS TYPE 1

Neurofibromatosis type 1 is an autosomal dominant disorder with an age-dependent penetrance caused by a defect in the *NF1* gene (neurofibromin) on chromosome 17q occurring with a frequency of about 1 in 4-5,000 (Table 18.1). Its frequency in Africa is likely to be similar. About 30-50% of cases are the result of new mutations. Clinically, it is characterised by neurofibromata lying on peripheral nerves, multiple cutaneous fibromas, and more than 5 hyperpigmented or café-au-lait (CAL) spots on the trunk (Fig. 18.1); see NIH clinical criteria and main clinical features NF1 (Table 18.2). The clinical picture can vary from very few to very many and distinctive skin lesions. Other clinical findings include axillary, neck and groin freckling, Lisch nodules on the iris and sometimes a scoliosis. Patients with type 1 may develop paraplegia secondary to an expanding intra axial neurofibroma arising from a nerve root pressing on the spinal cord (Fig. 18.1). They are also at risk for large deforming plexiform neuromas (Fig. 18.1), sarcomas, brain gliomas and pheochromocytoma.

Table 18.2 Diagnostic criteria for NF1

Criteria: *a diagnosis of NF type 1 is met if any two or more of the following is met.*
6 or more CAL* spots 1.5 cm or larger in post pubertal patients 0.5 cm or larger in prepubertal patients
2 or more neurofibromata of any type *or* 1 or more plexiform neurofibroma
freckling in axilla, neck or groin
optic glioma
2 or more Lisch nodules
a distinctive bone lesion dysplasia of the sphenoid bone dysplasia or thinning of long bone cortex (tibia)
first degree relative, independently diagnosed with NF1

* Café-au-lait

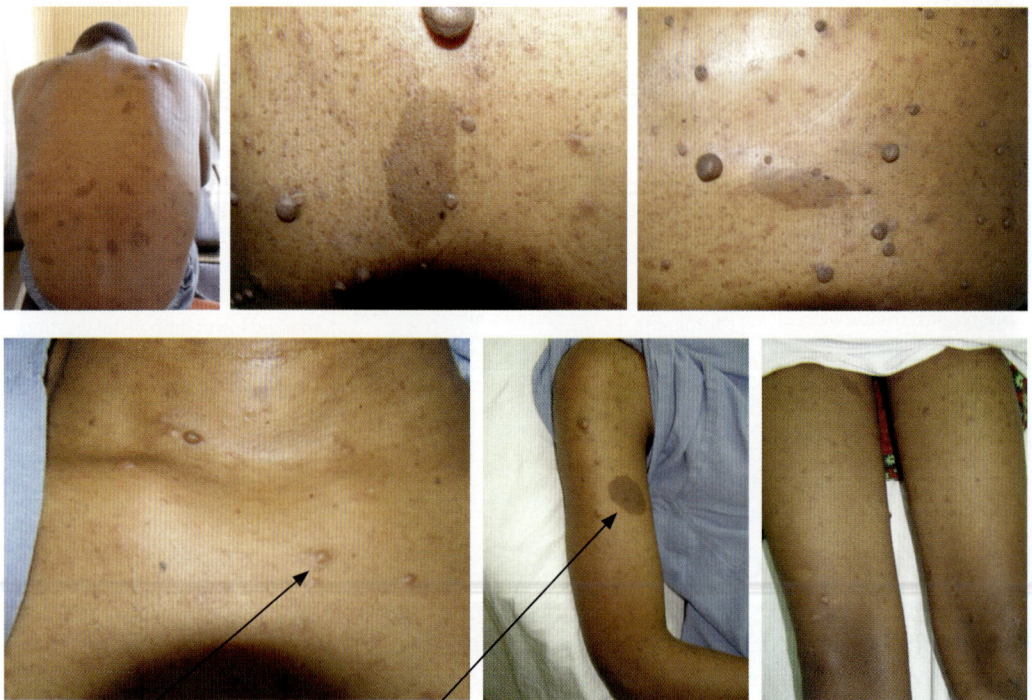

Multiple neurofibromata & cafe au lait spots

NF type 1 variant

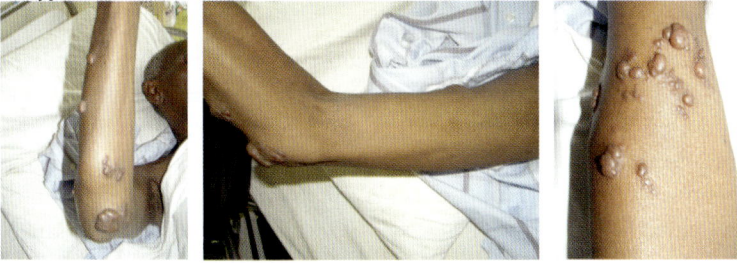

Segmental neurofibromata localised to dermatomes of right arm

Plexiform neurofibroma

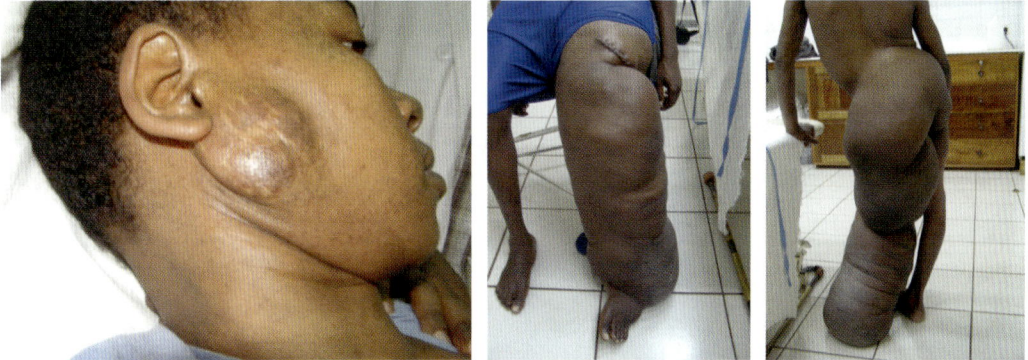

Involving the face

Gigantic plexiform neurofibroma of lower back & leg

CT chest

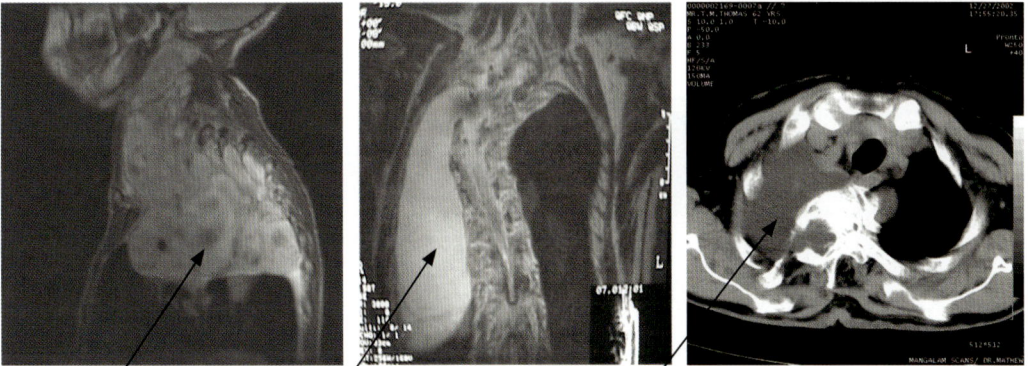

Giant plexiform neurofibroma involving upper mediastinum & right side of chest

Neurofibroma in NF1 compressing cervical cord & nerve roots

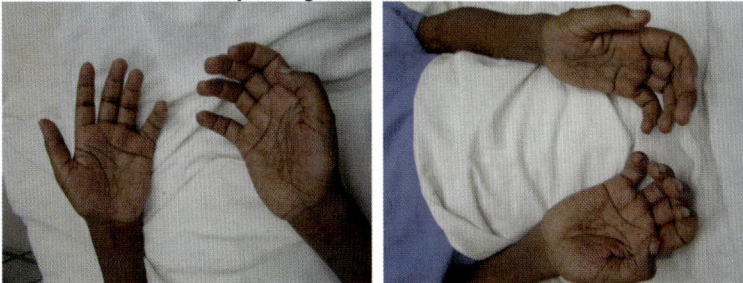

Clawing, wasting & weakness of hands

Figure 18.1 Clinical features NF type 1

NEUROFIBROMATOSIS TYPE 2

Neurofibromatosis type 2 is a much rarer autosomal dominant disorder affecting about 1 in 50,000 due to a defect in the *NF2* gene (merlin) on chromosome 22. It is characterised by few skin manifestations and the development of intracranial tumours, acoustic neuromas (vestibular Schwannoma) (Fig. 18.2) and meningiomas; see diagnostic criteria (Table 18.3). Deafness due to an acoustic neuroma involving the eighth cranial nerve is the main clinical presentation of type 2. This is usually accompanied by tinnitus, vertigo, ataxia, facial numbness and weakness. The clinical features at presentation are usually unilateral although the acoustic neuromas are commonly bilateral on neuroimaging. The diagnosis is confirmed by neuroimaging of the brain, usually MRI (Fig. 18.2). Management is either conservative by observation only or with deep X-ray therapy (DXT), or surgery for the tumours where possible. Genetic counselling is a very important part of management.

Table 18.3 Diagnostic criteria for NF2

Criteria: a diagnosis of NF2 is made if one of the following is met.
bilateral vestibular Schwannoma, (either histologically or by MRI with contrast)
a parent, sibling or child with NF2 and either a unilateral vestibular Schwannoma *or* 2 or more of meningioma, glioma, Schwannoma, posterior sub capsular lenticular opacities, cerebral calcifications
multiple meningiomas (2 or more) and one or more of glioma, Schwannoma, posterior sub capsular lenticular opacities, cerebral calcifications

MRI brain

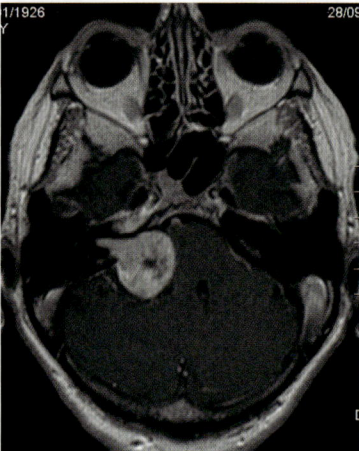

Unilateral Schwannoma (right sided)

Figure 18.2 NF type 2

TUBEROUS SCLEROSIS

This is an autosomal dominant condition, due to mutations in either *TSC1* on chromosome 9q (hamartin) or *TSC2* on chromosome 16p (tuberin) with a prevalence of 1/15,000. Its frequency is not known in Africa but is most probably the same. About 60% of cases are due to new mutations. The main clinical features are the characteristic facial angiofibromata or adenoma sebaceum lesions on the cheeks and nose (Fig. 18.3), in combination with a history of epilepsy. There may be associated cognitive impairment. Additional skin manifestations include ash leaf hypopigmented macular type patches and the shagreen patch, a 1-10cm patch of orange peel like sub epidermal fibrosis found most often over the lumbar sacral area and subungual fibromas. CT shows a characteristic pattern of paraventricular subependymal calcified nodules or tuberi. Complications include tumours in the brain, hamartoma (Fig. 18.3) and astrocytoma. There are frequently other affected family members, most commonly siblings. Epilepsy may be difficult to control.

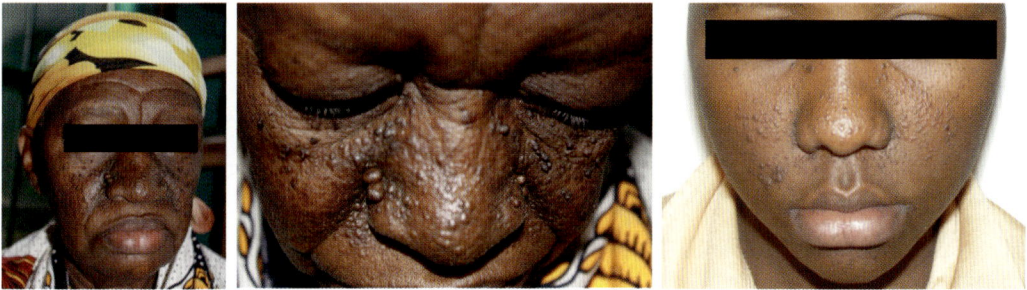

Adenoma sebaceum lesions on the cheeks and nose

Tuberous sclerosis & hamartoma

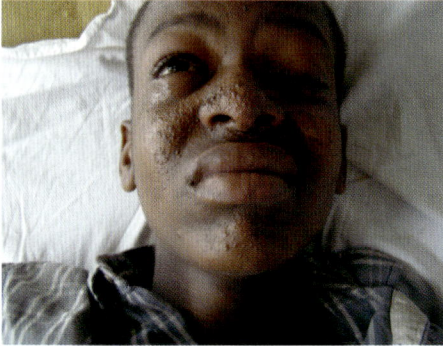

CT scan (with contrast)

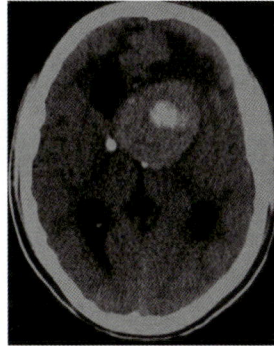

Adenoma sebaceum & left sided 3rd nerve palsy

Calcified tuberi & hamartoma in the same patient

Figure 18.3 Tuberous sclerosis

STURGE WEBER SYNDROME

This is an uncommon sporadic disorder affecting 1/50,000 in high income countries. It is a neurocutaneous syndrome characterized by a port wine staining affecting one half of the face (Fig. 18.4) usually in a V1 distribution and associated neurological abnormalities. The defining characteristic of the syndrome is an underlying intracranial vascular abnormality in the leptomeninges affecting the cortical regions of the hemispheres. The syndrome includes seizures, glaucoma, headaches, behavioural problems and stroke like episodes. It has its onset usually in early childhood and is usually progressive. However the clinical course is highly variable and it is important to note that not all children or adults with the characteristic port wine facial staining have the syndrome. Neuroimaging, usually CT confirms the presence of intracerebral calcifications affecting the parietal or occipital lobes on the affected side but they can be generalised. Management is largely symptomatic and supportive.

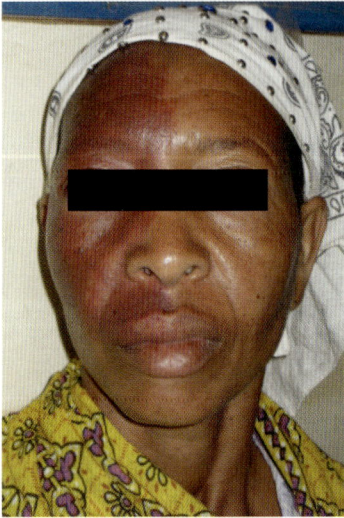

Port wine staining V1 & 2 distribution

Figure 18. 4 Sturge Weber syndrome

SPINOCEREBELLAR DISORDERS

These represent a wide but rare group of disorders with progressive cerebellar degeneration in combination with other neurological findings. Friedreich's ataxia is one of the main early onset ataxias.

FRIEDREICH'S ATAXIA

Friedreich's ataxia is an autosomal recessive condition caused by mutations in the *FDRA* gene (frataxin) on chromosome 9, mostly trinucleotide (GAA) repeat expansions (67–1700). It affects 1/50,000 with its onset usually in young persons under the age of 20 years (average 15.5 years with a range of 2-51 years). The severity of the disease depends on the number of abnormal trinucleotide repeats. The disease is characterized by progressive degeneration of the main cerebellar tracts with involvement of the corticospinal and posterior columns. The main clinical feature is gait ataxia which progressively worsens and may be accompanied by pyramidal findings and peripheral neuropathy (absent ankle jerks). Other less frequent findings include optic atrophy and deafness. There may be a scoliosis, pes cavus, diabetes mellitus and an associated cardiomyopathy as evidenced by widespread T inversion on ECG.

There is no treatment for the underlying genetic condition and management is mainly supportive and treatment of complications. The differential diagnosis includes the other hereditary cerebellar ataxias which are mainly the later onset type (>20 yrs) and are mostly autosomal dominant, mostly due to CAG repeat expansions and often characterized by anticipation. These may have associated spasticity, parkinsonism, neuropathy and retinopathy. A rare form of familial autosomal recessive isolated vitamin E deficiency is clinically very similar to Friedreich's ataxia and responds to high doses of vitamin E orally.

INHERITED NEUROPATHIES

These are also called the hereditary motor sensory neuropathies (HMSN). Charcot-Marie-Tooth disease (CMT1 = HMSN1) or peroneal muscular atrophy is the most common example in clinical practice. It is an autosomal dominant disorder, mostly due to 1, 5 Mb duplication, involving the *PMP22* gene on chromosome 17p. It affects about 1/3000 and the age of awareness of the disorder ranges from childhood to middle age, although it is already established in childhood but is subclinical. Patients present with a chronic distal wasting of the lower limbs (Fig. 18.5) which progresses very slowly over many years. Typically there is marked wasting of the calf and distal thigh muscles with bilateral pes cavus (high arched feet with clawed toes), reflexes are lost as may be distal sensation. When wasting is severe the leg is said to resemble an inverted champagne bottle with a long neck. This may be accompanied by wasting of forearms and clawing of the hands in about a third of patients (Fig. 18.5). The level of disability is less than expected for the degree of wasting.

There is no specific treatment for inherited neuropathies. Nerve conduction studies show severe slowing of motor conduction velocities consistent with neuropathy. The differential diagnosis includes other long standing neuropathies including leprosy and less common forms of hereditary neuropathies. These rarer forms of hereditary neuropathies may be accompanied by signs of spastic paraparesis, deafness, optic atrophy and retinitis pigmentosa.

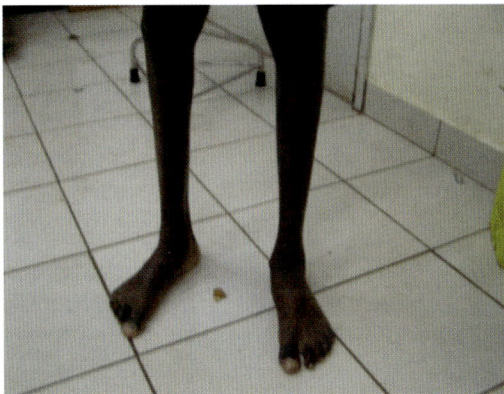

Characteristic wasting of the legs

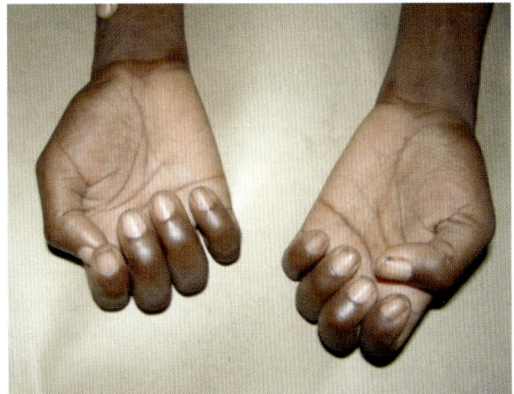

Clawing of hands

Figure 18. 5 Charcot-Marie-Tooth disease

HUNTINGTON'S DISEASE (HD)

This is an autosomal dominant inherited neurodegenerative disorder, affecting particularly the caudate nucleus and presenting in middle age with choreaform movements, progressive dementia and psychiatric symptoms. There is usually a positive family history. It affects about 1 in 10,000 persons and the causative gene lies on chromosome 4. It is an example of a trinucleotide repeat disorder with affected patients always having more than 36 cytosine-adenosine-guanosine (CAG) repeats. The normal number of repeats is <30, intermediate is 30-35, HD with reduced penetrance 36-39, and >39 in HD. The length of the repeats predicts the onset of the disease, the greater the number of repeats the earlier the onset and vice versa. Juvenile HD, characterized by rigidity rather than the chorea, is almost invariably paternally inherited with repeat sizes of 60 or more. Early features of HD include psychiatric and behavioural problems, characteristic fidgetiness, chorea and loss of intellectual function. The symptoms typically start insidiously in middle age at around the 4th and 5th decade and progress relentlessly to death within 15-20 years.

The diagnosis can be confirmed by diagnostic genetic testing, if available. Concerned relatives at risk need to be counselled carefully before presymptomatic or predictive DNA testing is performed. There is no effective treatment but the chorea and the anxiety may respond to treatment early on in the disease. If the patient's chorea is symptomatic tetrabenazine can be effective but parkinsonism and depression are adverse effects. Benzodiazepines can be used for anxiety and low dose haloperidol (0.5 mg bd) for aggression.

OTHER HEREDITARY NEUROLOGICAL DISORDERS

Muscular disorders
The main inherited myopathies are the dystrophies, Duchenne's (DMD), Becker's (BMD), limb girdle (LGMD), facioscapulohumeral (FSHD) and myotonic dystrophy. These are presented in chapter 13.

HEREDITARY SPASTIC PARAPARESIS (HSP)
This is an uncommon form of hereditary spastic paraparesis that usually follows an inheritance pattern of autosomal dominance and less frequently recessive and X-linked. Several genetic mutations occur involving over 20 different loci on different chromosomes with the spasmin gene on chromosome 2p22 accounting for 40-50% of cases. Two main age groups are affected, the more common one <35 yrs and the other with later onset (40-60 yrs) although the onset can be at any age. The time course is usually one of slow progression over many years.

The most common clinical phenotype is usually that of a slowly progressive spastic paraparesis beginning in childhood or teens characterized by hyperreflexia and up going toes with increasing difficulty in walking. If it occurs in childhood there may be pes cavus or arched feet coupled with tightening of the calf muscles which may result in heel-toe walking. Bladder and bowel function are not usually directly affected. The upper limbs are variably affected. HSP can occur in conjunction with other neurological abnormalities. These include cerebellar, optic atrophy, peripheral neuropathy, ocular palsies, macular degeneration and retardation and dementia.

The differential diagnosis includes the main causes of chronic spastic paraparesis in Africa including cord compression, primary lateral sclerosis, Konzo and HTLV-1. Management is by genetic counselling and the paraplegia measures already outlined in chapter 10.

WILSON'S DISEASE

This is a rare autosomal recessive disorder of copper metabolism which affects mainly teenagers and young adults. It occurs with a frequency of between 1/50-100,000. It is characterized by the accumulation of copper in various organs of the body including the liver and brain. This is caused by a deficiency of caeruloplasmin a copper transporting protein in the blood. In the brain, it chiefly affects the basal ganglia resulting in a range of movement disorders including tremor, chorea, dystonia and parkinsonism. Diagnosis clinically is by finding evidence of cirrhosis in the liver or deposition of copper on the cornea called the Kayser-Fleicher ring. This may need a slit lamp examination. In the serum the caeruloplasmin level is low and copper level high. Treatment is with copper chelating drugs penicillamine and a low copper diet.

Key points

- hereditary neurological disorders are uncommon but cause serious long-term disability
- follow genetic principles of inheritance: autosomal dominance, recessive & X-linked inheritance
- often start in childhood or during teenage years & other family members are affected
- no effective treatment for most hereditary neurological disorders
- genetic counselling is very important

Selected references

Ademiluyi SA, Ijaduola TG. *Neurofibromatosis in Nigerian children.* J Natl Med Assoc. 1988 Sep;80(9):1014-7.

Amir H, Moshi E, Kitinya JN. *Neurofibromatosis and malignant schwannomas in Tanzania. East Afr Med J. 1993 Oct;70(10):650-3.*

Bushby K, Finkel R, Birnkrant DJ, Case LE, Clemens PR, Cripe L, et al. *Diagnosis and management of Duchenne muscular dystrophy, part 1: diagnosis, and pharmacological and psychosocial management.* Lancet Neurol. 2010 Jan;9(1):77-93.

Bushby K, Finkel R, Birnkrant DJ, Case LE, Clemens PR, Cripe L, et al. *Diagnosis and management of Duchenne muscular dystrophy, part 2: implementation of multidisciplinary care.* Lancet Neurol. 2010 Feb;9(2):177-89.

Delatycki MB, Williamson R, Forrest SM. *Friedreich ataxia: an overview.* J Med Genet. 2000 Jan;37(1):1-8.

Evans DG, Huson SM, Donnai D, Neary W, Blair V, Teare D, et al. *A genetic study of type 2 neurofibromatosis in the United Kingdom. I. Prevalence, mutation rate, fitness, and confirmation of maternal transmission effect on severity.* J Med Genet. 1992 Dec;29(12):841-6.

Evans DG, Huson SM, Donnai D, Neary W, Blair V, Newton V, et al. *A genetic study of type 2 neurofibromatosis in the United Kingdom. II. Guidelines for genetic counselling.* J Med Genet. 1992 Dec;29(12):847-52.

Goldman A, Krause A, Ramsay M, Jenkins T. *Founder effect and prevalence of myotonic dystrophy in South Africans: molecular studies.* Am J Hum Genet. 1996 Aug;59(2):445-52.

Goldman A, Ramsay M, Jenkins T. *Ethnicity and myotonic dystrophy: a possible explanation for its absence in sub-Saharan Africa.* Ann Hum Genet. 1996 Jan;60(Pt 1):57-65.

McGaughran JM, Harris DI, Donnai D, Teare D, MacLeod R, Westerbeek R, et al. *A clinical study of type 1 neurofibromatosis in north west England.* J Med Genet. 1999 Mar;36(3):197-203.

Ramanjam V, Adnams C, Ndondo A, Fieggen G, Fieggen K, Wilmshurst J. *Clinical phenotype of South African children with neurofibromatosis 1.* J Child Neurol. 2006 Jan;21(1):63-70.

Pareyson D, Marchesi C. *Diagnosis, natural history, and management of Charcot-Marie-Tooth disease.* Lancet Neurol. 2009 Jul;8(7):654-67.

Roach ES, DiMario FJ, Kandt RS, Northrup H. *Tuberous Sclerosis Consensus Conference: recommendations for diagnostic evaluation. National Tuberous Sclerosis Association.* J Child Neurol. 1999 Jun;14(6):401-7.

Roos RA. *Huntington's disease: a clinical review.* Orphanet J Rare Dis. 2010;5(1):40.

Ginsberg Lionel, *Neurology, Lecture Notes,* Blackwell Publishing 8th edition 2005.

Wilmshurst JM, Ouvrier R. *Hereditary peripheral neuropathies of childhood: an overview for clinicians.* Neuromuscul Disord. 2011 Nov;21(11):763-75.

PART II – NEUROLOGICAL DISORDERS

CHAPTER 19
HEAD AND SPINAL INJURY

CONTENTS

CHAPTER 19

HEAD AND SPINAL INJURY

Trauma including head injury (HI) resulting in traumatic brain injury (TBI) and spinal injury is the leading cause of death and disability in 15-45 yr olds in high income countries. It is also a significant and increasing cause of morbidity and mortality in low and middle income countries, particularly in Africa. Road traffic accidents (RTAs) involving occupants and pedestrians account for the majority of cases and are increasing year on year. They are now a significant cause of disease burden in Africa. Head and spinal injuries occur as a consequence of the increasing numbers of vehicles, motorcycles, speeding, poor quality of the roads, and lack of enforcement of statutory safety regulations for driving and the lack of safety belts and helmets (Table 19.1). Other causes include falls and violence. Interpersonal violence is increasingly a cause of HI in some countries in Africa. The aim of this chapter is to present an overview of head and spinal injuries. The student should aim to know the increasing burden, clinical features, management and prevention of head and spinal injuries.

EPIDEMIOLOGY

The annual incidence of traumatic brain injury ranges from 150-500/100,000 per year depending on the individual country. It is estimated that 1-2% of high income populations live with a TBI disability. The incidence is high in some countries in Africa. In South Africa the mortality rate in TBI was reported to be 81/100,000 per year, with a >10% all case fatality rate. High risk groups for TBI include children, adolescents, young adults and the elderly, with males being affected 2-3 times more often than females.

Table 19.1 Main causes and risk factors for TBI in Africa

Cause	Risk factor	%	Risk
Road Traffic Accidents	speeding, driver sleepiness, lack of use of seat belts, poor roads, lack of law enforcement, alcohol, medications, drugs	>80	increasing
Falls	climbing trees, poor work place safety, age & co-morbidity	>10	static
Violence	urban poverty, unemployment, alcohol	<10	increasing

Pathology of head injury

The term HI includes injury to the brain, face, head and skull. Injury to the brain is called traumatic brain injury (TBI) and all grades can occur from mild to severe. Because the brain is a soft organ contained within a rigid box, any trauma to the skull will also cause movement of the brain inside the skull. This can result in TBI ranging from no visible signs in cases of mild head injury (concussion) to bruising, laceration, bleeding and oedema in severe head injury. Bleeding from torn blood vessels may result in a haematoma, either intracerebrally (intracerebral haematoma, ICH), or in the extradural space (extradural haematoma, EDH) and in the subdural space (subdural haematoma, SDH). If the resulting volume is too large there may be herniation of the brain or brain stem through the tentorium or foramen magnum and coning and death will follow. In addition to the primary brain injury there may be secondary brain injury as a result of hypotension and hypoxia. The main causes of these are blood loss, lung injury and seizures. Secondary infection may arise as a result of penetrating injuries or a fractured skull.

Clinical diagnosis

A history of the cause and the circumstances of the injury should if possible be obtained either from the patient or a witness. It is important to enquire if there was any period of loss of consciousness and the current state of consciousness of the patient. The main steps in the examination of head injury are outlined below in Table 19.2. The Glasgow Coma Scale (GCS) uses a point system out of a maximum of 15 to evaluate the best eye opening, verbal and motor response (Chapter 9). An underlying fracture of the skull is suspected if there is a CSF leak, bleeding from the ears, bruising around the eyes or ears, deafness or on the basis of a significant head wound. The severity of a head injury resulting in TBI is graded in terms of the following: *current level of consciousness, any period of unconsciousness, memory loss, focal neurological deficit* and *skull fracture*. The current level of consciousness of the patient is the most important indicator of the severity and progress of head injury.

Table 19.2 Summary of main steps in the examination of patient with head injury

Clinical finding (examine for the following)	Comments
STEP 1 level of consciousness	**most important of all assessments** *(repeat at regular intervals, usually every 15 mins)*
STEP 2 signs of HI	
lacerations, bruising or skull fractures	may be absent in TBI
injury to cervical spine	check neck & limbs
signs of basal skull fracture	
csf leak from nose/ear, usually clear	confirm by testing fluid for glucose
bleeding around eyes & subconjuctiva	no posterior limit indicates fractured skull
bleeding from external ear	exclude laceration of external ear
bruising over the mastoid (Battle's sign)	may take 48 hours to develop
STEP 3 focal neurological signs	
pupillary response to light	pupil may dilate on same side in expanding lesion
limb weakness	asymmetrical limb withdrawal to deep pain indicates focal brain lesion
eye movements	observe for spontaneous eye movements
cranial nerve lesions	may indicate a skull fracture
other observations	BP may rise & pulse rate fall in ↑ICP

Imaging

All head injuries should be considered for imaging. Imaging includes plain X-rays of skull and spine, CT of the head and occasionally MRI of the brain and spinal cord. Indications for urgent CT include depression/loss of consciousness, focal neurological signs, seizures, fractured skull and CSF leak. CT may reveal evidence of fractures, intracranial haematomas and cerebral contusion (Fig. 19.1).

Plain X-ray skull   **CT scans (without contrast)**

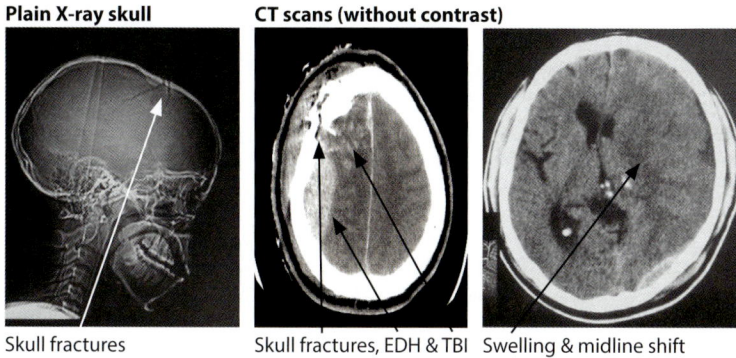

Skull fractures   Skull fractures, EDH & TBI Swelling & midline shift

Figure 19.1 Traumatic brain injury

DIFFUSE AXONAL INJURY (DAI)

This occurs from the shearing of axons as a result of a high impact closed HI. It is usually associated with an immediate LOC which persists after the injury. Imaging initially by CT is normal in >50-70% of cases and this may need to be repeated after 24/48 hours before showing haemorrhages and cerebral oedema. MRI is more sensitive than CT in the early stages of DAI. Management includes sedation, ventilation and measures for intracerebral pressure monitoring and control.

Classification

The classification or grading of HI is based on the initial history, clinical evaluation and GCS. This is made in order to identify and treat patients at risk. It is important to remember that the majority of cases of HI do not result in TBI. Of those that do, TBI is graded as mild if the GCS at assessment is >12, or the period of unconsciousness is <30 minutes. The majority, 85-90% of all TBIs are classified as mild. TBI is classified as moderate if the current GCS is 9-12 or there is persisting coma for >30 mins or there is a skull fracture but no evidence of brainstem malfunction (Table 19.3). TBI is categorised as severe if unconsciousness is greater than 24 hours or current GCS ≤8 or there are focal neurological signs or intracranial haematoma or failing brain stem function. Patients with moderate and severe TBI represent about 10-15% of all cases.

Table 19.3 Traumatic brain injury, summary of main clinical features

Grade	GCS	%	CT signs present*	Mortality %	Morbidity %	Disability
mild	13-15	85-90	in one third	1	50 (minor)	none/minor
moderate	9-12	5-10	in two thirds	2-5	60	disabled
severe	3-8	3-5	in all**	20-50	75	severely disabled

* includes fractured skull, contusion, bleeding, swelling
** except in diffuse axonal injury (DAI) when the initial CT of head may be normal

Key points

- main causes of HI are RTAs, falls & violence
- obtain a history of the cause of the head injury
- assess the level of consciousness
- examine for signs of head and neck injury& for neurological deficits
- TBIs are graded as mild, moderate and severe
- grade is the most important predictor of outcome

Management

The medical management of brain injured patients is complex. It involves 4 main sites/stages: *pre hospital care, transport to hospital, in hospital care* and *rehabilitation*. Any delay or failure at any of these stages results in increased mortality and morbidity.

Trivial and mild

Trivial head injuries and mild TBIs account for the majority of TBIs and most patients may be discharged home after initial examination with a warning about possible complications. The risk of complications for mild TBIs is low <1%. However patients with mild TBI and other clinical features of head injury should be admitted for 24 hours for closer neurological observations, care, possible CT scanning and a re-evaluation later. This group has an increased risk (1-5%), of serious neurological deterioration. The main indications for a CT scan in mild TBI include *alteration in level of consciousness, confusion, a history of transitory loss of consciousness, post traumatic amnesia, the presence of focal neurological signs* and *a possible skull fracture*. A skull X-ray should be performed if a CT scan is unavailable.

Moderate and severe injuries

This group represents 10-15% of all TBIs. Moderate and severe head injuries should all have a CT scan of the head, be admitted to an intensive care unit for observation and care and considered for any possible neurosurgical intervention.

Evaluation of moderate and severe TBIs

The first priority is to check that the airway is clear and that breathing and circulation are adequate. This may involve inserting an airway and ensuring that oxygen saturation is >95%. Circulation is maintained by starting emergency intravenous fluids and ensuring that ≤2 litres is given in the first 24 hours unless the patient is hypovolaemic for other reasons (Chapter 9). The next step is the evaluation of the extent and seriousness of the injuries. Many patients, in particular RTA cases, have concomitant injuries of the chest, abdomen, spine and extremities.

All patients with HI and altered consciousness should be assumed to have a neck injury and be immobilized until proven otherwise. This means a general evaluation in addition to measuring the level of consciousness, examining for neurological deficits and for evidence of head and spinal cord injury, and any skull or vertebral fractures. (Table 19.3) Check with family or friends for any history of any predisposing risk factors for head injury including loss of consciousness, stroke, seizures, alcohol and drugs. The GCS together with vital signs, pupil size and reaction to light should be checked every 15 minutes in unstable patients and then at 1-4 hourly intervals appropriate to the patient's condition. Special attention should be paid to avoiding the risk factors for secondary brain injury; this includes maintaining adequate blood pressure and oxygen saturation. If the patient's consciousness is deteriorating then mannitol 1 gm/kg/iv is given stat followed by iv boluses of 1-200 ml of 20% mannitol depending on the clinical situation. This may be helpful as a short term measure to reduce intracranial pressure. Prophylactic antibiotics and antiepileptics are indicated for all severe head injuries. Indicators of a poor prognosis are: *coma for >6 hours, fractured skull, non reacting pupils* and *focal neurological deficits*. The main indications for neurosurgical intervention are extradural and subdural haematoma, depressed skull fracture and occasionally intracerebral haemorrhage.

Key points

- 4 main stages, prehospital, transport, in hospital and rehabilitation
- aim is to prevent secondary complications of TBI
- brain damage is prevented by adequate evaluation & care
- this involves ABC & preventing seizures & infection
- CT head scan indicated in all moderate & severe TBI
- main indications for surgery are extradural & subdural haematomas and some ICH

OUTCOME

TBI accounts for up to half of all traumatic deaths with over half of these deaths occurring at the scene of the accident or on the way to hospital. The possible outcomes of TBIs are summarized in Table 19.3 and in the Glasgow Outcome Scale (Table 19.4). The initial grade of TBI after the primary injury is the most important predictor of outcome.

Table 19.4 Glasgow Outcome Scale

Classification	Description
dead	
persistent vegetative state	awake but unaware
severely disabled	conscious but dependent
moderately disabled	independent but disabled
good recovery	may have minor sequelae

Mortality

The overall case fatality rate (CFR) for all TBI is over 10%; however this varies from less than 1% in mild to 2-5% in moderate and 20-50% in severe TBI. The CFR for severe TBIs with coma lasting longer than 6 hours is >50%.

Morbidity

Most patients with mild TBI make a good recovery but about half have minor sequelae e.g. headache, lack of concentration etc which usually clear after a variable period of months to years. There is also increasing evidence that repeated episodes of mild TBI can lead to dementia and/or depression with lesions deep in the brain identified at post-mortem. In contrast, the majority of surviving patients with moderate and severe TBI will be permanently disabled from the onset. This is the leading cause of neurological disability in young persons (<40 yrs) worldwide. Moderate disability is 3-4 times more common than severe. The range of moderate and severe disabilities includes *personality changes, memory loss, dysphasia, paralysis* and *epilepsy*. Persistent vegetative state is uncommon. Over 90% of patients reach their maximum recovery by 6 months although some patients may continue to recover for years. Over 10% of patients with severe TBI develop epilepsy within 5 years of the injury.

REHABILITATION

Most patients with mild head injury make a good recovery without requiring any special measures or rehabilitation. Patients with moderate or severe head injury benefit most from rehabilitation. This may involve a considerable period of hospitalization, *usually >3 months* together with extensive inpatient and later outpatient rehabilitation while waiting for recovery of neurological function and healing of injuries. Recovery of function reaches a peak in about 90% of patients within the first six months after injury but may continue in some for years.

Post concussion syndrome

Post concussion syndrome may follow after mild or moderate head injuries. Patients can be disabled by recurrent symptoms including headaches, dizziness, poor concentration, impaired memory, fatigue and depression. These usually subside after a few months but can continue for as long as 6 months to 3 years. There are no abnormal neurological findings and no abnormalities on neuroimaging of the brain. Management is conservative and supportive.

Key points

- most patients with mild TBI eventually make a full recovery
- patients with moderate and severe TBI have high mortality & morbidity rates
- patients with moderate and severe TBI benefit most from rehabilitation

EXTRADURAL HAEMATOMA (EDH)

Extradural haematoma is a rapid collection of arterial blood occurring over minutes to hours in the extradural space as a result of a temporal/parietal skull fracture or a serious head injury. EDH results from a traumatic tear in the middle meningeal artery. The bleeding shells the dura mater from the inner table of the skull compressing the brain. The main cause is HI arising from RTA.

Clinical features

In EDH, characteristically there is a *lucid interval* between the patient waking up from the acute head injury and then becoming unconscious again. This lucid period is variable ranging from minutes to over 24 hours. It should be suspected whenever there is a sudden decline in the level of consciousness of a patient with a very recent head injury. The site of the extradural haematoma is on the same side as the underlying skull fracture and the pupillary dilatation.

Diagnosis

The diagnosis is suggested by the clinical presentation, neurological findings and a skull X-ray may show an underlying fracture. In EDH the CT scan of head shows on the affected side an area of increased density *biconvex inwards* with midline shift in severe cases (Figs. 19.2 & 3). However obtaining the CT scan should not be a reason to delay surgery, as any delay will inevitably result in the death of the patient.

CT scans (without contrast)

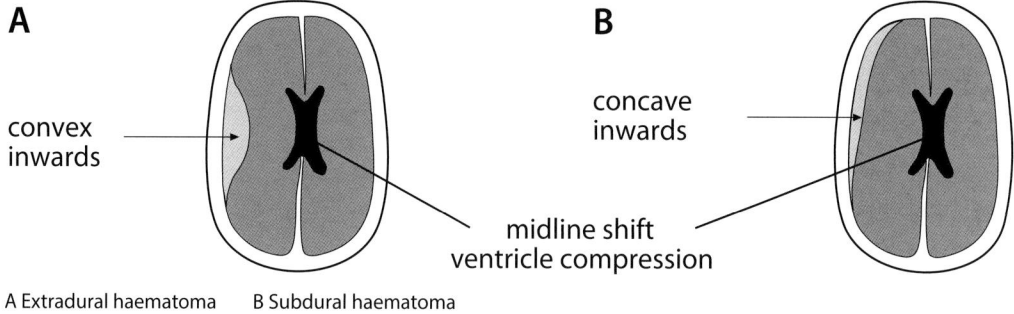

A Extradural haematoma   B Subdural haematoma

Figure 19.2 Illustrations of extradural and subdural haematoma

CT (without contrast)

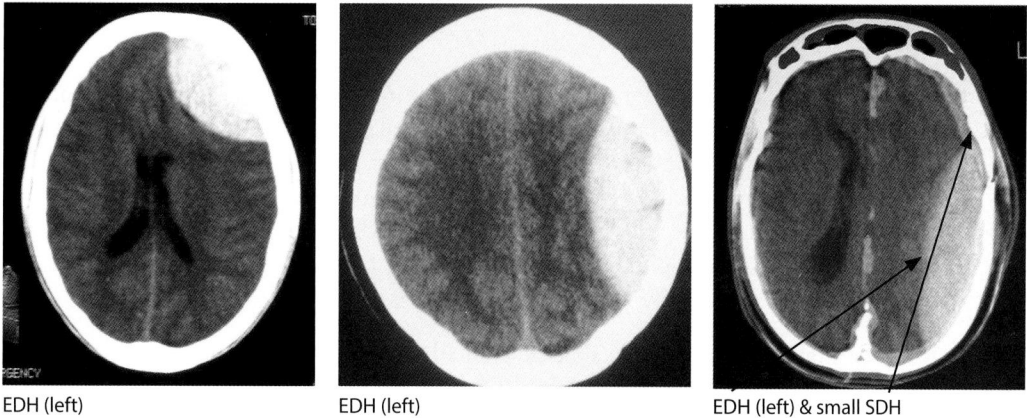

EDH (left)   EDH (left)   EDH (left) & small SDH

Figure 19.3 Extradural haematoma

Management

This is a true surgical emergency and management is by emergency craniotomy in order to establish urgent ligation of the bleeding vessel and surgical drainage of the EDH. Emergency resuscitation and a burr hole may provide temporary relief before the craniotomy.

Prognosis

Prognosis depends on the preoperative state of the patient. The presence of fixed dilated pupils is not a contraindication for surgery. If GCS ≤ 8 the mortality is >30%.

Key points

- EDH results from a meningeal artery tear outside the dura
- main cause is a fractured skull secondary to a RTA
- blood accumulates within minutes to hours in the extradural space
- lucid interval of minutes/hours followed by rapid onset of FND & LOC
- management is urgent craniotomy to ligate the bleeding vessel & drain the EDH

SUBDURAL HAEMATOMA (SDH)

Subdural haematoma (SDH) is a collection of blood which lies in the space between the dura and arachnoid layers of the meninges. It arises from an injury which causes rupture of bridging veins between the meningeal layers and can be *acute* or *chronic*.

Acute SDH

An acute SDH immediately follows a high energy head injury with just a short delay of hours or at most days between the injury and the onset of symptoms. Clinically this can lead to a rapid clinical deterioration due to the accumulation of blood with an immediate loss of consciousness and progressive or fluctuating decline in GCS. The source of the haemorrhage in acute SDH is both arterial and venous from contused cerebral cortex and blood vessels. If left untreated this may eventually lead to transtentorial herniation, coning, hemiparesis, coma and death. Management is by emergency surgical drainage usually involving a craniotomy. Cerebral swelling is common and may require decompression surgery. The prognosis is poor with 50-70% mortality.

Chronic SDH

A chronic SDH is a late complication which can follow any head injury but may occur after a relatively minor low energy or non reported head injury particularly in the elderly, in those on anticoagulants and in persons prone to falling e.g. alcoholics. The injury may be so minor that it is not remembered. Very occasionally chronic SDH is spontaneous without previous history of trauma. In chronic SDH there is a slow accumulation over weeks or months of venous blood over one or occasionally both cerebral hemispheres.

Clinical features

The clinical presentation is one of non specific gradual fluctuating drowsiness, confusion, and headache and only later followed by the onset of a focal neurological deficit, usually hemiparesis and progressing to alteration in level of consciousness, seizures and sometimes coma. The finding of a progressive hemiparesis or a recent onset confusional or dementia type illness is a feature in Africa because of late hospital presentation.

Imaging

The diagnosis of SDH is either confirmed or else newly discovered by a CT of the head. The SDH shows as a *crescent shaped concave inwards* area of increased density spreading round the surface of the cerebral hemisphere with or without an accompanying mid line shift (Figs. 19.2 & 4). Approximately 10-12 days after injury the appearance of SDH on CT becomes isodense and is then more difficult to notice. After about 3 weeks post HI the SDH becomes hypodense on non contrasted CT and is then more obvious.

Management

The management of chronic subdural haematoma depends on the size and clinical state of the patient. Small subdurals without focal neurological signs can be managed conservatively and these may resorb spontaneously. Larger subdurals with changing levels of consciousness and focal neurological signs need surgical drainage and evacuation. CT indications for surgery include *cortical compression, midline shift* and *hydrocephalus*. Drainage is established via burr holes in the skull with or without a surgical drain. This procedure is carried out by most general surgeons in Africa. Steroids, dexamethasone 4 mg qds may be helpful in the early stages.

CT scans (without contrast)

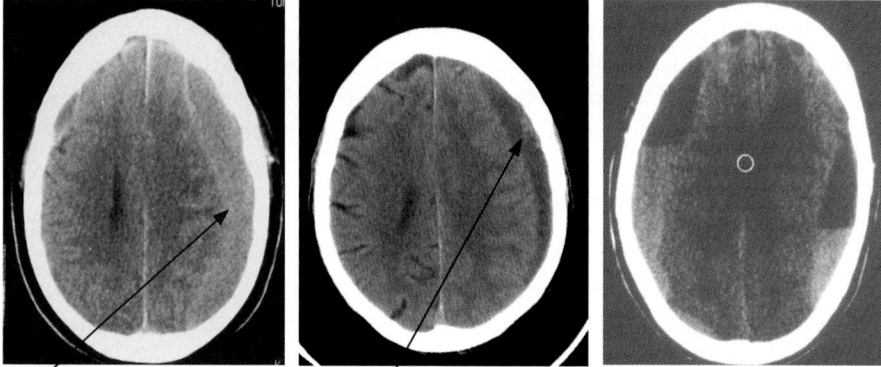

SDH (left) isodense   SDH (left) hypodense   SDH (bilateral, old)

Figure 19.4 Subdural haematoma (chronic)

Prognosis

The outcome is generally good in all age groups but 10-15% of patients may require a second drainage procedure and a subdural empyema occurs in <1%.

Key points

- in SDH there is usually a history of HI
- acute SDH occurs within hours or days of HI
- chronic SDH occurs within weeks/months of HI
- presentations include headache, confusion and coma, seizures & hemiparesis
- SDH is usually confirmed or diagnosed by CT of head
- management is mostly by surgical drainage

Intracerebral haematoma (ICH)

This arises from severe contusional HI or vascular injury. Common sites include the cerebral cortex, cerebellum and subarachnoid space (Fig. 19.5). Management depends on the severity, clinical condition and evidence of mass effect. Craniotomy and surgical evacuation is indicated in presence of focal neurological signs and decreasing GCS.

CT scans (without contrast)

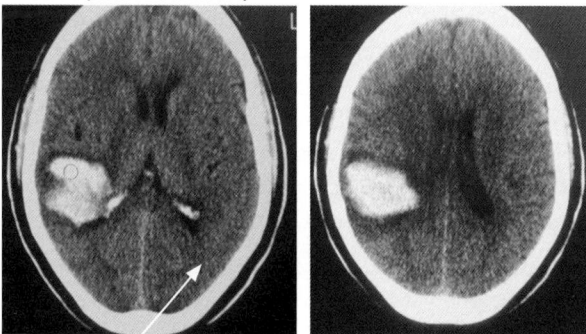

ICH & intraventricular extension

Figure 19.5 Intracerebral haematoma

SPINAL INJURY

Spinal injury arises mostly from road traffic accidents (RTAs) and falls and is a major cause of death and disability in Africa. It is often associated with HI and multiple trauma. Males in the age group 20-40 years are the main risk group affected. In Africa boys and adolescent males are frequently affected as a result of falls from trees and more recently RTAs. Females are also affected because of falls whilst carrying heavy loads on their heads. Early detection and immobilization are critical to avoid secondary damage.

Clinical features

The cervical and the lumbar spine are the most common sites of injury with the cervical spine being more frequently affected. Paraplegia and quadriplegia are the main neurological disorders resulting from spinal injury. Spinal injuries anywhere from the cervical spine down to the level of the first lumbar vertebra inevitably involve the spinal cord whereas injuries below L1 involve the cauda equina. In spinal cord injury there may be an initial period of *spinal shock* which can persist for *days* to *weeks* (usually 1-2 weeks) before the characteristic spasticity and upper motor neurone signs develop. Spinal shock is characterized by flaccid paralysis with no reflexes or sensation below the level of spinal cord injury. In contrast paraplegia resulting from spinal injury affecting the cauda equina remains permanently flaccid with characteristic lower motor neurone signs. Bladder and bowel dysfunction occurs with both types. The completeness of the lesion is the most important factor in determining prognosis and management. Incomplete lesions may recover to a variable extent.

Spinal stability

The stability of the spine at the level of injury plays a crucial role in further management. Instability is defined as the loss of ability of the spine to maintain normal alignment under normal loads. Instability increases the risk of further spinal cord damage. The Denis three column model (Table 19.5) is used to classify spinal stability.

Table 19.5 Denis three column model of the spine

anterior column	anterior one-half of the vertebral body and annulus fibrosus & the anterior longitudinal ligament (ALL)
middle column	posterior one-half of the vertebral body & annulus fibrosus & posterior longitudinal ligament (PLL)
posterior column	pedicles, laminae, spinous processes & ligaments

Spinal injuries are classified as stable when the interspinous ligaments are intact and as unstable when ligaments are disrupted. The spine is unstable if ≥2 columns on the Denis three column model are disrupted. The mechanism of injury helps to determine the degree of stability and type of cord injury. A shearing or hinge injury typically results in unstable spinal injury with cord involvement, whereas a compression injury results in stable fractures. Stable spinal injury occurs mostly without cord involvement. Typically the former arises from RTAs, whereas the latter arises from an object falling on to the head. However a severe or burst fracture from whatever cause results in an unstable spine and possible spinal cord injury.

The initial examination should be targeted at checking for local injury in the spine, particularly in the neck and looking for paralysis of limbs, being careful to avoid aggravating existing injuries by any movement. It is critical to emphasise *that the spine must be stabilized in any patient with evidence or suspicion of spinal injury before being moved.* This is done by means of using a *hard cervical collar*, putting the patient *lying on a back board* and using the *logrolling method* when turning the patient.

Key points

- RTAs and falls are the main causes of spinal injury
- neck and lower back are the sites most frequently affected
- spine should be stabilized in patients with spinal injury before being moved
- spinal shock lasting >24 hours is a bad prognostic sign
- death or paraplegia are the two main outcomes

X-rays spine

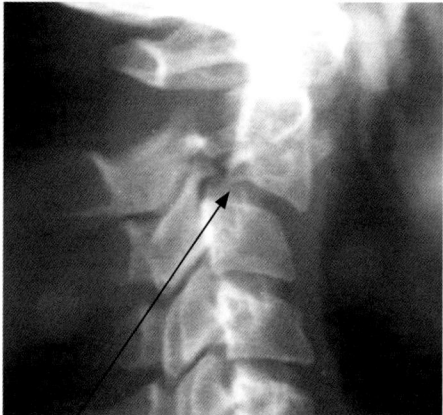
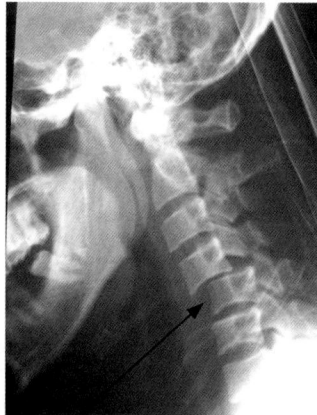

C2/C3   C4/5

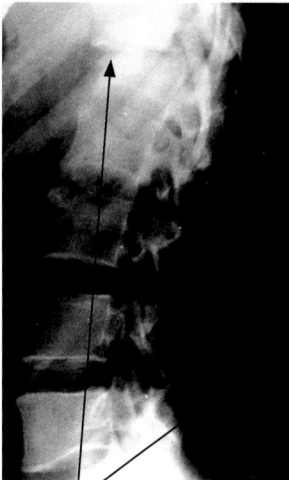
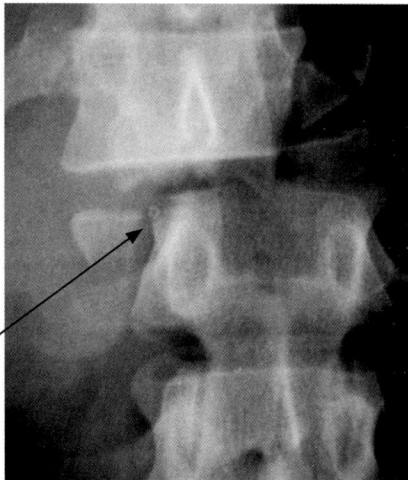
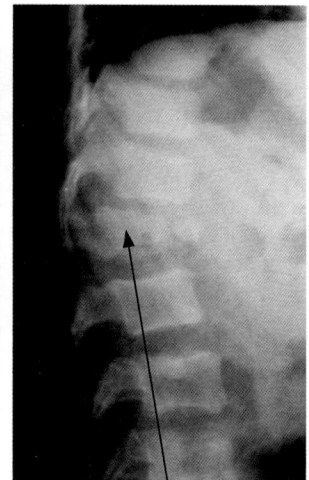

T12/L1   Compression fracture T9

Figure 19.6 Fracture dislocation of spine

Imaging

Management depends on the site and stability of the injury. Straight X-rays of the spine will confirm obvious fractures and dislocations (Fig. 19.6). X-rays, AP and lateral of the cervical spine should visualize C1 down to the upper border of T1. CT scan may reveal fractures not visible on plain X-rays.

Management

In principle, an unstable cervical fracture risks further damage to the spinal cord and requires immobilization before being moved or mobilized. This can be done by operative fixation or skull traction with a Halo or plaster jacket immobilization for 12 weeks. If a cervical fracture is stable without cord injury, then a cervical collar is used. Thoracolumbar fractures are managed along the same general principles, although internal fixation is used less frequently.

General management includes support of arterial oxygenation and adequate spinal cord perfusion pressure. The use of high dose steroids in acute cord injury is still common practice although its value is controversial. If methylprednisolone is given in doses of 2 grams intravenously within 8 hours of the spinal cord injury and continued over the first 24 hours it was considered previously to have a protective role. However recent evidence suggests that it not effective and may actually be deleterious. A urinary catheter should always be inserted. Very special attention from the onset should be paid to the prevention of respiratory complications, bedsores, urinary tract infections, DVT and limb contractures. Long term rehabilitation of paraplegia is already discussed in chapter 10.

Outcome

Patients with high cervical cord injuries seldom survive even with ventilatory support. Patients with a lesion above C7 remain dependent on others for continuous care. Patients with a lesion below C7 may be able to learn to transfer to wheelchair independently, while patients with lower spinal cord or cauda equina injuries gain complete wheelchair independence. Respiratory failure, infections and bedsores are the main complications of spinal cord injuries. Long initial periods of hospitalization of typically 3-6 months are usual, and mortality rates in Africa while recovering in hospital are frequently in the order of 20-30%.

Key points

- imaging is essential in the management of spinal injuries
- acute management includes stabilization of fractured spine & respiratory support
- scrupulous attention is needed to prevent bedsores and infection
- mortality rates are 20-30% and survivors need assistance with mobilization

PREVENTION

The main cause of head and neck injuries are RTAs. These are increasing at an alarming rate in Africa. They are mostly preventable by reducing both speed and dangerous driving. Measures to achieve these include adequate enforcing of traffic safety regulations, speed limits, road bumps, alcohol checks and ensuring that motor cyclists and cyclists wear helmets. Other causes of HI such as falls, work related accidents and violence are also partially preventable. General measures for prevention include better education and informed legislation.

Key points

· head and neck injury is a leading cause of death in Africa
· young adult males are a particularly high risk group
· main causes are RTAs and falls
· measures for primary prevention are now urgently needed

Selected references

Alexander T, Fuller G, Hargovan P, Clarke DL, Muckart DJ, Thomson SR. *An audit of the quality of care of traumatic brain injury at a busy regional hospital in South Africa*. S Afr J Surg. 2009 Nov;47(4):120-2, 4-6.

Benatar SR, Fleischer TE, Peter JC, Pope A, Taylor A. *Treatment of head injuries in the public sector in South Africa*. S Afr Med J. 2000 Aug;90(8):790-3.

Bruns J, Jr., Hauser WA. *The epidemiology of traumatic brain injury: a review*. Epilepsia. 2003;44 Suppl 10:2-10.

Casey ER, Muro F, Thielman NM, Maya E, Ossmann EW, Hocker MB, Gerardo CJ. *Analysis of traumatic injuries presenting to a referral hospital emergency department in Moshi, Tanzania*. Int J Emerg Med. 2012 Jun 8;5(1):28.

de Villiers JC. *Head injuries in South Africa*. S Afr J Surg. 1984 Feb-Mar;22(1):51-6.

Draulans N, Kiekens C, Roels E, Peers K. *Etiology of spinal cord injuries in Sub-Saharan Africa*. Spinal Cord. 2011 Dec;49(12):1148-54.

Fielingsdorf K, Dunn RN. *Cervical spine injury outcome--a review of 101 cases treated in a tertiary referral unit*. S Afr Med J. 2007 Mar;97(3):203-7.

Hart C, Williams E. *Epidemiology of spinal cord injuries: a reflection of changes in South African society*. Paraplegia. 1994 Nov;32(11):709-14.

Jennett B. *Epidemiology of head injury*. J Neurol Neurosurg Psychiatry. 1996 Apr;60(4):362-9.

Le Roux AA, Nadvi SS. *Acute extradural haematoma in the elderly*. Br J Neurosurg. 2007 Feb;21(1):16-20.

Leucht P, Fischer K, Muhr G, Mueller EJ. *Epidemiology of traumatic spine fractures*. Injury. 2009 Feb;40(2):166-72.

Lindsay Kenneth W, Bone Ian, *Neurology and Neurosurgery Illustrated,* Churchill Livingstone 4th edition 2004.

Neurological Disorders: *Global burden of neurological disorders*: WHO 2006

Nantulya VM, Reich MR. *The neglected epidemic: road traffic injuries in developing countries*. BMJ. 2002 May 11;324(7346):1139-41.

Nwadinigwe CU, Iloabuchi TC, Nwabude IA. *Traumatic spinal cord injuries (SCI): a study of 104 cases*. Niger J Med. 2004 Apr-Jun;13(2):161-5.

Omoke NI, Chukwu CO, Madubueze CC, Oyakhiolme OP. *Outcome of road traffic injuries received in the emergency room of a teaching hospital, Southeast Nigeria*. Trop Doct. 2012 Jan;42(1):18-22.

Seleye-Fubara D, Etebu EN. *Pathology of death from severe head injuries in Rivers State: a study of sixty eight consecutive cases in five years*. Niger J Med. 2011 Oct-Dec;20(4):470-4

Solagberu BA. *Spinal cord injuries in Ilorin, Nigeria*. West Afr J Med. 2002 Jul-Sep;21(3):230-2.

Tagliaferri F, Compagnone C, Korsic M, Servadei F, Kraus J. *A systematic review of brain injury epidemiology in Europe*. Acta Neurochir (Wien). 2006 Mar;148(3):255-68; discussion 68.

Umaru H, Ahidjo A. Pattern *of spinal cord injury in Maiduguri, North Eastern Nigeria. Niger* J Med. 2005 Jul-Sep;14(3):276-8.

Watters DA, Sinclair JR. *Outcome of severe head injuries in central Africa.* J R Coll Surg Edinb. 1988 Feb;33(1):35-8.

Wilson DA, Garrett MP, Wait SD, Kucia EJ, Saguda E, Ngayomela et al. *Expanding neurosurgical care in Northwest Tanzania: the early experience of an initiative to teach neurosurgery at Bugando Medical Centre.* World Neurosurg. 2012 Jan;77(1):32-8.

Winkler AS, Tluway A, Slottje D, Schmutzhard E, Hartl R. *The pattern of neurosurgical disorders in rural northern Tanzania: a prospective hospital-based study.* World Neurosurg. 2010 Apr;73(4):264-9.

CHAPTER 20
CARE IN NEUROLOGY

CONTENTS

CHAPTER 20

CARE IN NEUROLOGY

The burden of neurological disease in Africa is already evident from earlier chapters where they account for >5% of all deaths and >14% of all disabilities. Neurological disorders account for 10-20% of adult medical admissions to hospitals in Africa, 20-30% of whom die in hospital and >30% of whom are disabled at discharge. The leading neurological causes of death in hospitals are stroke, HIV disease, infections and head injury, and the leading causes of disability are stroke, paraplegia, trauma, and epilepsy. Most medical practice is concerned with the control of symptoms and this is particularly true when caring for patients with neurological disorders. The common symptoms and worries encountered in advanced neurological disorders are outlined below in Table 20.1. Neurological care invariably involves elements of palliative care. Palliative care is about caring for a patient when the disease no longer responds to curative treatment. This involves special attention to symptoms such as pain, and psychological, social and spiritual well-being. Palliative care regards dying as a normal process and offers practical support to help the patient and family. It is an integral part of patient care in hospital and is best delivered by a team approach. This includes family, nurses, doctors, physiotherapists, occupational therapists and spiritual advisors. The aim of this chapter is to present an overview of care and symptom control in patients with neurological disorders with an emphasis on palliative care. The student should aim to be familiar with this and in particular the relief of pain.

Table 20.1 Common symptoms and worries in patients with advanced neurological disorders

Physical	Psychological	Social	Spiritual
pain	depression	loss of income	religious
confusion/delirium	fear anxiety	fear for children spouse & dependants	non religious
loss of communication	stigma/guilt		why me?
dysphagia			
seizures			
nausea/vomiting			
spasticity			
dyspnoea			
immobility			
constipation			

MAIN SYMPTOMS

Pain

Pain is defined as *a subjective unpleasant sensory* and *emotional experience* associated with *actual or potential tissue damage*. Pain is a common disorder and WHO estimates that 5-30% of the world's population experience persistent pain depending on where they live. The most commonly affected sites worldwide are head, neck, knees and lower back. Pain is influenced by the patient's mood, morale and the underlying reason for the pain. Chronic pain may persist long after the tissue damage has been done and is defined as pain lasting for >3/12.

Total pain is an interaction of the physical, emotional, psychological and spiritual components. The consequences of pain include immobility, depression, poor sleep and nutrition and overdependence on family and carers. Longer term consequences affect employment, family, and social life. Chronic pain as a result of neurological disorders is a major and neglected cause of disability in Africa. The management of pain involves **non pharmacological measures, drug treatments, psychological** and s**piritual support**. The aim of drug treatment is to provide an effective and regular treatment which completely stops pain and prevents its recurrence. The commonly used drugs in pain control (Table 20.4) and the WHO steps in their use (Table 20.5) are outlined below.

Pathophysiology

Pain is broadly classified into two types: **nociceptive** and **neuropathic** (Table 20.2). The difference between nociceptive and neuropathic is not always clear-cut clinically and any one individual may suffer from one or both types of pain.

Nociceptive pain is caused by activation of primary pain receptors in tissues and is transmitted to the brain through slow non myelinated peripheral C fibres and faster conducting larger myelinated (A) fibres. It can be either somatic arising from skin, musculoskeletal (muscle spasticity, joint deformities) or visceral arising from internal organs (malignancy, stone) or bone (fracture). The type of pain depends on the site, origin and cause of pain. It ranges from the familiar pricking and burning pain in skin conditions to a dull, continuous, diffuse, aching as described in internal malignancy or the intermittent, sharp and colicky pain which occurs in gastrointestinal or ureteric colic.

Neuropathic pain by contrast is mostly neurological in origin arising from damaged neural tissue either in the peripheral or the central nervous system. The main sites of origin are peripheral nerves (HIV, diabetes), nerve roots (herniated disc, herpes zoster), spinal cord (paraplegia) and the brain (post stroke). The sensations that characterize neuropathic pain are variable and often multiple and are described as burning, gnawing, aching or lancinating (knife-like) or shooting in character. There is frequently numbness or dysaesthesia (altered unpleasant sensation) or allodynia (when a non painful stimulus is perceived as pain) in a superficial sensory distribution coupled with local autonomic dysfunction. Neuropathic pain can be either intermittent, lasting seconds or continuous, lasting hours, and can persist even without the stimulus. It generally responds poorly to treatment. Pain without identifiable tissue or nerve damage is termed idiopathic. The N-methyl–D aspartate (NMDA) channel receptor complex, substance P, bradykinin and serotonin are all involved in the pathophysiology of pain. These are found predominantly in the spinal cord and peripheral nervous system.

Table 20.2 Neurological types of pain

Classification	Main causes
Neuropathic	
peripheral	neuropathies: HIV, diabetes, neuralgia, injury, causalgia, complex regional pain syndromes (local limb injury)
central	thalamic stroke, paraplegia, spinal cord injury, disc disease, HIV, syphilis
Nociceptive	
spasticity & rigidity	strokes, quadriplegia/paraplegia, dystonia, tetanus, stiff person syndrome
others	headache, arthritis

Measurement

All types of pain should be described fully in terms of quality, severity, location, mode of onset, provoking and relieving factors, and time course. Pain is subjective but can be measured. The simplest measurement uses self reported severity in terms of mild, moderate, severe and very severe which can be recorded and graded on a corresponding scale of 1-4. In clinical practice however, there is widespread use of the verbal or written analogue scale. This is a scale of 1-10, where 1 is the least and 10 is the worst pain imaginable. The patient is asked *"where on this scale of 1-10 do you put your pain?"* The value of the pain scale is that it is independent of language, easy to understand and use and can be recorded and repeated at each patient visit and response to therapy monitored.

Major causes of neurological pain in Africa

- spinal cord injuries
- neuropathies
- myelopathies
- malignancies
- stroke
- chronic neurological disorders

MANAGEMENT OF PAIN

Relief of pain should be the responsibility of all health care workers. The main aim is to diagnose, treat and stop the pain. In chronic neurological disorders this frequently involves providing maximal pain relief, as complete alleviation is not always possible. The range of clinical treatments includes non pharmacological and pharmacological measures. The non pharmacological approach is summarised in Table 20.3. The drug treatment of pain of neurological origin is based on the distinction between the pain of nociceptive and neuropathic origin and is summarised in Table 20.4 In practice, although these may be difficult to distinguish, the pain of nociceptive origin responds better to non-opioid analgesics such as **paracetamol, aspirin** and **non steroidal anti-inflammatory drugs** whereas pain of neuropathic origin responds best to **tricyclic antidepressants** e.g. **amitriptyline** and the **anticonvulsants** e.g. **gabapentin** and **carbamazepine.** Opioids can be used in both types and their role in the management of pain is summarized below in Table 20.4. Pain due to local compression of peripheral nerves or nerve roots may be relieved by appropriate surgery. Nerve root blocks and epidural spinals provide temporary relief. Patients with chronic pain benefit from a multidisciplinary approach involving cognitive behaviour therapy, physiotherapy and occupational therapy.

Table 20.3 General and local measures used in pain management

Intervention	Indication	Comments
Non Pharmacological		
Explanation, relaxation, positioning	any pain	non invasive
Complementary therapies aromatherapy, massage	chronic pain	may improve pain relief *(no evidence for use in severe pain)*
Transcutaneous electrical nerve stimulation (TENS)	musculoskeletal, soft tissue	patient is in control
Acupuncture	chronic myofacial pain, migraine	pain relief *(no evidence for use in severe pain)*
Radiotherapy (palliative)	bony metastases particularly spinal	excellent pain relief
Local		
Invasive anaesthesia *spinal, regional blocks*	spinal & localised root/plexus lesions	very effective but needs skilled operator
Topical agents *heat/cold*	any pain	
capsaicin cream		burning, redness, cough. *(takes 2-6 weeks to work)*
lignocaine patch		few side effects, expensive

DRUG TREATMENT OF PAIN

Non-opioids

These include non steroidal anti-inflammatory drugs (NSAIDs) and paracetamol. The most commonly used NSAIDs are **aspirin, ibuprofen,** and **diclofenac**. Their doses, routes of administration and side effects are outlined in Table 20.4. These are the main first line treatment for most pain regardless of whether it is of nociceptive or neuropathic origin and are used at all 3 steps in the WHO analgesic ladder (Table 20.5). NSAIDs should be used cautiously in patients with renal impairment as they may further impair function and may provoke renal failure. In patients with a history of dyspepsia the concurrent prescription of **proton pump inhibitors** or **histamine-2 receptor blockers** help to reduce the symptomatic upper GIT side effects.

Opioids

Opioids include all drugs that act at opioid receptors. These receptors are scattered throughout the body though mainly in the central and peripheral nervous system. Opiates are either derived from the opium poppy **(morphine** and **codeine)** or synthesised in the laboratory

(pethidine). Opioids are indicated for pain at steps two and three of the WHO ladder (Table 20.5). This includes pain in patients with advanced disease and their short-term use to relieve breakthrough or severe acute pain of any origin.

The use of opioids for non-malignant chronic pain is controversial. In general, opioids on their own should be avoided for intractable chronic neurological pain (usually neuropathic) to reduce the risk of dependence. However their use in advanced or terminal disease should not be restricted as they are necessary and there is no risk of dependence in this setting. The biggest barriers to their use are availability and the stigma from both the doctor and the patient surrounding their use. Once these can be overcome they provide excellent pain relief. Whenever opioids are used, they should be given at regular intervals, e.g. morphine every 4 hours (**oxycodone** can be given 6 hourly), preferably via the oral route or when necessary via the parenteral route. The dose and frequency should be according to the needs of the patient and be reduced in renal or hepatic failure and in the elderly. Constipation is usually not a major issue in clinical practice.

It is important to realise that opioids are controlled drugs with strict regulations concerning their availability, prescription and use anywhere in the world. A major limitation to their use in many low income countries are the stringent national control policies regarding the accessibility and use of opioids for pain. However some countries in Africa have recently prioritized their use in pain control and opioids are available for medical use.

Adjuvants

These mainly include the antidepressants **amitriptyline** and the anticonvulsants **carbamazepine** and **gabapentin** or **pregabalin**. These are used in all three steps in the WHO analgesic ladder for the management of neuropathic pain. They are most commonly used as adjuvants in combination with opioids or non opioids depending on the severity of the pain. In some patients with chronic pain of neuropathic origin they are used on their own without analgesics. Examples of neurological disorders benefitting from their use include neuropathies (HIV & DM) and post herpetic and trigeminal neuralgias.

Their dose, route, frequency and side effects are outlined in Table 20.4. The main limitations are their side effects and frequency of administration which may limit patient compliance. It is always wise to start at the lowest dose and increase it slowly. In general antidepressants are taken once daily, often at night whereas anticonvulsants are prescribed twice or three times daily. The main side effects of tricyclics are anticholinergic and include sedation, dry mouth, postural hypotension and constipation among others. Side effects of the anticonvulsants include drowsiness (which often clears with regular usage), confusion and ataxia. Both antidepressants and anticonvulsants may be used together as they have different mechanisms of action in the nervous system.

Table 20.4 Drugs used in pain management

Indication	Drug/dose/route/frequency	Side effects
Minor pain *(non opioids)*	aspirin 300-500 mg tab, 1-2 po/6 hourly ibuprofen 400 mg tab, 1-2 po/pr/8-12 hourly diclofenac 50-75 mg, po/pr/im/12 hourly paracetamol 500 mg tab,1-2 po/pr/6 hourly	gastric irritation, peptic ulceration, GIT bleeding, nausea, renal dysfunction liver damage in over dosage
Intermediate pain *(opioids mild)*	codeine/dihydrocodeine 30-60 mg, po/pr/im/6 hourly tramadol 50-100 mg/po/pr/im/6 hourly	constipation
Major pain *(opioids strong)*	* pethidine 50-100 mg/po/im/4-6 hourly morphine 2.5, 5,10-20 mg/po/im/sc/4-6 hourly	constipation sedation, nausea, vomiting, respiratory depression (rare)
Chronic neurological pain *(adjuvant)*	amitriptyline 10-100 mg/po/nocte, starting dose is 10-25 mg increasing as tolerated	sedation, dry mouth, constipation, hypotension, blurred vision, confusion
	carbamazepine 2-300 mg/po/8-12 hourly *(main use is in trigeminal neuralgia)*	sedation, dizziness, ataxia, blood dyscrasias
	gabapentin 100 mg/po/8 hourly or 300 mg nocte increasing by 300 mg every 1-2 days to max of 2.4 3.6 gm daily as tolerated *or* pregabalin 75 mg/po/12 hourly increase to max of 600 mg daily as tolerated	sedation (transient) unsteadiness, oedema, headache

duration of action of pethidine is too short for use in chronic pain relief

Table 20.5 WHO analgesic ladder

Step 1	non-opioid ± **adjuvant**
Step 2	mild opioid for mild-moderate pain ± non-opioid ± **adjuvant**
Step 3	strong opioid for severe pain ± non opioid ± **adjuvant**

Key points

- adequate pain control is very important in patient care
- controlling pain, if done properly does not shorten & may allow normal life
- opioids are used for pain not responding to simple analgesics & NSAIDs
- opioids are indicated for pain control in advanced neurological disease
- neuropathic pain frequently responds to combinations of antidepressants & analgesics

OTHER MAIN SYMPTOMS

Impaired communication

Impaired communication occurs in many neurological disorders. It ranges from aphasia in stroke to dysarthria in motor neurone disease and the inability to understand or comprehend in dementia. In virtually all situations, communication with the patient switches from speech to a non verbal form. This may take the form of "fixed expressions", gestures, signs or written commands. The family should be encouraged to try anything they feel is acceptable as a way of communicating to the patient. A simple communication board with images or illustrations indicating a person's daily needs can be very helpful at this stage. It is also wise to advise health care workers, family members and carers to behave at the bedside as if the patient hears and understands what is being said. Impaired communication may be improved in certain circumstances. Measures include making certain the patient is comfortable and pain free, that the environment is conducive to communication, without outside noise or interference and with appropriate face to face seating. The help of a person trained in speech and language therapy should be sought where ever possible.

Key points

- make sure patient is pain free & comfortable
- encourage family to try to communicate
- communicate in a conducive environment without noise or interference
- sit in front so the patient can clearly see your face
- obtain help from a person experienced in speech and language therapy

Confusion/delirium

Neurological disorders have high rates of confusion and behavioural disturbances. The main causes include infections, stroke, anaemia/anoxia, metabolic disorders, neurodegenerative disorders e.g. dementia, extrapyramidal disorders, SOL, drugs and psychiatric disorders. The main causes of confusion/coma have already been outlined in chapter 9. Management depends on the clinical situation and the overall aim. In the early stages, it is important to retain a high index of suspicion for a reversible cause and the aim should be to screen for any underlying disorder. Simple bedside screening tests, include measuring oxygen saturation, glucose, malaria parasite and an HIV test. The patient should ideally be nursed in a quiet, dimly lit area or room away from other patients and surrounded by family. The health care worker should aim to be supportive and reassuring to the patient and family. If these measures do not succeed then drug treatment should be started with neuroleptics.

Drug treatment

Haloperidol is the drug of first choice starting with low dose 0.5-1.0 mg/po/im/bd increasing as required. In patients with acute delirium, it may be necessary to use higher starting doses, 1.5-3 mg stat po/im or sc and to repeat after the first 1-2 hours if necessary. The total 24 hour dosage of haloperidol ranges from 5-30 mg. **Chlorpromazine** 25-50 mg (or 50-100 mg if necessary) po/im/8 hourly is an alternative. In the later stages of an advanced or terminal disease treatment should start directly with neuroleptics.

If there is a major anxiety component, then an anxiolytic may be used in addition to neuroleptics. **Diazepam** 5-10 mg/po/im 8 hourly is usually the drug of first choice. If the cause is raised intracranial pressure, then steroids, usually **dexamethasone** 8 mg/po/iv is given twice or three times daily (steroids can be given once daily as a single dose) until symptoms are controlled and then it is reduced after 3-5 days to 4 mg twice or once daily or twice weekly as is necessary. The second dose should ideally not be later than early afternoon as steroids can sometimes cause insomnia. The drugs most commonly used to treat confusional states are outlined below in Table 20.6.

Table 20.6 Drugs commonly used for confusion/delirium

Class	Drug/dose/route/duration	Indication	Side effects
Neuroleptics	haloperidol 0.5-3 mg/po/sc/12 hourly increasing to 5-10 mg 12 hourly if necessary	delirium/insomnia	drowsiness, dry mouth, parkinsonism
	chlorpromazine 25-50 mg/po/im/ or 100 mg/po/8 hourly	psychosis	dyskinesia, parkinsonism
	thioridazine 10-75 mg/po/nocte	confusion/insomnia	arrhythmias, parkinsonism
Anxiolytics	diazepam 10-20 mg/po/rectally/8 hourly	anxiety	drowsiness
	lorazepam 0.5-2 mg/po/im/iv/od	anxiety	drowsiness
	midazolam 5-10 mg/sc/im/or rectally /8 hourly	anxiety	drowsiness
	oxazepam/temazepam 10-15 mg/po/nocte	insomnia	drowsiness

Key points

- neurological disorders have high rates of confusion & delirium
- it is important to exclude a treatable cause
- main antipsychotic drugs used are haloperidol & chlorpromazine
- it is important to treat with an adequate dose
- main anxiolytics are the benzodiazepines

Seizures

Epileptic seizures are a common complication in terminal neurological disorders and are usually self limiting. Acute management is directed at protecting the patient from immediate injury and aspiration and the emergency drug treatment and prevention of recurrences. **Benzodiazepines** followed by **phenytoin** or **phenobarbitone** are the drugs of first choice for active or prolonged tonic clonic seizures. The choice of drug, dosage and frequency may have to be adjusted according to the age of the patient and the underlying disorder and these have already been outlined in chapter 4.

Dysphagia

This is a frequent and very disabling symptom in patients with neurological disease. The main causes include all causes of coma, stroke, motor neurone disease, myasthenia gravis and acute neuropathies. The main presenting complaints are inability or difficulty eating, drinking or swallowing safely. Quite apart from the practical difficulties is the loss of enjoyment of eating and drinking. The main aim is to support safe oral feeding for as long as possible while avoiding aspiration, dehydration, malnutrition and patient exhaustion. Good nursing/family care is needed as these patients are more difficult to feed and usually take longer. Some practical measures to deal with dysphagia include upright positioning whilst feeding, physical therapy with chewing and swallowing exercises, a high calorie diet with food/liquids thickened and regular oral hygiene every 2-4 hourly. Nasogastric tube feeding is a useful temporary or short term measure but should be avoided where death is inevitable as occurs in dementia. A percutaneous endoscopic gastrostomy (PEG) feeding tube may be used in patients with long term disorders presenting with intractable dysphagia. Measures used to treat dysphagia in neurological disorders are summarised in Table 20.7

Table 20.7 Measures used to treat dysphagia in neurological disorders

Indication	Intervention	limitations
Partial dysphagia	physical therapy with chewing and swallowing exercises, head & neck position, increased frequency of swallowing	aspiration pneumonia
Dehydration	fluids >2-3 litres/daily	aspiration pneumonia
Malnutrition	diet: food/liquids thickened, high calorie diet	dehydration/aspiration
Excess saliva/ drooling	oral hygiene 2-4 hourly anticholinergics: amitriptyline 10-25 mg/day/po, scopolamine 0.4 mg/sc/patches prn	mouth too dry and saliva more difficult to swallow
Dysphagia	nasogastric tube feeding (NGT)	aspiration pneumonia, (usually a short term intervention but can save lives)
	percutaneous endoscopic gastrostomy (PEG)	perforation, infection, (used in long term dysphagia)

Nausea and vomiting

This is a common symptom complicating intracranial disorders. The main aim in treatment is to maintain adequate fluid and calorie intake and good oral hygiene. The antiemetics **metoclopramide** and **domperidone** are useful for nausea of gastrointestinal origin. **Ondansetron** is helpful for chemotherapy and drug induced nausea and **cyclizine** in combination with dexamethasone for vomiting in patients with raised intracranial pressure. The commonly used drugs to treat nausea and vomiting are presented in Table 20.8.

Table 20.8 Drugs commonly used for nausea and vomiting

Indication	Drugs/dose/route/duration	Side effects
Nausea vomiting	metoclopramide10 mg/po/iv/8 hourly prochloperazine 5 mg/po/im/8 hourly domperidone10-20 mg/po/pr/8 hourly	dystonic reactions, parkinsonism, drowsiness
	cyclizine 25-50 mg/iv/im/6 hourly	drowsiness, dystonic reactions, parkinsonism
	ondansetron 8-16 mg/po/pr/iv 12 hourly	constipation, headache
Raised intracranial pressure	dexamethasone 4-16 mg/po/iv/bid	indigestion, insomnia, mood disturbance, hyperglycaemia, (perforation increased with NSAIDs), bone necrosis

Spasticity

Spasticity is a common and complex problem in neurological care particularly in patients with stroke and paraplegia. The aim of treatment is to increase mobility and avoid pain, contractures and bedsores. The management of spasticity mainly involves physiotherapy, occupational therapy and drug treatment (Chapter 10). Physiotherapy involves passive stretching exercises and local measures including joint supporting and splinting. The antispasmodics most widely available in Africa are **diazepam** and **baclofen**. The starting dose of diazepam is 2-5 mg three times daily increasing gradually over weeks to a maximum of 20 mg three times daily. **Clonazepam** once daily is an alternative to diazepam. The starting dose of baclofen is 5 mg twice daily orally increasing slowly over weeks to 20-30 mg twice daily as required. These can be used either as monotherapy or in combination if monotherapy fails. Both drugs are started at a low dose titrating slowly upwards against response. The limiting adverse effects of both are drowsiness and fatigue.

Other oral drugs used for spasticity include **dantrolene** and **tizanidine**. These are mainly second line antispasmodics but are often used in conjunction with first line drugs. Baclofen can be administered intrathecally by injection or pump for intractable spasticity and **botulinum toxin** is used by local injections for intractable spasticity, but both of these measures are only available at specialised centres. Pain resulting from spasticity or spasms can be very severe and is sometimes opioid refractory and needs high doses of muscle relaxants. The main drugs used to treat spasticity are outlined in Table 20.9.

Table 20.9 Drugs used for spasticity

Indication	Drugs/dose/route/duration	Side effects
Spasticity	diazepam 2.5-5 mg/po/8 hourly increasing to 10-20 mg/8 hourly	drowsiness, fatigue
	baclofen 5-10 mg/po/12 hourly increasing to 20-30 mg/12 hourly	muscle weakness, drowsiness, headache, nausea, insomnia
	dantrolene 25 mg/po/daily increasing slowly to 50-100 mg/6 hourly	drowsiness, fatigue, hepatocellular damage
	tizanadine 2 mg/po/6-8 hourly increasing slowly to 6 mg/6-8-hourly	drowsiness, GIT symptoms, allergy, hepatocellular damage

Immobility

Immobility occurs in most patients with advanced or terminal neurological disorders. The main aim of management of the immobile patient is to prevent pain, bed sores and contractures and to make the patient comfortable. To help achieve this aim it is necessary to keep the skin dry and clean. This may involve urinary catheterization when there is a non-functioning bladder or the patient is unable to mobilise to the toilet. Care of paralysed or immobile limbs involves frequent passive movements and ensuring the patient's position is regularly changed. This task is best done initially by a physiotherapist with the aid of antispasmodics and analgesics and the methods later taught to a family carer.

Dyspnoea

Breathlessness and cough are common and distressing symptoms in patients with neurological disorders. The main causes include stroke, infections, neuromuscular disorders and neurodegenerative disorders such as motor neurone disease. It is important to exclude acute reversible causes of respiratory failure such as myasthenia gravis, Guillain-Barre syndrome, medications or infection. Non pharmacological management includes the use of oxygen and relaxation techniques. Ventilatory support is usually not a realistic option unless there is a reversible component.

Management therefore in advanced neurological disorders involves the use of **morphine** initially 2.5-5 mg orally 6 hourly increasing the dose and frequency as required to relieve patient distress. The route of administration may be changed to parenteral depending on the patient's overall condition. Increasing dyspnoea in neurological disorders is frequently a sign of underlying pneumonia.

Constipation

Constipation is a frequent complication of neurological disorders, in particular those with spinal cord dysfunction, paralysis and immobility. Early intervention is important to prevent this. Measures include ensuring a satisfactory fluid intake, adequate high bulk and roughage diet and the careful use of laxatives. This includes the combined use of stool softeners (liquid paraffin), osmotic laxatives e.g. **magnesium salts** and **lactulose** and/or **colonic stimulants including senna** and **bisacodyl**. Rectal stimulants include **glycerine** and/or **bisacodyl** suppositories or enemas with **phosphate** or **soap** and water. Suppositories and enemas may be the best method of dealing with chronic neurological constipation and manual evacuation may be necessary in cases of faecal impaction.

PALLIATIVE CARE

Palliative care can be involved at any stage of a life-threatening condition, including at the time of diagnosis even if the survival prognosis is fairly long. A large part of palliative care is the provision of adequate relief of pain and other distressing symptoms. The most common problem identified in persons with advanced and terminal neurological disease in Africa is a lack of pain relief. Economic loss caused by lack of earnings, spiritual loss caused by a feeling of loss of God's help, emotional loss caused by a loss of hope and the social stigma of the disease and of feeling isolated in the community have all been identified as problems. Difficulties identified for care givers in Africa are lack of finance, loss of time from work and other activities and the practical aspects of caring for an often bedbound patient. Their main activities include the provision of food, drugs, and consolation needed for the day to day care of the patient. Palliative care aims to provide practical measures to support both patient and family. These include provision of food, drugs, consolation and assisting with the day to day care for the patient.

General care and support

Care in Africa is done mostly by the patient's family and they should always be involved in all major decisions concerning the patient. Both patient and family need understanding of their difficult situation. The health care worker should aim to be informed, gentle, honest, and to be aware of the range of emotions that may be encountered including fear, denial, grief, sadness, worry and finally acceptance. Carers should also be sensitive to and respect the cultural and spiritual needs of the patient. These may involve traditional healers, alternative medicines and religious support depending on the patient's wishes, needs and beliefs. It is important to ask the patient directly concerning the need for spiritual support.

Needs of patients

Palliative care emphasises the importance of alleviation of symptoms particularly in the final stages of disease process. In the last days, weeks and months of life the patient's main needs are symptom relief including pain, anxiety, secretions and nausea. Most people at this stage benefit from combinations of **morphine/antiemetic/anxiolytic ± antimuscarinic**. These can delivered either orally or parenterally by injection. A syringe pump driver is the preferred method of delivery in very ill people. A good death occurs when the patient is cared for where he wishes to die which is usually at home and is free from pain, worry and other distressing symptoms. Palliative care aims to help patients and their carers achieve this (Table 20.10).

Table 20.10 Aims & possible interventions with palliative care

Main Aim	Intervention
Relieve pain & other symptoms	provide analgesics and medications that are accessible, affordable & available (AAA)
Provide resources necessary to care	financial support
Provide an infrastructure to deliver care	teach, train health care workers & involve family members
Include palliative care as part of the continuum of health care and living	make palliative care a right for everyone

Selected references

Birbeck GL. *Barriers to care for patients with neurologic disease in rural Zambia.* Arch Neurol. 2000 Mar;57(3):414-7.

Chetty S, Baalbergen E, Bhigjee AI, Kamerman P, Ouma J, Raath R, Raff M, et al. *Clinical practice guidelines for management of neuropathic pain: Expert panel recommendations for South Africa.* S Afr Med J. 2012 Mar 8;102(5):312-25.

Clark D, Wright M, Hunt J, Lynch T. *Hospice and palliative care development in Africa: a multi-method review of services and experiences.* J Pain Symptom Manage. 2007 Jun;33(6):698-710.

Collins K, Harding R. *Improving HIV management in sub-Saharan Africa: how much palliative care is needed?* AIDS Care. 2007 Nov;19(10):1304-6.

Frohlich E, Shipton EA. *Can the development of pain management units be justified in an emerging democracy?* S Afr Med J. 2007 Sep;97(9):826-8.

Hall EJ, Sykes NP. *Analgesia for patients with advanced disease:* I. Postgrad Med J. 2004 Mar;80(941):148-54.

Hall EJ, Sykes NP. *Analgesia for patients with advanced disease: 2.* Postgrad Med J. 2004 Apr;80(942):190-5.

Harding R, Gwyther L, Mwangi-Powell F, Powell RA, Dinat N. *How can we improve palliative care patient outcomes in low- and middle-income countries? Successful outcomes research in sub-Saharan Africa.* J Pain Symptom Manage. 2010 Jul;40(1):23-6.

Harding R, Higginson IJ. *Palliative care in sub-Saharan Africa.* Lancet. 2005 Jun 4-10;365(9475):1971-7.

Kikule E. *A good death in Uganda: survey of needs for palliative care for terminally ill people in urban areas.* BMJ. 2003 Jul 26;327(7408):192-4.

Logie DE, Harding R. *An evaluation of a morphine public health programme for cancer and AIDS pain relief in Sub-Saharan Africa.* BMC Public Health. 2005;5:82.

Louw QA, Morris LD, Grimmer-Somers K. *The prevalence of low back pain in Africa: a systematic review.* BMC Musculoskelet Disord. 2007;8:105.

O'Brien T, Welsh J, Dunn FG. *ABC of palliative care. Non-malignant conditions.* BMJ. 1998 Jan 24;316(7127):286-9.

Sepulveda C, Habiyambere V, Amandua J, Borok M, Kikule E, Mudanga B, et al. *Quality care at the end of life in Africa. BMJ.* 2003 Jul 26;327(7408):209-13.

Sepulveda C, Marlin A, Yoshida T, Ullrich A. *Palliative Care: the World Health Organization's global perspective.* J Pain Symptom Manage. 2002 Aug;24(2):91-6.

INDEX

INDEX

Names of main infecting organisms in *italics*
Page number in **bold face** indicates major discussion

ABBREVIATIONS

ABBREVIATIONS

ABM	acute bacterial meningitis		CV	conduction velocity
AC	air conduction		CVS	cardiovascular system
ACA	anterior cerebral artery		CXR	chest X-ray
AChR	acetylcholine receptor		DA	dopamine
AD	Alzheimer's disease		DAI	diffuse axonal injury
ADC	AIDS dementia complex		DALYs	disability adjusted lost years
ADEM	acute disseminated encephalomyelitis		d4T	stavudine
ADL	activities of daily living		ddi	didanosine
AED	antiepileptic drug		DHE	dihydroergotamine
AF	atrial fibrillation		DLB	dementia with Lewy bodies
AIDP	acute inflammatory demyelinating polyneuropathy		DM	diabetes mellitus
			DMD	Duchenne muscular dystrophy
AIDS	acquired immune deficiency syndrome		DOT	directly observed treatment
ALS	amyotrophic lateral sclerosis		DSN	distal sensory neuropathy
ART	antiretroviral therapy		DVT	deep vein thrombosis
AVM	arteriovenous malformation		EBV	Epstein-Barr virus
AZT	zidovudine		ECG	electrocardiogram
BB	borderline leprosy		EDH	extradural haematoma
BC	bone conduction		EEG	electroencephalogram
BET	benign essential tremor		EMG	electromyography
bd	twice daily		ENL	erythema nodosum leprosum
BIH	benign intracranial hypertension		ESR	erythrocyte sedimentation rate
BMD	Becker muscular dystrophy		FBC	full blood count
BP	blood pressure		FC	febrile convulsion
BPPV	benign paroxysmal positional vertigo		FH	family history
BTL	borderline tuberculoid leprosy		FLRSs	frontal lobe release signs
CATT	card agglutination trypanosomiasis test		FND	focal neurological disorder/deficit
CBD	corticobasal degeneration		FSH	facioscapulohumeral dystrophy
CDH	chronic daily headache		FTP	frontotemporal dementia
CFR	case fatality ratio/rate		FTA	fluorescent treponemal antibody absorption (FTA)
CIDP	chronic inflammatory demyelinating polyneuropathy			
			FVC	forced vital capacity
CM	cryptococcal meningitis		GABA	gamma-aminobutyric acid
CMTD	Charcot–Marie-Tooth disease		GBS	Guillain-Barre syndrome
CMV	cytomegalovirus		GCS	Glasgow Coma Scale
CNS	central nervous system		GTCS	generalized tonic clonic seizure
COW	circle of Willis		HAART	highly active antiretroviral therapy
CPA	cerebellopontine angle		HAD	HIV associated dementia
CR	controlled release		HAM	HTLV associated myelopathy
CRAg	cryptococcal antigen		HAND	HIV associated neurocognitive dysfunction
CSF	cerebrospinal fluid			
CT	computerized tomography		HAT	human African trypanosomiasis
CTS	carpal tunnel syndrome		Hb	haemoglobin

HCW	health care worker	MRI	magnetic resonance imaging
HD	Huntington's disease	MSA	multiple system atrophy
HI	head injury	MUP	motor unit potential
Hib	haemophilus influenza	NAP	nerve action potential
HIV	human immunodeficiency virus	NCD	non communicable disease
HMSN	hereditary motor sensory neuropathy	NCS	nerve conduction study
HSE	herpes simplex encephalitis	NF1	neurofibromatosis type 1
HSP	hereditary spastic paraparesis	NF2	neurofibromatosis type 2
HSV	herpes simplex virus	NGT	nasogastric tube
HTLV-1	human T-cell lymphotropic virus type 1	NMJ	neuromuscular junction
IBM	inclusion body myositis	NMO	neuromyelitis optica
IAC	internal auditory canal	NSAID	non-steroidal anti-inflammatory drug
ICA	internal carotid artery	NTP	non traumatic paraplegia
ICH	intracerebral haemorrhage	od	once daily
ICP	intracranial pressure	OI	opportunistic infection
ICT	intracranial tumour	ON	optic neuritis
ICU	intensive care unit	OP	opening pressure
IFA	immunofluorescent antibody	OT	occupational therapist
IVIG	intravenous immunoglobulin	PBP	progressive bulbar palsy
im	intramuscular	PCL	primary cerebral lymphoma
INO	internuclear opthalmoplegia	PC	posterior column
INR	international normalized ratio	PCA	posterior cerebral artery
IPD	idiopathic Parkinson's disease	PCP	pneumocystis pneumonia
IRIS	immune reconstitution inflammatory syndrome	PCR	polymerase chain reaction
		PD	Parkinson's disease
iv	intravenous	PE	plasma exchange
JME	juvenile myoclonic epilepsy	PHB	phenobarbitone
LCST	lateral corticospinal tract	PHCW	primary health care worker
LFT	liver function test	PHT	phenytoin
LGMD	limb girdle muscular dystrophy	PLS	primary lateral sclerosis
LMNL	lower motor neurone lesion	PM	polymyositis
LOC	loss of consciousness	PMA	progressive muscular atrophy
LL	lepromatous leprosy	PMH	past medical history
LP	lumbar puncture	PML	progressive multifocal leucoencephalopathy
MAOI	monoamine oxidase inhibitors		
MAP	muscle action potential	PND	peripheral nerve disorder
MCA	middle cerebral artery	PNS	peripheral nervous system
MD	myotonic dystrophy	po	per oral
MDT	multidrug therapy	PP	paraplegia
MG	myasthenia gravis	PSP	progressive supranuclear palsy
MMSE	mini mental state examination	qds	four times a day
MND	motor neurone disease	RAPD	relative afferent pupil defect
MR	mortality rate	RDT	rapid diagnostic test
MRC	Medical Research Council	RRT	rapid reagent test

RTA	road traffic accident
Rx	treatment
SACD	subacute combined degeneration of spinal cord
SAH	subarachnoid haemorrhage
sc	subcutaneous
SDH	subdural haematoma
SNAP	sensory nerve action potential
SOL	space occupying lesion
SSA	sub Saharan Africa
STT	spinothalamic tract
SUDEP	sudden unexpected death in epilepsy
SVP	sodium valproate
TA	temporal arteritis
TAN	tropical ataxic neuropathy
TB	tuberculosis
Tbg	*Trypanosoma brucei gambiense*
TBI	traumatic brain injury
TBM	tuberculous meningitis
Tbr	*Trypanosoma brucei rhodesiense*
tds	three times daily
TE	toxoplasma encephalitis
TIA	transient ischaemic attack
TLE	temporal lobe epilepsy
TN	trigeminal neuralgia
TPHA	Treponema pallidum haemagglutination assay
TPI	treponemal pallidum immobilization test
TT	tuberculoid leprosy
U&E	urea and electrolytes
UMNL	upper motor neurone lesion
VA	visual acuity
VDRL	Venereal Disease Research Laboratory
VM	vacuolar myelopathy
ZN	Ziehl-Neelsen
VZ	varicella zoster
WHO	World Health Organization
WKS	Wernicke-Korsakoff-syndrome
YLD	years lived with disability
YLL	years life lost

USEFUL WEBSITES

USEFUL WEBSITES

General Medical Websites

1. www.healthnet.org/essential-links
   Highly systematic listing of health care websites aimed at professionals in the developing world.

2. www.pubmedcentral.nih.gov
   "Large number of full-text biomedical journals available at publication date or after six months or one year." John Eyers.

3. extranet.who.int/hinari/en/journals.php
   A highly useful resource for researchers; medical students may require initial formal instruction.

4. www.unaids.com
   Useful resource covering both the socio-economic and medical aspects of HIV/AIDS.

5. www.cdc.gov
   High yield resource for infectious disease; rapid response to on-line queries.

Neurology Websites

1. emedicine.medscape.com/neurology
   Excellent link to neurology articles on a wide range of topics. Detailed yet concise information.

2. hardinmd.lib.uiowa.edu/neuro.html
   Contains links to neurology websites chosen for quality; useful resource.

3. www.freebooks4doctors.com/fb/NEURO.HTM
   Free downloads of various high quality neurology texts; excellent resource.

4. www.freemedicaljournals.com/fmj/IP_NEURO.HTM
   Free access to world-renowned neurology journals such as "Brain" and "Archives of Neurology".

5. www.neuroexam.com/neuroexam
   Videos on neurologic exam from Yale New Haven Hospital; excellent website.

6. www.med.harvard.edu/AANLIB/home.html
   Very useful resource; serves as an introduction to neuro-imaging for medical students.

7. www.who.int/topics/meningitis/en
   Simple but relevant information on bacterial meningitis; fact sheet is a must read for students.

8. www.refbooks.msf.org/MSF_Docs/En/Meningitis/Mening_en.pdf
   Useful resource on case detection and management of epidemic meningococcal meningitis.

9. www.ilep.org.uk
   Very useful for introducing leprosy diagnosis and treatment.

10. www.epilepsy.org.uk
    Useful for introduction to epilepsy; med students may need additional information.